INFECTION AND PREGNANCY

RCOG Press

Since 1973 The Royal College of Obstetricians and Gynaecologists has regularly convened Study Groups to address important growth areas within obstetrics and gynaecology. An international group of eminent scientists and clinicians from various disciplines is invited to present the results of recent research and to take part in in-depth discussions. The resulting volume, containing the papers presented and also edited transcripts of the discussions, is published within a few months of the meeting and provides a summary of the subject that is both authoritative and up to date.

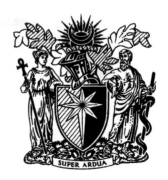

Previous Study Group publications available

HRT and Osteoporosis
Edited by JO Drife and JWW Studd

Antenatal Diagnosis of Fetal Abnormalities
Edited by JO Drife and D Donnai

Prostaglandins and the Uterus
Edited by JO Drife and AA Calder

Infertility
Edited by AA Templeton and JO Drife

Intrapartum Fetal Surveillance
Edited by JAD Spencer and RHT Ward

Early Fetal Growth and Development
Edited by RHT Ward, SK Smith and D Donnai

Ethics in Obstetrics and Gynaecology
Edited by S Bewley and RHT Ward

The Biology of Gynaecological Cancer
Edited by R Leake, M Gore and RHT Ward

Multiple Pregnancy
Edited by RHT Ward and M Whittle

The Prevention of Pelvic Infection
Edited by AA Templeton

Screening for Down Syndrome in the First Trimester
Edited by JG Grudzinskas and RHT Ward

Problems in Early Pregnancy: Advances in Diagnosis and Management
Edited by JG Grudzinskas and PMS O'Brien

Gene Identification, Manipulation and Treatment
Edited by SK Smith, EJ Thomas and PMS O'Brien

Evidence-based Fertility Treatment
Edited by AA Templeton, ID Cooke and PMS O'Brien

Fetal Programming: Influences on Development and Disease in Later Life
Edited by PMS O'Brien, T Wheeler and DJP Barker

Hormones and Cancer
Edited by PMS O'Brien and AB MacLean

The Placenta: Basic Science and Clinical Practice
Edited by JCP Kingdom, ERM Jauniaux and PMS O'Brien

Disorders of the Menstrual Cycle
Edited by PMS O'Brien, IT Cameron and AB MacLean

Infection and Pregnancy

Edited by

Allan B MacLean, Lesley Regan and David Carrington

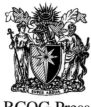

RCOG Press

It was not possible to refer all the material back to the authors or discussants but it is hoped that the proceedings have been reported fairly and accurately.

Allan B MacLean MD FRCOG
Professor of Obstetrics and Gynaecology, University Department of Obstetrics and Gynaecology, Royal Free Hospital, Rowland Hill Street, Hampstead, London NW3 2PF, UK

Lesley Regan MD FRCOG
Department of Reproductive Science and Medicine, Imperial College School of Medicine at St Mary's Hospital, Mint Wing, South Wharf Road, London W2 1NY, UK

David Carrington DTMH FRCPath
Regional Virus Laboratory, Public Health Laboratory, Myrtle Road, Bristol BS2 8EL, UK

First published 2001

ISBN 1 900364 44 1

DECLARATION OF INTEREST
All contributors to the Study Group were invited to make a specific Declaration of Interest in relation to the subject of the Study Group. This was undertaken and all contributors complied with this request. Professor Griffiths acts as an occasional consultant for GlaxoWellcome on treatment of herpes simplex virus, cytomegalovirus and varicella-zoster virus during pregnancy. Dr Hay has acted as a consultant to and has received a research grant from 3M. He has been involved in clinical trials with 3M, Pharmacia & Upjohn, Core Technologies and Osmetech. Dr Holliman is an unpaid consultant to the charity Community Hygiene Concern. Professor McIntyre acted as a consultant to Boehringer-Ingelheim South Africa on nevirapine in pregnancy in 1999. Professor Regan is a professional adviser to the Miscarriage Association, Tommy's Campaign and Save the Baby Charity. Dr Ridgway acts as a consultant for Abbott Diagnostics and other pharmaceutical companies. Dr Smith holds a patent for the Smiths Safety Needleholder, which is manufactured by Femcare. Professor Soothill has a patent pending on mucinase inhibitor in relation to preterm labour.

Published by the **RCOG Press** at
The Royal College of Obstetricians and Gynaecologists
27 Sussex Place, Regent's Park
London NW1 4RG, UK

Registered Charity No. 213280

RCOG Press Editor: Andrew Welsh
Cover designed by Geoffrey Wadsley
Printed by FiSH Books, London

Contents

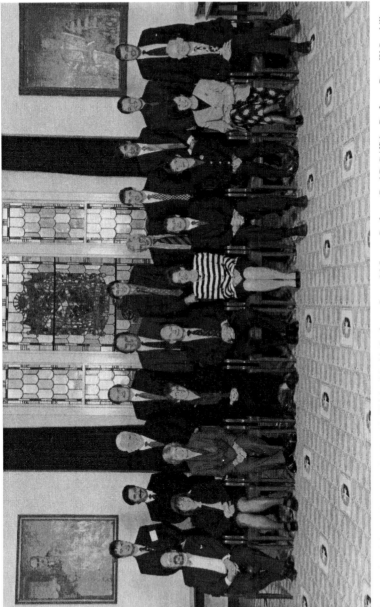

Top row (from left to right): Dr Phillip Hay, Mr J Richard Smith, Professor James McIntyre, Professor Paul D Griffiths, Professor Peter W Soothill, Dr Eric Jauniaux, Professor Harold Fox, Dr Richard E Holliman, Professor John Collinge, Dr Peter Brocklehurst, Dr Geoffrey L Ridgway

Bottom row (from left to right): Professor James Drife, Dr Caroline E Shulman, Professor Catherine Peckham, Dr Marie-Louise Newell, Professor Allan B MacLean, Professor Lesley Regan, Dr David Carrington, Dr Rhona G Hughes, Dr Nicola S Brink, Dr Geoff M Scott,

Participants

Dr Nicola S Brink
Consultant Virologist, Lead Clinician, Virology, and Honorary Senior Lecturer, Department of Virology, University College London Hospitals, Windeyer Building, 46 Cleveland Street, London W1T 4JF, UK

Dr Peter Brocklehurst
Consultant Clinical Epidemiologist, National Perinatal Epidemiology Unit, Institute of Health Sciences, Old Road, Oxford OX3 7LF, UK

Dr David Carrington
Consultant Medical Virologist, Regional Virus Laboratory, Public Health Laboratory, Myrtle Road, Bristol BS2 8EL, UK

Professor James Drife
Professor of Obstetrics and Gynaecology, Division of Obstetrics, Clarendon Wing, The General Infirmary at Leeds, Belmont Grove, Leeds, LS2 9NS, UK and Vice President, The Royal College of Obstetricians and Gynaecologists, UK

Professor David Edwards
Chairman, Division of Paediatrics, Obstetrics and Gynaecology and Weston Professor of Neonatal Medicine, Imperial College School of Medicine, Hammersmith Hospital, Du Cane Road, London W12 0NN, UK

Professor Harold Fox
Emeritus Professor of Reproductive Pathology, Department of Pathological Sciences, Stopford Building, University of Manchester, Manchester M13 9PT, UK

Professor Paul D Griffiths
Professor of Virology, Department of Virology, Royal Free and University College Medical School, Rowland Hill Street, London NW3 2PF, UK

Dr Phillip Hay
Senior Lecturer in Genitourinary Medicine, Courtyard Clinic, St George's Hospital Medical School, Blackshaw Road, London SW17 0QT, UK

Dr Paul T Heath
Senior Lecturer and Honorary Consultant, Department of Child Health, St George's Hospital Medical School, London SW17 0RE, UK

Dr Richard E Holliman
Consultant and Reader in Clinical Microbiology, Department of Medical
Microbiology, St George's Hospital Medical School, Blackshaw Road, London
SW17 0QT, UK

Dr Rhona G Hughes
Consultant and Honorary Senior Lecturer in Obstetrics and Gynaecology, Simpson
Memorial Maternity Pavilion, Lauriston Place, Edinburgh EH3 9YW, UK

Dr Eric Jauniaux
Reader in Obstetrics and Gynaecology, Department of Obstetrics and Gynaecology,
University College London, 86–96 Chenies Mews, London WC1E 6HX, UK

Mr Ronald F Lamont
Consultant, Department of Obstetrics and Gynaecology, Northwick Park Hospital,
Watford Road, Harrow HA1 3UJ and Visiting Reader, Imperial College, London,
UK.

Professor James McIntyre
Director, Perinatal HIV Research Unit, Department of Obstetrics and Gynaecology,
Chris Hani Baragwanath Hospital, PO Bertsham, Johannesburg 2013, South Africa

Professor Allan B MacLean
Professor of Obstetrics and Gynaecology, University Department of Obstetrics and
Gynaecology, Royal Free Hospital, Rowland Hill Street, London NW3 2PF, UK and
Convenor of Study Groups, The Royal College of Obstetricians and Gynaecologists,
UK

Dr Elizabeth Miller
Head, Immunisation Division, Communicable Disease Surveillance Centre, Public
Health Laboratory Service, 61 Colindale Avenue, London NW9 5EQ, UK

Dr Marie-Louise Newell
Reader in Epidemiology, Department of Paediatric Epidemiology and Biostatistics,
Institute of Child Health, 30 Guilford Street, London WC1N 1EH, UK

Professor Catherine Peckham
Head, Department of Paediatric Epidemiology and Biostatistics, Institute of Child
Health, 30 Guilford Street, London WC1N 1EH, UK

Professor Lesley Regan
Professor of Obstetrics and Gynaecology in the Department of Reproductive Science
and Medicine, Imperial College School of Medicine at St Mary's Hospital, Mint
Wing, South Wharf Road, London W2 1NY, UK

Dr Geoffrey L Ridgway
Consultant Microbiologist, Department of Clinical Microbiology, University College
London Hospitals, Grafton Way, London WC1E 6DB, UK

Dr Geoff M Scott
Consultant Clinical Microbiologist, Department of Clinical Microbiology, University
College London Hospitals, Grafton Way, London WC1E 6DB, UK

Dr Caroline E Shulman
Senior Lecturer, Gates Malaria Programme, London School of Hygiene and Tropical
Medicine, Keppel Street, London WC1E 7HT, UK

Professor Peter Simmonds
Laboratory for Clinical and Molecular Virology, University of Edinburgh,
Summerhall, Edinburgh EH9 1QH, UK

Mr J Richard Smith
Consultant and Honorary Senior Lecturer, Chelsea and Westminster Hospital, Fulham
Road, London SW10 9NH, UK

Professor Peter W Soothill
Professor of Maternal and Fetal Medicine and Head of Division of Obstetrics and
Gynaecology, University of Bristol, St Michael's Hospital, Southwell Street, Bristol
BS2 8EG, UK

Additional contributors

Mr Sherif A Abdel-Fattah
Lecturer and Senior Registrar, Division of Obstetrics and Gynaecology, University of
Bristol, St Michael's Hospital, Southwell Street, Bristol BS2 8EG, UK

Professor Bernard Brabin
Professor of Tropical Paediatrics, Emma Kinderziekenhuis, Academic Medical
Centre, Meibergdreef 9, Postbus 22660, 1100 DD Amsterdam, The Netherlands and
Tropical Child Health Group, Liverpool School of Tropical Medicine, Pembroke
Place, Liverpool L3 5QA, UK

Dr Natasha S Crowcroft
Consultant Epidemiologist, Immunisation Division, Communicable Disease
Surveillance Centre, Public Health Laboratory Service, 61 Colindale Avenue, London
NW9 5EQ, UK

Mr Edgar K Dorman
Consultant Obstetrician and Gynaecologist, Homerton Hospital, Homerton Row,
London E9 6SR, UK

Dr Phil Duggan
Clinical Research Fellow, Weston Laboratory, Department of Paediatrics, Imperial
College School of Medicine, Hammersmith Hospital, Du Cane Road, London W12
0NN, UK

Dr Shehnaaz Jivraj
Clinical Research Fellow, Department of Reproductive Science and Medicine,
Imperial College School of Medicine at St Mary's Hospital, Mint Wing, South Wharf
Road, London W2 1NY, UK

Dr Steven Kaye
Senior Research Fellow, Department of Virology, Royal Free and University College
Medical School, Windeyer Building, 46 Cleveland Street, London W1T 4JF, UK

Dr Nigel L Kennea
Clinical Research Fellow, Weston Laboratory, Department of Paediatrics, Imperial College School of Medicine, Hammersmith Hospital, Du Cane Road, London W12 0NN, UK

Dr Naomi Low-Beer
Clinical Research Fellow, Clinical Trials Centre, Winston Churchill Building, St Mary's Hospital, Praed Street, London W2 1NY, UK

Dr A Christine McCartney
Deputy Director, Central Public Health Laboratory, 61 Colindale Avenue, London NW9 5NT, UK

Professor Peter Morgan-Capner
Medical Director, Preston Acute Hospitals NHS Trust and Chorley and South Ribble Trust, Trust Headquarters, Preston Road, Chorley PR7 1PP, UK

Preface

Infection has always been a major threat for both the pregnant woman and her fetus or neonate. So, what is new? This 40th RCOG Study Group has brought together experts in infectious diseases, microbiology, virology, epidemiology, pathology, obstetrics and paediatrics to assess what is new and relevant to our current practice, including:

- techniques now available in the laboratory for rapid and accurate diagnosis
- the use of high-resolution ultrasound and amniotic fluid or fetal sampling to assess the fetus for the effects of infection
- the recognition that certain more common or epidemic infections still have serious sequelae for the pregnant woman or fetus
- criteria for screening for infection and lessons from the past
- the importance of food preparation and eating patterns during pregnancy
- the fact that air travel allows pregnant women to visit parts of the world where they may be exposed to infection
- the implications of immigration, which brings women of reproductive age to the UK who either have infection or are more susceptible to infection prevalent in the UK
- new organisms, e.g. hepatitis C, or diseases, e.g. prion disease, and the possibility of vertical transmission
- the availability of antiviral agents that are suitable for use in pregnancy.

This Study Group may have identified more questions than answers, but it has certainly defined opportunities for further research, multicentre studies and the need for continuing support to pursue infection and its impact on pregnancy.

Allan B MacLean
Lesley Regan
David Carrington

SECTION 1

EPIDEMIOLOGY OF INFECTION AND PREGNANCY

Chapter 1

Infections in pregnancy: past and present

Catherine Peckham

This chapter provides an overview, largely from a population perspective, of the salient issues that arise in relation to the detection and management of infections in pregnancy. Infections in pregnancy are common but few specific infections have been shown to have serious consequences for the fetus or infant. Although pregnancy *per se* does not usually affect the incidence and severity of infection, some physiological changes associated with pregnancy can result in an increased risk of certain infections, particularly urinary tract infections, pneumonia and chorioamnionitis. There is also some evidence that hepatitis B infection and possibly varicella-zoster virus may be more severe in the pregnant than the nonpregnant woman.

The number and type of maternal infections associated with adverse pregnancy outcomes continues to increase and the emphasis on particular infections has changed over the years. Infections in pregnancy that can result in adverse fetal or neonatal outcome are listed below:

- rubella
- cytomegalovirus (CMV)
- herpes simplex virus (HSV)
- varicella-zoster virus
- parvovirus B19
- hepatitis B and C
- papillomavirus
- HIV-1 and HIV-2
- human T-cell leukaemia virus (HTLV) 1 and 2
- *Toxoplasma gondii*
- *Treponema pallidum*
- group B streptococcus
- *Listeria monocytogenes*

In 1983, the situation was somewhat different and a comparable list included not only rubella but rubella vaccine, Epstein–Barr virus and vaccinia and variola viruses as agents causing fetal infection, and mumps, influenza, hepatitis A, coxsackieviruses, echoviruses, measles and non-A, non-B hepatitis listed as suspected agents.[1] There was no mention of HIV, HTLV-1, parvovirus B19 or papillomavirus. In the 1970s and

Table 1.1.   Congenital rubella reviewed

Year	Developments
1941	Association between syndrome and maternal rubella infection[34]
1950s	Prospective epidemiological studies confirmed this association and estimated the risk[35,36]
1962	Rubella virus isolated[37,38]
1963	Extensive rubella epidemic in the USA with an estimated 20000–30000 infants damaged by the virus[2]
1970	Rubella vaccine introduced in the UK for girls aged 11–14 years
1978	896 therapeutic abortions for rubella in the UK (148/100000), 66 for inadvertent vaccination in pregnancy
1988	Measles, mumps and rubella (MMR) vaccine introduced for all children in their second year of life
1994	Mass measles and rubella vaccination programme in the UK for children aged 5–16 years
1996	MMR preschool booster introduced and schoolgirl programme discontinued

1980s, rubella was regarded as the model for many studies investigating the potential effects of other viruses in causing adverse fetal outcome, with the focus largely on congenital abnormalities.

The prevalence of some maternal infections has changed substantially and rubella infection provides a good example (Table 1.1). In the 1960s, rubella infection was a major concern, with between 20000 and 40000 infants born with congenital rubella damage following the extensive rubella epidemic that occurred in the USA in 1962.[2] This epidemic added to the stimulus to develop a rubella vaccine and eight years after the virus had been isolated rubella vaccine programmes were already being introduced. Nearly a decade later the situation had changed dramatically and congenital rubella had become a rare disease in countries with a rubella vaccination policy.[3] The absence of maternal rubella, due to the high population immunity resulting from the vaccine and the low prevalence of susceptibility among pregnant women, has led to a decline in cases of congenital rubella and termination of pregnancy for rubella in the UK (Figure 1.1). There is no evidence that rubella vaccination in pregnancy is detrimental to the fetus, despite initial concerns.[4] Nevertheless, it is important not to become complacent as sporadic cases do still occur; three cases of congenital rubella were reported to the National Congenital Rubella Surveillance Programme in 2000. Immigrants and asylum seekers from countries where there is no rubella vaccination programme remain a potential source of infection. High levels of measles, mumps and rubella immunisation in the second year of life will need to be maintained so that the pool of susceptible individuals remains small and outbreaks do not occur. Continued surveillance of congenital rubella is essential.

After the discovery that rubella was an important teratogen it was speculated that other viral infections would also cause congenital defects, but this has not proved to be the case. In the 1970s and early 1980s, infections such as mumps, influenza and the enteroviruses (particularly echo 9 virus and coxsackie B3 and B4 infection) had been incriminated as causes of congenital malformation but evidence for this was usually based on isolated observations that were likely to have been chance associations. During this period, viruses in pregnancy were the particular focus of attention, with the emphasis on adverse outcome focusing on congenital malformations rather than perinatal disease, as it was assumed that the damage following exposure to maternal infections would be evident early in life.

Influenza was regarded for many years as a potential teratogenic agent for the human

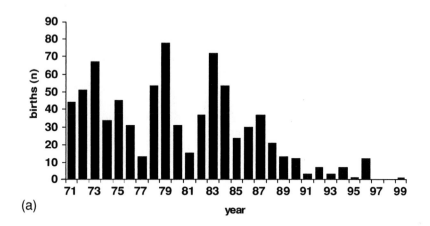

(a)

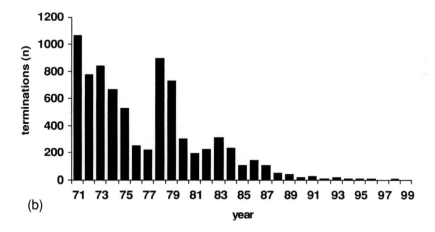

(b)

Fig. 1.1   (a) Congenital rubella births registered with the National Congenital Rubella Surveillance Programme 1971–99;   (b) Rubella-associated terminations reported to the Office for National Statistics 1971–99

fetus and although there is little evidence that the influenza virus can cross the placenta there is a growing literature on the long-term effects of influenza in pregnancy. These studies usually relate to specific epidemics, particularly that in 1957, and the variable effects reported make generalisations difficult. Influenza has been associated with congenital abnormalities, childhood malignancy and schizophrenia.[5-7] However, results from studies are conflicting and causality is mainly based on temporal association between births during an epidemic and specific conditions in later life, such as schizophrenia. It has been suggested that some of the reported associations could be due to hyperthermia associated with maternal influenza, or to its treatment.

In the 1980s, following an increase in notifications of genital herpes simplex in the population, there was concern that an increase in maternal infection could pose a risk for the newborn. As little was known about the prevalence of maternal infection in the UK and even less about the prevalence of neonatal herpes infection, a national study was set up to establish the incidence of neonatal herpes.[8] At that time, weekly antenatal screening for virus shedding in the cervix in late pregnancy was recommended in the USA for women with a history of recurrent genital HSV infection. A caesarean section was recommended if virus shedding was detected in the week of delivery or if lesions were present.[9] This policy was subsequently abandoned, as it became evident from prospective studies that recurrent maternal genital HSV infection posed a low risk of transmission and that most cases of neonatal herpes resulted from a primary, often asymptomatic, infection acquired in late pregnancy.[10,11] The earlier screening strategies were likely to have prevented few cases of neonatal infection at the cost of large numbers of additional caesarean deliveries.[12]

In the late 1970s, there was an increasing awareness of the importance of congenital CMV infection as a cause of childhood disability, particularly mental impairment, and some experts were recommending antenatal screening for the detection of a primary infection and the termination of affected pregnancies.[13] Data to support this view were lacking, no prospective data were available at the time and the assumption was based on information from studies in selected populations referred to special units in the USA that was then extrapolated to the UK population. It is misleading to extrapolate the long-term risks derived from a relatively small group of children, many of whom presented with obvious impairment or were in poor condition at birth, to the general population. This editorial stimulated research and large prospective studies were soon set up in Europe and elsewhere to obtain the information necessary to inform decisions about the management of this infection in pregnancy. Data from these large prospective studies established reasonably accurate estimates of transmission risk and risk of fetal damage and demonstrated considerably lower rates than those that had been reported previously.[14-16]

The infection that poses the greatest challenge at the present time is HIV infection. This is one of the few maternal infections for which there is a treatment of proven efficacy to prevent mother-to-child transmission.[17] With prophylactic anti-retroviral therapy to the mother, together with the avoidance of breastfeeding and increased use of caesarean delivery, transmission rates as low as 1% are now being reported in Europe and North America. The key issue in the UK has been to ensure that all women are offered an antenatal HIV test so that those who are infected can be offered interventions to reduce transmission and they themselves can benefit from early treatment and care. The dilemma worldwide is that most HIV infections occur in populations where access to health care is limited and where treatment is neither feasible nor affordable and alternatives to breastfeeding are not an option. The scientific effort and resources that have gone into the understanding of the mechanisms of mother-to-child transmission of HIV infection and to furthering knowledge of the underlying biological and immunological factors that influence transmission have been enormous. The development of these new technologies has stimulated research efforts into a better understanding of the 'old' infections.

Mode of acquisition of fetal or neonatal infection

Infections of the newborn may be acquired *in utero* (congenital infection), around the time of delivery (intrapartum infection) or in the neonatal period (postpartum infection). Intrauterine infection follows systemic blood-borne maternal infection with placental infection and/or transplacental transmission to the fetus. Sometimes the placenta may be infected without fetal spread. Infections may also reach the fetus from the genital tract by the cervical amniotic route, or they may be acquired during birth as a result of exposure to infected cervical secretions or to maternal blood or faeces. Delayed delivery after rupture of the membranes may increase the risk of infection. Postpartum infection may be acquired through breastfeeding, transfused blood, by hands or instruments or via the respiratory route from infected contacts such as the mother, other babies, medical attendants or other family members. Abrasions of the infant's skin due to birth trauma may provide a portal of entry and the risk of infection may be enhanced by the application of invasive procedures such as scalp electrodes. The nature of the infecting organism, its portal of entry, the time and length of exposure, the dose and the maternal and fetal immune status are likely to influence outcome.

Pregnancy outcome

The effects of maternal infection on the fetus may be due to the direct actions of toxins or organisms, as is the case for congenital rubella or toxoplasmosis infection, or they may be indirect and a consequence of interference with placental or uterine function. The effect of a specific infection on fetal development is likely to depend on multiple maternal and fetal factors, including genetic make-up, nutritional status and the stage of fetal development, as well as anatomical factors such as the site or the structure of the placental vessels. Placental failure due to placental infection could affect function, as in the case of malaria, or cause fetal malnutrition. Infection can also result in premature labour and delivery and the long-term damage associated with congenital or perinatal infection with non-persisting organisms appears to be non-specifically due to prematurity. Long-term effects on immunological competence of the fetus could also be important. Possible adverse outcomes associated with infections in pregnancy include:

- spontaneous abortion
- congenital abnormality
- stillbirth
- intrauterine growth restriction

- prematurity
- acute illness or death in neonatal period
- damage that may be obvious at birth, or may not manifest or even develop until later in life
- subsequent infertility or ectopic pregnancy.

Long-term effects

Developmental abnormalities have been associated with specific infections such as rubella, CMV and toxoplasmosis whereas other infections, such as HSV, are associated with acute infection in the newborn and a high risk of mortality and subsequent morbidity in survivors. Some infections pose particular problems because the organism persists in the host and continues to replicate and may cause tissue destruction after birth. Such chronic infection occurs with rubella, CMV, toxoplasmosis, syphilis, HIV and HTLV-I. Exposure to chickenpox in pregnancy, for example, may result in subclinical infection with reactivation of the virus in the early months or years of life, manifesting as herpes zoster.[18] It has been suggested that the varicella syndrome that occurs following exposure to infection in early gestation is the result of virus reactivation in later pregnancy rather than the result of the initial infection.[19]

Long-term effects are those that become evident or develop long after the neonatal period (Table 1.2). They may be caused directly by irreversible damage inflicted at the time of the initial infection or by damage resulting from persistent infection or reactivation of infection during childhood or adult life. Damage may also occur as a result of interference with fetal growth producing disturbances in developmental pattern or structure, as in the case of congenital rubella. There may be a diminution of the normal number or a change in the form of fetal cells, which interferes with the structure, or function of selected organs or whole systems. Changes may be subtle: in

Table 1.2. Possible long-term outcomes of infections acquired prenatally

Infection	Possible long-term outcome
Rubella	Sensorineural deafness
	Diabetes mellitus
	Thyroid disease
	Growth hormone deficiency
	Vascular effects
	Encephalitis
Cytomegalovirus	Sensorineural deafness
Toxoplasmosis	Visual impairment
Mumps	Diabetes
Hepatitis B	Liver cirrhosis
	Hepatocellular carcinoma
HTLV-I	T-cell leukaemia
	Tropical spastic paralysis
Non-specific viral infection (herpesviruses)	Malignant disease
Influenza A2	Schizophrenia
	Childhood malignancies

the brain, for example, they could affect later perception or learning ability. The changes produced may not manifest themselves unless the affected individual meets a specific challenge late in life, many years after the initial infection.

Most infants congenitally infected by these agents have no clinical illness at birth but may later develop signs and symptoms in infancy, childhood or adult life because of the persistence of viable organisms. This phenomenon was first demonstrated in the follow-up of children identified at birth to have congenital rubella. Children with no apparent defect, and whose language was developing normally, were later found to have a profound sensorineural hearing loss.[20] Late-onset diabetes mellitus and thyroid disease have also been reported, presenting in late adolescence or early adult life.[21] Toxoplasmosis is another infection where long-term effects, particularly visual impairment, have been demonstrated as a result of the persistence of the toxoplasmosis cyst, which subsequently ruptures.[22]

Epidemiological data

The management of an infection in pregnancy and the development of appropriate prevention strategies depend on a sound knowledge of the epidemiology of the infection. Epidemiological information required includes:

- background prevalence of the infection
- incidence of the infection in pregnancy
- risk of mother-to-child transmission
- timing of mother-to-child transmission
- risk factors for maternal and perinatal infection
- consequences of congenital/perinatal infection, both short-term and long-term.

Not only is it difficult to establish a link between an infection in pregnancy and a condition presenting in the infant or child, or even in later life, but it is difficult to establish estimates of risk of vertical transmission or fetal or newborn damage. To estimate the maternal prevalence and gestational effects of an infection that is subclinical or non-specific and mild, and can only be diagnosed if serological screening is carried out, requires a prospective study. This necessitates the serological follow-up of women through pregnancy to identify those who become infected and the investigation of fetal or neonatal samples for evidence of congenital infection. Where the sensitivity of the laboratory investigation of the neonate is in doubt (as for toxoplasma immunoglobulin M) or unknown, infants must be followed clinically and serologically for at least the first year. The significance of non-specific outcomes such as abortion, prematurity and neurological or sensory organ sequelae can only be assessed by comparison with a control group of pregnancies matched for confounding variables such as age, parity, social class and ethnic background. Large numbers of women have to be studied because even the most common congenital infection, CMV, occurs in only 1% of pregnancies and in only a proportion of these will transplacental infection take place. Associating an infection with fetal damage is particularly difficult if the infection is uncommon in pregnancy, even if the maternal infection is symptomatic. The likelihood of an association is increased if the organism can be recovered from the fetus or infant, or if there is serological evidence of infection in the neonate. However, unless a series of cases with similar defects or with a characteristic syndrome is reported, as with congenital varicella, evidence of vertical transmission does not necessarily confirm that the agent was responsible for the defect. It is only in recent years that it has been possible to estimate the risk of damage following maternal varicella infection from data collected in prospective studies.[19]

Most congenitally infected infants are not diagnosed as such, since the majority have no clinical manifestations of the infection at birth. Signs and symptoms relating to the infection may develop later in infancy, childhood or even adult life, at which stage microbiological investigations cannot distinguish congenital from postnatal infection. By that time it may no longer be possible to determine whether the damage was the result of an infection acquired *in utero* or an unrelated problem. For example, a diagnosis of congenital infection cannot be made in a three-year-old child presenting with severe developmental delay and excreting CMV in the urine. Demonstrating the possible role of infections in pregnancy as a cause of fetal damage can therefore be difficult and open to misinterpretation.

Population prevalence

Infectious agents that induce protective immunity, such as rubella or measles, can only survive in communities large enough to ensure a reasonable pool of susceptible individuals; herd immunity prevents transmission. In contrast, organisms that are capable of persisting, such as herpes simplex, can survive indefinitely, even in small communities. The vertical transmission of an infection such as hepatitis B can also influence the population prevalence and clinical impact of the infection. In some populations where CMV infection is acquired early in life through vertical or horizontal transmission, the seroprevalence is high among the pregnant population. Subsequent changes in lifestyle, such as the avoidance of breastfeeding and smaller families, could result in fewer children being exposed to CMV in early life and subsequently a reduced maternal seroprevalence, with more women susceptible to a primary infection in pregnancy. The prevalence of toxoplasmosis is low in the UK, compared with many other countries, and congenital infection is rare. There is also some evidence for a decline in the prevalence of toxoplasmosis in northern Europe, which suggests a reduction in exposure to the parasite in these countries and an anticipated reduction in congenital toxoplasmosis.[23] The geographical pattern of specific infections in different populations, both between countries and within a country, highlights the need for accurate information about the prevalence of an infection and risk factors for acquisition of infection when making decisions about management and policy.

Timing of infection

Knowledge about the timing of infection in pregnancy will influence decisions about screening and treatment and will also be important for the development of appropriate interventions to reduce vertical transmission.

The gestational age of the pregnancy when infection occurs may influence the risk of vertical transmission and/or the fetal or perinatal consequences. For example, fetal infection is highest following exposure to maternal rubella in early and late gestation but exposure in the first trimester is associated with a high risk of serious congenital defects whereas exposure to infection late in pregnancy or in the postpartum period poses little risk. In contrast, exposure of the fetus to a primary CMV infection at any stage of pregnancy poses a risk of adverse outcome, although the risk is probably higher following exposure in early rather than late gestation. With maternal toxoplasmosis infection, the overall reported rate of transmission is low (10%) following infection acquired in the first two weeks after conception and increases to over 90% following infection in the last two weeks of pregnancy. In contrast, the risk of serious adverse sequelae is much higher following exposure to infection in early pregnancy rather than later exposure.[24] It is still not clear whether the timing of treatment after maternal toxoplasmosis will influence the risk of transmission and this is obviously important in reaching decisions about the role of antenatal screening. Maternal infection with parvovirus B19 in the first 20 weeks of gestation can lead to intrauterine death and hydrops fetalis. These consequences usually occur three to five weeks after the onset of maternal infection. Although congenital infection may occur, there is no evidence that this is associated with abnormalities.[25]

In contrast to infections where intrauterine transmission is the major route of infection, the risk of neonatal herpes infection is high and associated with a significant risk of mortality and morbidity when a primary maternal herpes infection is acquired at the time of delivery. Maternal infection in early pregnancy poses little risk for the fetus. Similarly, varicella at the time of delivery or just before may cause overwhelming infection in the newborn but infection in earlier pregnancy is associated with a low risk of defects, about 1%. Infection in mid-trimester poses no risk but is associated with the development of herpes zoster in early life.

Intrapartum and neonatal acquisition of CMV is common in infants exposed to seropositive mothers as a result of exposure to infected cervical secretions, or to infected breast milk.[26] There is no evidence to date, however, that infection acquired at this time is associated with adverse effects, except in the very premature or immune-compromised infant. In a non-breastfed population, about two-thirds of mother-to-child transmission of HIV occurs during the intrapartum period and, in contrast to CMV, infection acquired at this stage has serious consequences for the infant.[27]

Type of infection – primary or recurrent

Infections that affect the fetus or newborn may follow a primary maternal infection, reactivation of a latent maternal infection, or result from exposure to infectious agents that constitute part of the lower genital tract flora. A primary infection in pregnancy usually presents a more serious threat to the fetus or infant than a recurrent or secondary infection. This is related to the mother's immune status and the level of exposure to the organism. This is exemplified by the example of perinatal HSV and varicella-zoster virus infection where the presence of maternal antibodies at the time of exposure provides some protection.[10] For some infections, such as rubella, it is the primary infection that results in maternal viraemia with subsequent fetal infection and damage. The rationale for the prevention of congenital rubella through immunisation is based on this assumption although a few cases of congenital infection have been reported following a reinfection of rubella in pregnancy. Although congenital CMV infection may result from primary maternal infection or recurrent infection, evidence until recently has shown that fetal damage results from primary infection, with only a few anecdotal reports of damage following recurrent infection. However, reports in 1999 from the USA and Sweden showed that an equal number of congenitally infected children with damage had been exposed to recurrent maternal infection as to primary infection.[28,29] This observation is important and likely to influence any screening policy. Congenital syphilis is more common following fetal exposure to primary or secondary infection than latent or tertiary infection.

Risk factors for acquisition of maternal and fetal or newborn infection

With the development of more-sophisticated laboratory methods and well-designed epidemiological studies, risk factors for vertical transmission of infection are now being elucidated. This clearly has implications for the management of infection. Examples include maternal factors such as viral load, maternal immune status, stage of disease and the woman's general health and nutritional status. Associated genital infections, prematurity and low birthweight may also be important, as are as obstetric factors and interventions in labour, such as the use of scalp electrodes (HSV and HIV), length of rupture of the membranes and mode of delivery. The maturity of the fetal immune system is another factor. For each infection, risk factors for acquisition of infection or fetal/newborn damage need to be considered, as they are likely to influence the management of pregnancy.

Treatment in pregnancy

As new treatments become available it is essential that they be evaluated in randomised controlled trials. Until now, little has been available for the treatment of viral infections in pregnancy but, with the development of new and promising antiviral drugs, the situation may well change. There is now good evidence for the effectiveness of anti-retroviral drugs to prevent HIV infection[17] and women have been treated for HSV infection with aciclovir to reduce the viral shedding in the genital tract. With the increase in maternal anti-retroviral therapy to prevent perinatal transmission of HIV, there has been a marked decline in vertically acquired infection.[30] However, these uninfected infants have been exposed to combination anti-retroviral therapy and it will be essential for them to be followed up so that any potential adverse effects can be identified.

The treatment of women with toxoplasmosis in pregnancy with spiramycin, or the more potent regimen of pyrimethamine and sulphadiazine, has been the standard practice for many years. The efficacy of these drugs in reducing transmission has never been evaluated in a randomised clinical trial and such a trial would no longer be considered ethical. However, there is now increasing evidence to suggest that this treatment is unlikely to reduce mother-to-child transmission or to reduce the subsequent complications of congenital toxoplasmosis.[31] Treatments for bacterial sepsis such as group B streptococcal infection and bacterial vaginosis have implications for screening programmes and need to be evaluated carefully before they are introduced into practice.

Conclusion

With the development of new technologies and the availability of improved laboratory diagnostic tests, the diagnosis of many infections in pregnancy is becoming more feasible and more reliable. This progress has been accompanied by a tendency to assume that the detection of an infection *per se* can only be beneficial. This is not necessarily the case if the infection has little impact on pregnancy outcome or maternal wellbeing. It is not the number of women with a positive test that measures the effectiveness of a screening programme but the reduction in harm to the infant that will ensue and the impact that such an intervention will have in the prevention of handicap and disabilities. There is some evidence to suggest that certain ultrasound appearances are suggestive of an infectious aetiology. This observation needs to be confirmed in more rigorous scientific studies before women are subjected to detailed investigations, particularly as there is often no treatment available for the infection in question and the only intervention is pregnancy termination.

The recent speculation that subclinical infections in pregnancy may be important in the aetiology of cerebral palsy is challenging.[32] This hypothesis needs further investigation and, if shown to be true, could have huge implications. A meta-analysis reported in 2000 indicated that chorioamnionitis is a risk factor for cerebral palsy and cystic periventricular leucomalacia which is believed to be a precursor of cerebral palsy in premature infants.[33]

Infections for which routine testing in pregnancy has recently been proposed include HTLV-1 infection, hepatitis C infection, parvovirus infection and streptococcus B infection. The management of a woman who presents with clinical signs of an infection poses different issues to the active screening of all pregnant women to identify those who have the infection. The complex issue of screening will be addressed in the next chapter.

Much is now known about the adverse perinatal outcomes resulting from the classic infections such as rubella, CMV infection, toxoplasmosis, syphilis and hepatitis B. The possible association of bacterial vaginosis and occult intrauterine infections with premature delivery and cerebral palsy could contribute further to the overall burden of adverse pregnancy outcome and needs to be addressed.

References

1. Peckham C, Marshall WC. Infections in pregnancy. In: *Obstetrical Epidemiology.* London: Academic Press; 1983. p. 209–59.
2. Katz RG, White LR, Sever JL. Maternal and congenital rubella. *Clin Pediatr (Phila)* 1968;**7**:323–30.
3. Tookey PA, Peckham C. Surveillance of congenital rubella in Great Britain, 1971–1996. *BMJ* 1999;**318**:769–70.
4. Tookey PA, Jones G, Miller BH, Peckham CS. Rubella vaccination in pregnancy. *CDR (Lond Engl Rev)* 1991;**1**:R86–8.
5. McGrath J, Castle D, Murray R. How can we judge whether or not prenatal exposure to influenza causes schizophrenia? In: Melnick SA, Hollister JM, editors. *Neural Development and Schizophrenia.* New

York: Plenum; 1995. p. 203–14.

6. Leck I. Incidence of malformations following influenza epidemics. *Br J Prev Soc Med* 1963;**17**:70–80.
7. Fedrick J, Alberman ED. Reported influenza in pregnancy and subsequent cancer in the child. *BMJ* 1972;**2**:485–8.
8. Tookey P, Peckham C. Neonatal herpes simplex virus infection in the British Isles. *Paediatr Perinat Epidemiol* 1996;**10**:432–42.
9. American College of Obstetricians and Gynecologists. *Perinatal Herpes Simplex-Virus Infections.* Washington DC: ACOG; 1988. ACOG Technical Bulletin 122.
10. Prober CG, Sullender WM, Yasukawa LL, Au DS, Yeager AS, Arvin AM. Low risk of herpes simplex virus infections in neonates exposed to the virus at the time of vaginal delivery to mothers with recurrent genital herpes simplex virus infections. *N Engl J Med* 1987;**316**:240–4.
11. Brown ZA, Benedetti J, Ashley R, Burchett S, Selke S, Berry S, *et al.* Neonatal herpes simplex virus infection in relation to asymptomatic maternal infection at the time of labour. *N Engl J Med* 1991;**324**:1247–52.
12. Binkin NJ, Koplan JP, Cates W. Preventing neonatal herpes: the value of weekly viral cultures in pregnant women with recurrent genital herpes. *JAMA* 1984;**251**:2816–21.
13. Anonymous. Cytomegalovirus in adults. *Lancet* 1977;**ii**:541.
14. Peckham C, Coleman JC, Hurley R, Chin KS, Henderson K, Preece PM. Cytomegalovirus infection in pregnancy: preliminary findings from a prospective study. *Lancet* 1983;**i**:1352–5.
15. Ahlfors K, Ivarsson SA, Johnsson T, Svanberg L. Primary and secondary maternal cytomegalovirus infections and their relation to congenital infection. Analysis of maternal sera. *Acta Paediatr Scand* 1982;**71**:109–13.
16. Larke RPB, Wheatly E, Saigal S, Chernesky MA. Congenital cytomegalovirus infection in an urban Canadian community. *J Infect Dis* 1980;**142**:647–53.
17. Connor EM, Sperling RS, Gelber R, Kiselev P, Scott G, O'Sullivan MJ. Reduction of maternal–infant transmission of human immunodeficiency virus type 1 with zidovudine treatment. *N Engl J Med* 1994;**331**:1173–80.
18. Higa K, Dan K, Manabe H. Varicella zoster virus infections during pregnancy: hypothesis concerning the mechanisms of congenital malformations. *Obstet Gynecol* 1987;**69**:214–22.
19. Enders G, Miller E, Cradock-Watson J, Bolley I, Ridehalgh M. Consequences of varicella and herpes zoster in pregnancy: prospective study of 1739 cases. *Lancet* 1994;**343**:1548–51.
20. Peckham C. Clinical and laboratory study of children exposed *in utero* to maternal rubella. *Arch Dis Child* 1972;**47**:571–7.
21. Forrest JM, Menser MA, Burgess JA. High frequency of diabetes mellitus in young adults with congenital rubella. *Lancet* 1971;**ii**:332–4.
22. Koppe JG, Rothova A. Congenital toxoplasmosis. a long-term follow-up of 20 years. *Int Ophthalmol* 1989;**13**:387–90.
23. Walker J, Nokes DJ, Jennings R. Longitudinal study of toxoplasma sero-prevalence in south Yorkshire. *Epidemiol Infect* 1992;**108**:99–108.
24. Dunn D, Wallon M, Peyron F, Petersen E, Peckham C, Gilbert R. Mother-to-child transmission of toxoplasmosis: risk estimates for clinical counselling. *Lancet* 1999;**353**:1829–33.
25. Miller E, Fairley CK, Cohen BJ, Seng C. Immediate and long term outcome of human parvovirus B19 infection in pregnancy. *Br J Obstet Gynaecol* 1998;**105**:174–8.
26. Reynolds DW, Stagno S, Mosty TS. Maternal cytomegalovirus excretion and perinatal infection. *N Engl J Med* 1980;**302**:1073–6.
27. Newell M-L. Mechanisms and timing of mother-to-child transmission of HIV-1. *AIDS* 1998;**12**:831–7.
28. Ahlfors K, Ivarsson SA, Harris S. Report on a long-term study of maternal and congenital cytomegalovirus infection in Sweden. Review of prospective studies available in the literature. *Scand J Infect Dis* 1999;**31**:443–57.
29. Boppana SB, Fowler KB, Britt WJ, Stagno S, Pass RF. Symptomatic congenital cytomegalovirus infection in infants born to mothers with pre-existing immunity to cytomegalovirus. *Pediatrics* 1999;**104**:55–60.
30. European Collaborative Study. Maternal viral load and vertical transmission of HIV-1: an important factor but not the only one. *AIDS* 1999;**13**:1377–85.
31. Foulon W, Villena I, Stray-Pedersen B, Decoster A, Lappalainen M, Pinon J-M, *et al.* Treatment of toxoplasmosis during pregnancy: a multicenter study of impact on fetal transmission and children's sequelae at age 1 year. *Am J Obstet Gynecol* 1999;**180**:410–15.
32. Nelson KB, Dambrosia JM, Grether JK, Phillips TM. Neonatal cytokines and coagulation factors in children with cerebral palsy. *Ann Neurol* 1998;**44**:665–75.
33. Wu YW, Colford JM. Chorioamnionitis as a risk factor for cerebral palsy. *JAMA* 2000;**284**:1417–24.

34. Gregg NM. Congenital cataract following German measles in the mother. *Trans Ophthalmol Soc Aust* 1941;**3**:35–46.
35. Lundström R. Rubella during pregnancy: a follow-up study of children born after an epidemic of rubella in Sweden, 1951, with additional investigations on prophylaxis and treatment of maternal rubella. *Acta Paediatr Scand Suppl* 1962;**133**:1–110.
36. Manson MM, Logan WPD, Loy RM. Rubella and other virus infections during pregnancy. *Rep Public Health Med Subj (Lond)* 1960;101.
37. Weller TH, Neva FA. Propagation in tissue culture of cytopathic agents from patients with rubella-like illness. *Proc Soc Exp Biol Med* 1962;**111**:215–25.
38. Parkman PD, Buescher E L, Artenstein M S. Recovery of rubella virus from army recruits. *Proc Soc Exp Biol Med* 1962;**111**:225–30.

Chapter 2

Antenatal screening for infections

Marie-Louise Newell

Introduction

Screening is the systematic application of a test or enquiry to identify individuals at sufficient risk of a specific disorder to benefit from further investigation or direct preventive action, among people who have not sought medical attention on account of symptoms of that disorder.[1] Screening tests thus aim to distinguish apparently healthy people from those who may have a disease or an infection requiring treatment. Screening may involve the whole population (routine screening approach) or it may target groups with specific exposure. Case-finding or opportunistic screening is restricted to patients who consult a clinician for some other purpose.

The UK Department of Health, through the National Screening Committee, reviews the appropriateness of introducing antenatal screening programmes for various conditions, using standard requirements. In the UK, all pregnant women are screened for specific conditions on a routine basis. There is no condition for which selective screening is recommended, although in the past hepatitis B virus (HBV) screening was targeted at women at increased risk of being infected.[2,3] Decisions to introduce targeted screening were based on the finding that the prevalence of HBV varies between populations and within countries. In South-East Asia and Africa, up to 20% of pregnant women are chronic carriers of HBV. In Eastern Europe, Japan, Russia and the Mediterranean countries, 20–30% of women have evidence of past infection and 2–7% are carriers. In Northern Europe and North America, the prevalence is low and less than 1% of pregnant women are chronic carriers. Although information about HBV prevalence in specific populations could thus serve as a basis for selective screening programmes, it has now been recognised that this approach fails to identify a substantial proportion of infected women. This recognition has led to a change in approach and the recommendation of routine antenatal screening for HBV.[4,5] However, primary screening for risk factors to identify those at increased risk of being infected, who could then be offered further screening tests, has never been formally evaluated as a policy.

Infections in pregnancy can be transmitted from mother to child and result in congenital or perinatal infection with adverse sequelae for the infant. Maternal infections with potential infection of the fetus or newborn infant are discussed in Chapter 1. The justification of screening for specific infections in pregnancy is to prevent or reduce the adverse consequences of these infections for the fetus or newborn, through treatment, or for the mother through termination of the pregnancy. Most congenital infections occur after an asymptomatic infection during pregnancy in the mother and there are usually no symptoms or signs of infection in the newborn either. It may be weeks, months or even years before damage in the child first becomes apparent, complicating the diagnosis of the congenital nature of the infection. For example, in a child with progressive sensorineural deafness, it is not possible to attribute the cause of the deafness to congenital cytomegalovirus (CMV) infection if samples taken from the infant shortly after birth are not available for investigation.[6] Acquisition of CMV infection in the first year of life is common, especially in breastfed infants. In children with virological or serological evidence of infection after six months of age, it is not possible to distinguish congenital from acquired infection.[7]

The role of screening for infections during pregnancy

One of the major, possibly preventable, causes of perinatal morbidity and mortality is infection. Infection during pregnancy is relatively common. Although most infections do not have serious consequences for obstetric or perinatal outcomes, some do. The National Screening Committee recommends antenatal screening of all women for syphilis, HBV, HIV and rubella, and other conditions are currently being reviewed by this committee. The aim in screening for syphilis, HBV and HIV infection is to prevent fetal abnormalities by identifying women early in pregnancy so that treatment can be initiated to reduce transmission of infection from mother to child, or to prevent an adverse outcome in the infant.

Screening for rubella is different in that it does not aim to reduce damage in the current pregnancy but to identify susceptible women who require postpartum vaccination to protect a subsequent pregnancy. Fetal exposure to rubella in the first trimester of pregnancy is associated with a high risk of serious congenital defects, whereas exposure to infection late in pregnancy or in the postpartum period poses little risk.[8] It has been estimated that less than 2% of all pregnant women in the UK are susceptible to rubella.[9] Screening for rubella in pregnancy cannot influence the prevalence of congenital rubella in that pregnancy, since susceptible women cannot be immunised until after the pregnancy during which they are screened. A targeted approach with screening of high-risk women has been suggested, but this alternative is generally dismissed.

The National Screening Committee has recommended universal screening of all pregnant women for syphilis, despite suggestions from some quarters that this may no longer be necessary as so few infections among women are reported in the UK (about 50–60 cases a year). However, it was argued that this low level of infection might not be maintained.[3,10,11] With the increased immigration from Eastern Europe, where the prevalence of syphilis is relatively high, there have been outbreaks in the UK. This highlights the need for continued vigilance and the justification of the decision at national level to continue the antenatal programme. Untreated syphilis in pregnancy may result in significant perinatal mortality and morbidity, depending on the stage of the infection in the mother. In order to prevent congenital syphilis, pregnant women are tested serologically and those who are seropositive are treated with penicillin. This approach, when taken in early pregnancy, prevents most cases of congenital syphilis. Detection in late pregnancy is less effective but may still prevent some of the sequelae. The diagnosis of congenital syphilis is difficult and there is a lack of reliable data on the number of pregnant women with syphilis. Based on information from Oxford and Merseyside, it has been estimated that the prevalence nationally is about 70 per million deliveries. If this figure applied to England and Wales as a whole, and if the children of nearly all untreated women with active syphilis and of 60% with early latent syphilis die in fetal or neonatal life or are damaged by the infection, syphilis may be associated with adverse outcome in 50–60 per million pregnancies in the absence of screening.

Requirements for the introduction of a screening programme

There is a continuing public and professional debate as to the relative merits of extending antenatal screening programmes to include other infections such as toxoplasmosis, CMV, herpes simplex, chlamydia, hepatitis C virus (HCV) and streptococcal B infection.[12,13] The development and wider availability of laboratory tests together with advances in prenatal diagnoses have increased the scope and pressure for possible interventions to reduce the consequences of congenital and perinatal infections.

However, screening can only be justified for infections that are serious, a significant health problem and for which a treatment or intervention is available. The following are typical requirements of a successful screening programme:

1.   The condition is an important public health problem;

2.   The natural history of the infection is clear;

3.   Primary prevention should have been implemented if possible;

4.   The screening test is safe, valid and reliable;

5.   The screening test, and available treatment, should be acceptable to the population;

6.   Agreed policy and adequate facilities to confirm the diagnosis and for treatment;

7.   Treatment, or intervention, is of proven effectiveness;

8.   There is evidence that early treatment is associated with better outcome than late treatment;

9.   The risk of harm to those being screened is less than the chance of benefit;

10.   Objectives of the screening programme justify its costs;

11.   The screening programme should be monitored.

Specific information required in reaching a decision to screen antenatally for any infection includes:[14]

1.   The prevalence of the infection in the pregnant population;

2.   The rate of mother-to-child transmission of that infection;

3.   The reliability of the screening and subsequent diagnostic tests;

4.   The assessment of disease burden in both symptomatic and asymptomatic congenitally infected infants;

5.   The effectiveness, acceptability and safety of the interventions and treatment.

In order to estimate the burden of disease resulting from a specific infection in pregnancy, detailed epidemiological information is required. An understanding of the epidemiology of individual infections is also essential for counselling women about the risk of adverse effects, the development of appropriate management and prevention strategies and for the evaluation of available interventions. The natural history of the disease should be understood.

In the UK, the National Screening Committee has been established to develop screening policies based on all available evidence, including an economic analysis. The Population Screening Panel is an advisory committee of the National Health Service R&D Health Technology Assessment programme that commissions reviews of new and existing programmes. The pressure to screen is often considerable. A major requirement for the introduction of a screening programme is the availability of a suitable and acceptable screening test, with high sensitivity and specificity. A substantial number of diagnostic or screening tests have been accepted in clinical practice before their effectiveness has been demonstrated, although the reverse is also found.[15] The identification of a specific infection in pregnancy is complicated by the fact that maternal infections are generally asymptomatic or present with non-specific signs and symptoms, which usually do not warrant clinic attendance. This is the reason for the introduction of screening programmes that can be applied to all women or to a relevant subgroup to identify those who have evidence of past infection and those who remain susceptible for acquisition of infection during pregnancy. Another complication is that women remain at risk of acquiring an infection throughout their pregnancy and it may thus be necessary to offer repeat testing to women who screened negative on the first antenatal sample. This is especially important where acquisition of infection at different times during pregnancy is associated with severity of outcome for the infant. For example, in toxoplasmosis, the risk of vertical transmission increases with gestational age of maternal infection, while the risk of serious adverse effects decreases.[16,17]

The screening test

A screening programme has several clear components, including the identification of women likely to have infection, the confirmation of the infection and the subsequent management and treatment, although much attention focuses on the screening test itself. Any test will find true and false positives, and true and false negatives. Although ideally the test used would only find those truly with the infection and would correctly identify those truly without the infection, in practice this is rarely possible. No screening test can guarantee a true result in all cases and there will therefore be false reassurance for some and false anxiety for others. In deciding on the test to be used, there is thus a trade-off between not missing real cases and not finding false cases. For women who are truly infected, there may be treatment benefit or at least the opportunity of preventing transmission to the unborn child. However, women who are positive on the screening test, but where further investigations exclude true infection, will be exposed to unnecessary treatment, or even pregnancy termination, and anxiety.[18]

Terms commonly used when assessing particular programmes include: the detection rate, sensitivity, specificity, false positivity and false negativity rate, and positive and negative predictive value. The detection rate is the number of people identified with the disease in the population screened. The sensitivity is the proportion of affected individuals identified through screening, and the specificity is the proportion of unaffected women correctly identified as being negative. High specificity would be desirable if:

1.   The diagnosis is associated with stigma or anxiety;

2.   Further investigations would be time-consuming, painful or expensive;

3.   Cases are likely to be detected by other means at a time when treatment can still be instigated;

4.   Treatment is to be offered without further investigations.

High sensitivity would be desirable if there are serious adverse consequences of a missed diagnosis for the individual or for society and if the diagnosis is to be confirmed by other investigations, so that the period of anxiety is short and the correct diagnosis is given before treatment is started.[18] The false positivity rate is the proportion of non-infected women identified as infected through the screening, and the false negativity rate the proportion of infected women identified as uninfected through screening. The rarer the condition, the smaller the chance that those with a positive screening test are truly infected. A reduction in the false positivity rate is usually only achieved at the expense of a rise in the false negativity rate. A screening test, even when of high sensitivity, will give some false negative results when applied to a large number of people. It should be understood by the health carer and by the patient that a negative result does not necessarily guarantee absence of infection. The positive predictive value is the probability of disease in a woman with a positive test result, while the negative predictive value relates to the probability of absence of disease in a woman with a negative test result.

Sensitivity and specificity have limited value in clinical practice, where all that is known is the test result. Clinicians will want to know what proportion of women with abnormal test results are truly abnormal. Although the probability of the test's giving the correct diagnosis is reflected in the negative and positive predictive values, these measures are strongly influenced by the prevalence of the infection in that population. A commonly used alternative is the likelihood ratio.[15] The likelihood ratio of a positive result is the probability of a positive test in an infected woman divided by the probability of a positive test in an uninfected woman. It can be calculated from the sensitivity and specificity of a test.[15]

Subsequent to a positive screening test, further investigations involving, for example, repeat blood samples or amniocentesis will be needed to confirm the diagnosis. Even if subsequently shown not to have the infection these women for whom further investigations were deemed necessary are potentially at risk of anxiety, misdiagnosis, unnecessary interventions and the adverse effects of the test procedures. The consequences of a false positive or a false negative diagnosis must not be underestimated and have become increasingly important with the increase in litigation.

Information for health professionals and parents

Information giving and obtaining consent has been a particular issue in the management of HIV infection during the 1990s in the UK. The diagnosis of HIV infection is often associated with stigma, fear and other negative experiences. Initially, there was little to balance these negative aspects. However, the emergence of interventions to prevent mother-to-child transmission and the acceptance of early therapy to delay progression of disease have resulted in wider acceptance of the offer of antenatal testing. Nevertheless, it has been shown that the most important determinant of whether a woman accepts antenatal testing for HIV is the midwife she sees rather than the information she receives.[19-21] The provision of leaflets and other means of information dissemination relating to HIV infection has been integrated with those of other infections routinely screened for antenatally. This has had a positive effect on knowledge about these other infections, for example, syphilis, rubella, and HBV infection.

In London, of the 18 antenatal units that had implemented a policy of recommending and offering an HIV test in 1999, 13 obtained verbal consent and five obtained written consent.[22] The lack of information for healthcare professionals was identified as one of the major issues hindering the success of an antenatal screening programme. The importance of involvement of members of relevant ethnic groups was also highlighted. The InterCollegiate Working Party recommends that testing for all infections and conditions in pregnancy should continue to be with the women's knowledge and verbal consent. These recommendations stress the importance of giving pre-test information and post-test counselling.

Ethical considerations

Screening is different from most other forms of health care, as apparently healthy people are being convinced to take up testing and then treatment if found to be infected. It is thus essential to demonstrate that there is benefit from the programme, and that the collective benefit will outweigh any adverse effects. Ethical considerations have an important role to play in decisions regarding the appropriateness of specific screening programmes. The pressure to introduce a programme may be because the problem is a major one, and because of the intuitive assumption that prevention is better than cure. It may also be driven by technology, the ability to carry out the screening or the development of new treatment. The costs of screening can be substantial and need to be balanced against alternative approaches to the problem, such as primary prevention programmes. The outcome of the programme may be clearer in population terms than on an individual basis. The nature of the infection itself can also cause problems. For example, a diagnosis of HIV infection carries stigma, which can create social problems, and may affect the ability to obtain life assurance and a mortgage. For all infections, facilities need to be in place for the management of those women and children diagnosed with a particular infection.

Infections not included in the UK screening programme

There has been some pressure from the public and from professionals to introduce routine antenatal screening for CMV and toxoplasmosis infection[12] and the appropriateness or otherwise of their inclusion in the current programme is under review. In the early 1990s, the Royal College of Obstetricians and Gynaecologists concluded that, in the light of available knowledge, screening for acute toxoplasmosis was not of proven benefit, and noted the possibility that such a programme might cause more harm than good.[22] A subsequent review confirmed the original recommendations. In 1994, a Chief Medical Officer's report stated that antenatal screening for CMV was not appropriate in the UK based on the information available. As the pattern of infection and the distribution of disease may differ between countries, national decisions taken regarding antenatal screening for these infections are also likely to differ.

Exposure of the fetus to a primary CMV infection poses a risk of adverse outcome at any stage of pregnancy. Infection can be acquired *in utero*, in the intrapartum period or postpartum through breastfeeding. About 50% of pregnant women in the UK are susceptible to CMV infection, with considerable age-specific variation in seroprevalence by ethnic group, which would mean that about half of pregnant women would have to be tested serologically repeatedly throughout pregnancy. About one in every 100 women found to be susceptible in early pregnancy will acquire a primary infection during pregnancy, and about 40% of infected women are likely to transmit the infection to their fetus. Long-term sequelae occur in about 6% of all infants whose mothers experience a primary CMV infection during pregnancy. Both primary and recurrent infection during pregnancy can result in fetal damage, although the risk is thought to be small after recurrent infection. There is currently no effective treatment for either maternal or fetal CMV infection and the only intervention to prevent congenital CMV is termination of a fetus believed to be infected.

The overall rate of fetal infection following exposure to maternal toxoplasmosis infection depends on the time of acquisition of maternal infection. The rate is low following infection acquired in the first two weeks after conception and increases to over 90% following infection in the last two weeks of pregnancy.[16,17] In contrast, the risk of serious adverse sequelae following toxoplasmosis infection is much higher following exposure to infection in early pregnancy than following exposure in later pregnancy. It is generally accepted that fetal infection is associated with acute toxoplasmosis infection in the mother rather than with chronic infection, and screening programmes are based on this principle. There are marked differences in the prevalence of past toxoplasmosis infection in pregnant women. For example, about 10% of women in the UK and Norway have evidence of past infection, whereas the figure in France and Greece is more than 50%.[17]

The aim of screening would be to identify women at risk of becoming infected during pregnancy, so that maternal infections arising after conception can be treated. No maternal screening test will identify fetal infection, but women with a positive screening test can be offered amniocentesis or cordocentesis to establish whether fetal infection has occurred. However, these investigations carry a risk of associated pregnancy loss. If maternal infection is diagnosed, the use of antibiotic spiramycin to reduce the risk of fetal infection is widely recommended, although its efficacy has never been tested in a randomised controlled trial. In research carried out within the

European Network on Toxoplasmosis, evidence is starting to emerge that treatment does not reduce vertical transmission risk, probably because of the delay between infection, diagnosis and initiation of therapy, even if pregnant women are screened every month.[24]

Antenatal toxoplasmosis screening programmes have been set up in some European countries and there has been continued pressure in the UK to follow this option. However, there is insufficient evidence to recommend routine screening for toxoplasmosis in the UK, where 80–90% of women would have to be repeatedly tested throughout pregnancy for a primary toxoplasmosis infection. Furthermore, there is no reliable information regarding the efficacy of therapeutic intervention in preventing vertical transmission. The natural history of congenital toxoplasmosis is inadequately described.

It has been suggested that all pregnant women should be offered testing for HCV infection. The prevalence of HCV in antenatal populations in the UK is low and the risk of mother-to-child transmission is about 5% in the general population. There is currently no intervention available to prevent vertical transmission and indeed interferon, which may be used in the treatment of HCV infection in adults, is contraindicated during pregnancy. HCV infection has not yet been considered by the National Screening Committee and HCV is not included in the national programme.

Also under consideration is screening for infections such as group B streptococcus, which is an important cause of neonatal bacterial sepsis.[25] Healthy women may carry group B streptococci and be a source of peripartum infection of their offspring. There is considerable variation in colonisation rates between and within countries.[13,26] In the USA, the high prevalence of the carrier state and the economic burden this imposes has led to the recommendation that, except where the prevalence is high, women with risk factors such as onset of labour before 37 weeks, prolonged rupture of the membranes or maternal fever during labour should have swabs taken from the genital tract and tested, so that women with positive results could receive intrapartum antibiotics.[13,25,26] In the UK, the low prevalence of group B streptococcal disease in neonates provides a strong argument against routine antenatal screening.

Monitoring the efficacy of a screening programme

Once established, all screening programmes need to be kept under review and, if necessary, modified to ensure that they are achieving their objectives. Monitoring of antenatal screening programmes requires computerised databases linking the laboratories to clinical information such as the offer of a test, its uptake, the proportion of women who are positive and their subsequent management at hospital level. Measuring the success of antenatal screening programmes in identifying women with an infection is essential. For example, national targets have been set for the reduction in number of infants with vertically acquired HIV infection and the uptake of antenatal HIV testing offers. However, the success of the HIV screening programme depends on the acceptability and uptake of the interventions to reduce the risk of mother-to-child transmission. Similarly, the effectiveness of the HBV antenatal screening programme depends heavily on the adequate follow-up of infants born to mothers with hepatitis B surface antigen and the immediate administration of immunoglobulin and vaccination.[3,5] It has been shown in some programmes that many infants at risk of acquiring hepatitis B in the perinatal period are not receiving the appropriate treatment.[4] Unless attention is given to the allocation of responsibility for the infant follow-up, antenatal screening for HBV infection cannot be successful.[5] There is a lack of information regarding the proportion of pregnant women susceptible to rubella and the number of susceptible women who are vaccinated. The antenatal rubella screening programme can thus not be adequately monitored.

Conclusion

In the UK, the current antenatal screening programme includes syphilis, rubella, HIV and HBV, and the justification for inclusion of these infections is clear-cut. Debate is continuing about whether toxoplasmosis, CMV and streptococcal B infection should also be included, but to date there have been insufficient grounds to do so. As tests for new conditions, for example, HCV and chlamydia infection, are developed their inclusion or otherwise in an antenatal screening programme will be considered by the National Screening Committee. Monitoring of existing programmes ensures continued assessment of their effectiveness. An informed decision, based on all available evidence, can then be taken.

References

1. Peckham CS, Dezateux C. Issues underlying the evaluation of screening programmes. *Br Med Bull* 1998;**54**:767–78.
2. Law M, Jordan R. An appraisal of the efficacy and cost effectiveness of antenatal screening for hepatitis B. *J Med Screen* 1997;**4**:117–27.
3. Newell ML, Thorne C, Pembrey L, Nicoll A, Goldberg D, Peckham C. Antenatal screening for hepatitis B infection and syphilis in the UK. *Br J Obstet Gynaecol* 1999;**106**:66–71.
4. Kohn MA, Farley TA, Scott C. The need for more aggressive follow-up of children born to hepatitis B surface antigen-positive mothers: lessons from the Louisiana perinatal hepatitis B immunization program. *Pediatr Infect Dis J* 1996;**15**:535–40.
5. Mortimer PP, Miller E. Commentary: Antenatal screening and targeting should be sufficient in some countries. *BMJ* 1997;**314**:1036–7.
6. Ahlfors K, Ivarsson SA, Harris S. Report on a long-term study of maternal and congenital cytomegalovirus infection in Sweden. Review of prospective studies available in the literature. *Scand J Infect Dis* 1999;**31**:443–547.
7. Peckham CS. Cytomegalovirus infection: congenital and neonatal disease. *Scand J Infect Dis Suppl* 1991;**80**:82–7.
8. Miller E, Cradock-Watson JE, Pollock TM. Consequences of confirmed maternal rubella at successive stages of pregnancy. *Lancet* 1982;**ii**:781–4.
9. Miller C, Miller E, Begg N. Rubella vaccination policy: a note of reassurance. *Lancet* 1987;**ii**:210.
10. Nicoll A, Moisley C. Antenatal screening for syphilis. *BMJ* 1994;**308**:1253–4.
11. Snowise N. Antenatal screening for syphilis is not justified [letter]. *BMJ* 1994;**309**:194.
12. Peckham CS, Logan S. Screening for toxoplasmosis during pregnancy. *Arch Dis Child* 1993;**68**:3–5.
13. American Academy of Pediatrics Committee On Infectious Diseases and Committee on Fetus and Newborn: Guidelines for prevention of group B streptococcal (GBS) infection by chemoprophylaxis. *Pediatrics* 1992;**90**:775–8.
14. Wilson JM, Junger G. *Principles and Practice of Screening for Disease*. Geneva: WHO; 1968.
15. Abalos EJ, Gulmezoglu M, Carroli G. Assessing the scientific value of screening for antenatal infections. In: Newell ML, McIntyre J, editors. *Congenital and Perinatal Infections: Prevention, Diagnosis and Treatment*. Cambridge: Cambridge University Press; 2000. p. 64–79.

16. Dunn D, Foulon W, Peyron F, Petersen E, Peckham CS, Gilbert RE. Mother to child transmission of toxoplasmosis: risk estimates for clinical counselling. *Lancet* 1999;**353**:1829–33.
17. Gilbert RE. Toxoplasmosis. In: Newell ML, McIntyre J, editors. *Congenital and Perinatal Infections: Prevention, Diagnosis and Treatment*. Cambridge: Cambridge University Press; 2000. p. 305–20.
18. Shickle D, Chadwick R. The ethics of screening: is 'screeningitis' an incurable disease? *J Med Ethics* 1994;**20**:12–18.
19. MacDonagh SE, Masters J, Helps BA, Tookey PA, Ades A, Gibb DM. Descriptive survey of antenatal HIV testing in London: policy, uptake, and detection. *BMJ* 1996;**313**:532–3.
20. Chrystie IL, Wolfe CDA, Kennedy J, Zander L, Tilzey A, Banatvala JE. Voluntary, named testing for HIV in a community based antenatal clinic: a pilot study. *BMJ* 1995;**311**:928–31.
21. MacDonagh SE, Masters J, Helps BA, Tookey PA, Gibb DM. Why are antenatal HIV testing policies in London failing? *Br J Midwifery* 1996;**4**:466–70.
22. Bedford H, Chapple J. *Review of Antenatal HIV Testing Services in London*. London: Kensington & Chelsea and Westminster Health Authority; 1999.
23. Royal College of Obstetricians and Gynaecologists. *Prenatal Screening for Toxoplasmosis in the UK. Report of a Multidisciplinary Working Group*. London; 1992.
24. R Gilbert, personal communication.
25. Shah V, Ohlsson A. Perinatal group B streptococcal infections. In: Newell ML, McIntyre J, editors. *Congenital and Perinatal Infections: Prevention, Diagnosis and Treatment*. Cambridge: Cambridge University Press; 2000. p. 96–121.
26. Boyer KM, Gotoff SP. Prevention of early-onset neonatal group B streptococcal disease with selective intrapartum chemoprophylaxis. *N Engl J Med* 1986;**314**:1665–9.

Chapter 3

Investigation of rash illness, and exposure to rash illness, in pregnancy

Peter Morgan-Capner, Natasha S Crowcroft and
Elizabeth Miller

Introduction

This chapter considers the management of the pregnant woman with or exposed to rash illness, with a particular focus on rubella and parvovirus B19 infection. Previous guidance[1-3] has been published; this chapter also addresses aspects for which there was previously no consensus advice. It does not include localised skin disease, such as herpes zoster (see Chapter 19) and that caused by herpes simplex virus (see Chapter 20), but uses as a definition of a rash illness 'a rash compatible with a systemic viral illness'.

A Joint Working Party of the Advisory Committees of Virology and Vaccines and Immunisation was convened by the Public Health Laboratory Service (PHLS) to provide guidance based upon evidence where this is available and consensus where it is not.

The chapter does not attempt to embrace all aspects of management; those areas for which management is well established are only briefly considered, if at all, but relevant sources of further and background information are given.

Background

Although rubella, parvovirus B19 and varicella-zoster virus are the infections that are of most relevance because of their potential impact on the fetus and neonate, pregnant women will present with a generalised rash (or contact with a rash), the cause of which may not be clinically apparent. It is acknowledged, however, that often, particularly for varicella-zoster virus, clinical and/or epidemiological features may be sufficiently suggestive of the aetiology to form the basis of investigation and management.

Infections that may present with a rash illness in pregnant women in the UK include:

- rubella
- parvovirus B19
- varicella-zoster virus
- measles
- enterovirus
- infectious mononucleosis (Epstein–Barr virus or, very rarely, cytomegalovirus)
- syphilis
- streptococcus
- meningococcus
- a range of other infections not endemic within the UK and that only need consideration if there is a relevant history of recent travel (e.g. dengue).

Syphilis, streptococcal disease, meningococcal disease and imported infections are not considered further, as clinical and epidemiological information would focus appropriate investigation and diagnosis.

Table 3.1 shows the characteristic features and incidence of those infections in the UK of particular significance for the fetus – rubella and parvovirus B19.

All requests for laboratory investigation must give the following information to enable the results to be reported with the correct interpretation:

- full demographic details
- gestation of pregnancy (date of last menstrual period)
- date of onset, clinical features, type and distribution of any rash illness
- past history of rubella and any other antibody testing and/or rubella vaccine administration (and dates/places)
- any known contacts with rash illness, and dates of contact.

Antenatal sera should be retained for at least one year to assist in diagnosis/exposure in later pregnancy and investigation of the neonate. This may include exposure to varicella-zoster virus and parvovirus B19, when the availability of such sera for testing can be invaluable in rapidly assessing susceptibility.

Information for the pregnant woman

Information and advice concerning rashes should be given to all pregnant women. At booking, midwives should:

- enquire if women have previously had chickenpox or shingles and, if they have not, advise that they seek urgent medical attention if they develop chickenpox-type vesicles in pregnancy or have contact with chickenpox or shingles
- advise women to inform their midwife, GP or obstetrician urgently if they develop a rash in pregnancy
- advise women that they should inform their midwife, GP or obstetrician if they have 'contact' (see below) in pregnancy with someone who has a rash.

Women should be provided with unbiased information regarding screening and diagnostic tests, the meaning and consequences of both, what to expect in terms of results, and further options for management. Women should feel free to exercise whatever options they choose. Minimum standards of information prior to any screening or diagnostic tests to differentiate the origin of rash in pregnancy should include:

Table 3.1.   Characteristics of rubella and parvovirus B19 infections in the UK

	Rubella	Parvovirus B19
Proportion susceptible in young adult females	1–2%	40–50%
Infectivity – risk of transmission from close contact (household attack rate)	High (90%)	Medium (50%)
Risk of intrauterine transmission by gestational age	<11 weeks: 90% 11–16 weeks: 55% >16 weeks: 45%	<4 weeks: 0% 5–16 weeks: 15% >16 weeks: 25–70% (increasing with gestation)
Risk of adverse fetal outcome by gestational age	<11 weeks: 90% 11–16 weeks: 20% 16–20 weeks: minimal risk of deafness only >20 weeks: no increased risk	<20 weeks: 9% excess fetal loss; 3% hydrops fetalis, of which about 50% die
Adverse maternal outcome	Arthritis	Arthritis
Interventions	Termination of pregnancy	Fetal hydrops: intrauterine transfusion reduces odds of death to 0.14
Incubation period	14–21 days	13–18 days
Infectivity period	7 days pre to 10 days post onset of rash	10 days pre to day of onset of rash
Infections in pregnancy	Currently rare	1 in 400 pregnancies[17] or seroconversion of 1.5–13% per annum among susceptible women
Terminations of pregnancy (*n*)	1995–96: 18 1997: 2	Unknown – not recommended
Babies with congenital infection (proven) (*n*)	1994–96: 20 1997–2000: 1	Unknown
Babies with congenital damage (proven) (*n*)	1994–96: 19 1997–2000: 1	Unknown
Babies with congenital infection (estimate)	Rare (see text)	See below
Babies with congenital damage (estimate)	Rare (see text)	2–8 fetal hydrops per 100 000 pregnancies (14–56 cases per year) 12–48 per 100 000 spontaneous abortions (84–336 cases per year)

- informing the woman that all tests to establish the initial diagnosis will be on blood samples obtained by phlebotomy. More-invasive tests, such as amniocentesis, are only required in rare situations, detailed below. All tests may uncommonly give inconclusive results and further testing may be necessary, which may prolong the time to result. Occasionally, further later sera may be required. If investigation is commenced some weeks after rash or contact, it may not be possible to confirm or refute a possible diagnosis.

- how long the results will take (consult local laboratory)
- who will give the test results
- who will discuss future management of the pregnancy
- who they can contact if they have any unanswered queries or concerns.

Written information should be provided to back up verbal advice or information given. The use of an interpreter for women who do not speak English and the use of audiotapes to reiterate verbal discussions indicates good practice. All discussions, advice and care management plans should be documented.

All pregnant women with rash illness, or contact with rash illness, should be referred for medical management.

Specific infections

Rubella

The clinical features and consequences for the fetus of primary rubella in pregnancy are well established.[4] The unreliability of a clinical diagnosis of rubella is accepted.[5] The risk to the fetus of primary rubella in the first 16 weeks of gestation is substantial (Table 3.1), with major and varied congenital abnormalities being associated with infection in the first trimester, and a lesser risk, limited to deafness, in the fourth month.[4] Rubella infection prior to the estimated date of conception or after 20 weeks carries no documented risk,[4,6] and primary rubella contracted between 16 and 20 weeks of gestation carries a minimal risk of deafness only.[7]

A rubella reinfection is defined as rubella infection in someone who has previously had either documented natural rubella virus infection or successful rubella immunisation.[8] Maternal reinfection is usually subclinical and diagnosed by changes in immunoglobulin G (IgG) and/or immunoglobulin M (IgM) antibody concentration only. The risk to the fetus of subclinical maternal reinfection in the first 16 weeks of gestation has not been precisely determined but an overview would suggest that the risk of congenital damage is less than 10%, and probably less than 5%.[9] Maternal rubella reinfection, with fetal infection and damage, made a substantial contribution to the incidence of congenital rubella in the UK in the late 1980s and early 1990s[9] but has declined as the incidence of rubella has fallen. Maternal reinfection with a rash is rare but can be presumed to present a significant, but not quantified, risk to the fetus as viraemia will have occurred.

The epidemiology of rubella in the UK has changed substantially since the introduction in 1988 of mumps, measles and rubella (MMR) vaccine for males and females in the second year of life, with an early 'catch-up' programme in preschool years, and the measles/rubella (MR) vaccine campaign of 1994. Since the early 1990s, rubella has largely affected young adult males, with only a few cases in pregnant women:[10,11] the National Congenital Rubella Surveillance Programme's records indicate that the last year in which several cases of confirmed congenital rubella acquired in England and Wales occurred was 1996 (total 12), although occasional sporadic cases acquired from importations have been reported since then.[12]

Parvovirus B19

There is a wide range of potential consequences of parvovirus B19 infection, from minor febrile illness to erythema infectiosum (fifth disease or slapped-cheek syndrome), generalised rash illness clinically indistinguishable from rubella, aplastic crises in patients with shortened red cell life, arthralgia and persistent infection in the immunocompromised.[13] Infection in the first 20 weeks of pregnancy can lead to intrauterine death (risk 15% versus 5% in control group; excess risk 9%) and hydrops fetalis (risk 3%, of which about half die and are included in the excess risk of 9%, if infection occurs at between 9 and 20 weeks of gestation).[14] These consequences usually occur three to five weeks after the onset of maternal infection, but can be later. Permanent congenital abnormality has not been identified as a consequence of intrauterine infection, although persistent neonatal infection and anaemia occurs rarely.[15]

Parvovirus B19 reinfection and reactivation has been shown in volunteer studies[16] and in the immunocompromised. However, there is no evidence to suggest reinfection is a risk to the fetus. Parvovirus B19 infection is common, with 50–60% of adults having been infected.[17] No vaccine or preventive measures are available and an increased incidence typically occurs every three to four years, primarily in schoolchildren. In 1998, guidance on the management of parvovirus B19 infection was issued by the PHLS after consultation with a range of authorities.[2]

Measles

The clinical features and complications of measles in the child and adult are well established and include disseminated rash, coryza, conjunctivitis, pneumonia, otitis media and encephalitis.[18] Infection in pregnancy can lead to intrauterine death and preterm delivery[19] but is not associated with congenital infection or damage.

Indigenous measles is rare in the UK as a result of the introduction of the MMR vaccine in 1988 and the MR vaccine campaign of 1994,[20] except in unvaccinated people or in communities with low coverage.[21] Most cases are now noted in people who move to the UK from countries where measles is still endemic. Recent falls in vaccine coverage have contributed to a rise in susceptible individuals, which may eventually accumulate to the point where an epidemic will occur, as seen in Dublin in 1999/2000.[22] Human normal immunoglobulin (HNIG) may not prevent measles but has been shown to attenuate the illness. There is no evidence that it prevents intrauterine death or preterm delivery.

Enteroviruses

Enteroviruses (coxsackieviruses A and B, echovirus, enteroviruses 68–71) can cause a wide range of manifestations, such as meningitis, hand, foot and mouth disease, febrile illness, myocarditis and Bornholm disease. Infection during pregnancy is not associated with any particular fetal consequence, although rarely can result in abortion (as can any febrile illness).[23] Neonatal infection is usually acquired from the mother or by cross-infection. Neonatal infection, particularly with selected echoviruses, can have multisystem life-threatening complications.[24]

Sporadic enterovirus infection is not uncommon but major summer epidemics have not been seen in the UK for some years. Except for poliovirus, no vaccines are available. Immunoglobulin has been advised for prophylaxis in exposed neonates.[24]

Hand, foot and mouth disease is characterised by vesicular lesions of hands, feet and mouth; the latter soon break down to ulcers. The disease is a commonly recognised manifestation of enterovirus infection. Pregnant women presenting with the characteristic features may be investigated by viral cultures of faeces and throat swab (serology is of little value), but can be reassured that there are no adverse consequences for the fetus. Pregnant women in contact with cases of hand, foot and mouth disease should be reassured.

Infectious mononucleosis

Infectious mononucleosis (IM) is a common presentation of primary Epstein–Barr virus (EBV) in young adults. IM is characterised by generalised lymphadenopathy, fever, sore throat and typical haematological and serological findings, including the detection of heterophil antibody. A generalised maculopapular rash is an associated feature,[25] particularly if ampicillin or a similar antibiotic has been taken.

Primary EBV infection in pregnancy (whether clinically apparent as IM or asymptomatic) carries no specific risk to the fetus.[26] EBV infection results in a latent infection with persistent excretion in the throat in a proportion (approximately 20%) of individuals. Hence, exposure to EBV can occur irrespective of whether the contact patient has IM; exposure to IM does not require investigation and the patient can be reassured.

Some 50% of young adults are susceptible to EBV, with higher rates in more affluent social groups, and 2% or more of those susceptible become infected annually. About 50% of these infections will present with IM.

Cytomegalovirus (CMV) can cause an IM-like syndrome with a generalised maculopapular rash, and must be considered if heterophil antibody is not detected. Primary infection with CMV may lead to intrauterine infection.[27] It is not considered further as occurrence of a rash is rare and no effective intervention exists.

The pregnant woman with a non-vesicular rash illness

Care must be taken in assessing the rash in a patient with a dark skin, as the appearance may not be the same as that seen in those with a lighter skin. Those whose first language is not English may not be familiar with common terms such as 'chickenpox' and thus relevant history obtained must be interpreted with care. Patients who have spent their childhood years in other countries may not have had the same exposure to natural infection or vaccination opportunities as those brought up in the UK; consequently, the risk estimates presented here may not apply to these groups as they may have a higher or lower level of susceptibility.

Apart from varicella in the seven days prior to delivery, the infections that may have a specific impact on the fetus (rubella, parvovirus B19, varicella-zoster virus) only do so if infection occurs in the first 20 weeks of gestation. Hence, it is left to the managing clinician to decide whether investigation after 20 weeks is warranted, but it is strongly advised, irrespective of gestation, as:

- specific diagnosis would help in managing potential risk to contacts (e.g. in healthcare situations such as GP surgeries and antenatal clinics)
- it would confirm the date of infection related to gestational age
- the estimate of the gestation may be wrong
- the mother may be reassured that a specific diagnosis has been reached or excluded, which may be helpful in the management of subsequent exposure.

Investigation will be directed by clinical/epidemiological information:

- a disseminated vesicular rash is highly suggestive of varicella
- the probability of streptococcal and meningococcal infection, measles, enterovirus, syphilis and infectious mononucleosis should be suggested by clinical features, and would instigate appropriate specific investigation and management
- any doubt as to one of these diagnoses or failure to confirm by laboratory investigation must result in initiating specific investigation for rubella and parvovirus B19.

If features are compatible with rubella or parvovirus B19, appropriate laboratory investigation should be initiated, irrespective of past testing for these agents or, for rubella, past immunisation (Figure 3.1). There is a remote possibility of past laboratory or documentation error, failed immunisation, symptomatic rubella reinfection or parvovirus B19 reinfection.

It is recommended that, irrespective of a request for specific rubella or parvovirus B19 infection, all sera from women with rash illness be simultaneously investigated for both infections.

Current methods developed for use on saliva are not suitable for individual patient diagnosis in pregnancy.

The pregnant woman in contact with a rash illness

Contact is defined as being in the same room (e.g. house or classroom or two- to four-bed hospital bay) for a significant period of time (15 minutes or more) or face-to-face contact.

This definition is based on experience with varicella-zoster virus exposure and errs on the side of caution. This definition of contact is probably sensible for all nosocomial exposures. In community exposures, which are probably more frequent and less likely to be well defined, it may be more practicable to consider a less stringent definition of contact, especially for parvovirus B19 infections, where household exposure is overwhelmingly the most important source of infections in pregnancy (followed by intense occupational exposure).

The aetiology of the rash in the contact may be diverse and include non-infective causes. The possible causes that warrant consideration include measles, rubella and parvovirus B19. Consideration of other possible infective causes in the contact (e.g. enterovirus) should await development of illness in the pregnant woman. Investigation is recommended for rubella and parvovirus B19 in all cases unless there is a strong reason to suspect measles and susceptibility to rubella is unlikely.

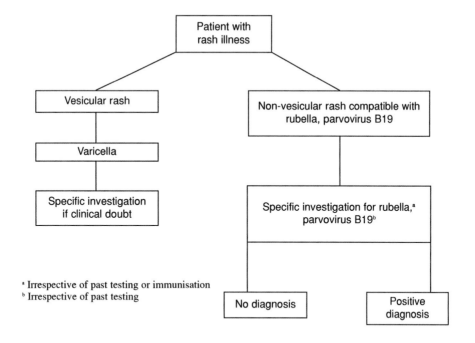

Fig. 3.1.   Management of pregnant women with rash illness

Rubella

If a woman has had one of the following, she should be reassured that the likelihood of rubella is extraordinarily remote and that specific rubella investigation is not required, but she should be advised to return if a rash develops:

- at least two previous rubella antibody screening tests that have detected antibody
- at least two documented doses of rubella vaccine
- one documented dose of vaccine followed by one previous rubella antibody screening test that has detected antibody.

If rubella susceptibility is possible (i.e. the criteria above are not present), a serum should be obtained as soon after contact as possible. Full details must be given on the request form to ensure correct interpretation of results.

The laboratory should simultaneously test for rubella-specific IgG and IgM, and the advice given in Figures 3.2 and 3.3 followed. If rubella-specific IgG is detected but rubella-specific IgM is not detected, women will be reported as 'No evidence of recent primary rubella'. There may be rare occasions when detection of rubella-specific IgG may precede by one to two days the development of specific IgM in the evolution of the antibody response in primary rubella. In a pregnant patient with a rash of onset in

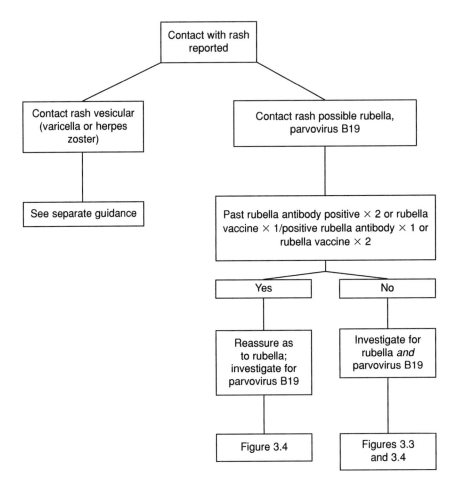

Fig. 3.2.   Management of pregnant women in contact with rash illness

the previous ten days, if a low concentration (< 10 iu/ml) of rubella-specific IgG is detected, a further serum screening should be requested even if rubella-specific IgM is not detected.

Active investigation for reinfection by obtaining and testing later sera is not indicated, given the low incidence of rubella in the UK (and hence it being unlikely that the contact had rubella) and the low risk to the fetus of reinfection in the absence of a maternal rash.

If rubella-specific IgM reactivity is detected, similar caveats as to the specificity of this result, and procedures to be followed, are as detailed in the next section.

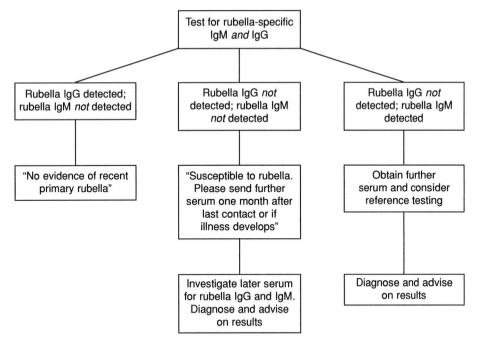

Fig. 3.3. Investigation for rubella in pregnant women in contact with rash illness

Parvovirus B19

The pregnant woman should be investigated for asymptomatic parvovirus B19 infection (Figures 3.2 and 3.4). Investigation should not be delayed to ascertain if symptomatic infection occurs as:

- maternal asymptomatic parvovirus B19 infection is at least as likely to infect and damage the fetus as symptomatic infection[15]
- active management of the infected fetus may reduce the risk of adverse outcome[28] (see later).

Serum should be collected as soon after contact as possible and submitted to the laboratory with full clinical and epidemiological details. Serum should be tested for both parvovirus B19-specific IgG and IgM. If specific IgG or IgM are not detected, further serum should be collected and tested one month after last contact. If specific IgM is detected but specific IgG not detected, a further serum sample should be collected and tested immediately. If specific IgG is detected (approximately 50% probability) but specific IgM not detected, the woman can be reassured that she has had a parvovirus B19 infection at some time, but not recently. If, after testing of the one-month sample, specific IgG and IgM are not detected, the woman can be reassured that no evidence of recent parvovirus B19 infection as a consequence of the contact investigated has been found, although she is still susceptible.

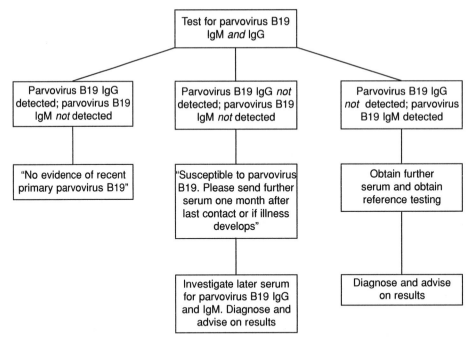

Fig. 3.4.   Investigation for parvovirus B19 in pregnant women in contact with rash illness

Measles

If the source patient is suspected of having measles, based on epidemiology and clinical features, consideration should be given to passive prophylaxis with intramuscular HNIG as soon as possible after exposure, but within six days.[29] There is no evidence that post-exposure prophylaxis with HNIG confers any benefit for the fetus, although it may attenuate maternal illness. Factors that would increase the likelihood of measles are that:

- the rash contact took place when the woman was abroad
- the contact had travelled abroad
- the contact has not received measles vaccine in the past
- the contact has been hospitalised recently
- the contact is linked epidemiologically to a confirmed measles case.

If the woman has received two doses of measles vaccine in the past, and in view of the low incidence of measles infection in the UK, she should be reassured as to the low probability of her becoming infected. If there is no or poorly documented history of vaccination, serum should be collected and administration of HNIG should await an urgent determination of measles-specific IgG. If measles-specific IgG is detected within ten days of contact (there is a greater than 95% probability of being 'immune' in the UK, particularly if born before 1970) further action is unnecessary. Failure to detect measles-specific IgG would warrant administration of HNIG and serological follow-up three weeks after last contact: HNIG may attenuate but not prevent measles. If contact was more than ten days prior to presentation, serum should be collected and stored. Management would be expectant and specific measles serological investigation only performed if rash illness develops.

Laboratory investigation

Rubella

The purpose of routine antenatal testing for rubella antibody is to determine susceptibility and to identify those for whom vaccine is advised post delivery; it does not determine whether rubella may have occurred in the current pregnancy. If such investigation is required, the request should clearly state that recent rubella is a possibility, and full clinical and epidemiological details given. The serological diagnosis of rubella is well established.[30] A serum must be collected at first presentation and sent for laboratory testing. It is recommended that the laboratory investigate all cases of possible rubella by simultaneous testing for rubella-specific IgG (or total rubella antibody) and IgM. When reporting the results of rubella serology, the laboratory must advise on any further sera/follow-up required, and give a definitive conclusion of their investigations; for example, 'No evidence of recent primary rubella'.

Problems arise when investigation commences four weeks or more after the onset of rash illness. If rubella-specific IgG is detected and specific IgM is not detected, rubella as a cause of the rash illness cannot be excluded serologically unless past sera can be tested to determine whether seroconversion has occurred recently. An assessment of probabilities has to be made based on recent epidemiology of rubella in the community, past history of vaccine and testing, characteristics of illness, etc.

Some women present significant problems in diagnosis, particularly in those who give a positive result for rubella-specific IgM. Although positive rubella IgM results that do not reflect recent rubella (primary or reinfection) ('false positive') are infrequent, the control of rubella in the UK means that most rubella-specific IgM positive results do not reflect recent rubella. No woman in the first 20 weeks of pregnancy should have rubella diagnosed on the basis of a positive rubella-specific IgM alone. Results must be interpreted in relation to full clinical and epidemiological information. Unless seroconversion has been shown, further testing by alternative rubella-specific IgM tests and measuring the strength of binding of specific IgG (avidity)[30] is advised. IgG avidity is low soon after a primary infection but matures over a few weeks to become more strongly binding. If rubella-specific IgM positivity reflects a recent rubella episode (whether primary or reinfection), the degree of reactivity will usually change over the period of a few weeks, rather than persisting at a similar level.

Parvovirus B19

Recent parvovirus B19 infection can be confirmed or excluded by testing for parvovirus B19-specific IgM on the first serum obtained. Failure to detect parvovirus B19-specific IgM excludes infection in the four weeks prior to collection of the serum. Hence, infection cannot be excluded if investigation commences more than four weeks after onset of rash illness.

If parvovirus B19 IgM is detected in the first 20 weeks of pregnancy, confirmation is required by alternative assay, for example M-capture radioimmunoassay, IgM-specific immunofluorescence or IgG seroconversion using an antenatal booking blood sample. Repeat testing will demonstrate a decline in IgM reactivity and provide an additional confirmation method.

Hydrops fetalis

In a pregnant woman presenting with hydrops fetalis without a rash history, the diagnosis of recent parvovirus B19 infection can only occasionally be achieved by testing for parvovirus B19-specific IgM, as the acute infection was usually some weeks prior to presentation. Infection with parvovirus B19 as the cause of hydrops fetalis can be investigated by testing the antenatal booking sample in parallel with the sample at presentation for parvovirus-specific IgG to show seroconversion.

Following confirmation of parvovirus B19 in a pregnant woman presenting with hydrops fetalis, referral to a regional unit for fetal medicine is recommended if this has not already occurred. If a fetal blood sample is collected, examination by molecular methods (polymerase chain reaction or dot-blot hybridisation) and/or electron microscopy for parvovirus B19 virus particles to confirm fetal infection can be arranged by virology laboratories. Proven parvovirus B19 infection in the hydropic fetus will influence the management of the woman as it is important in establishing the aetiology of the hydrops and in excluding other causes so allowing appropriate counselling of the patient.

Management of proven infection

Rubella – primary and reinfection

The management of primary rubella or symptomatic rubella reinfection depends on the gestation of pregnancy at which rubella occurred and the individual circumstances of the woman (Table 3.1).

If a case of asymptomatic rubella reinfection is identified or suspected, management depends, as for primary rubella, on the gestation of pregnancy and the individual circumstances of the woman. Given the low but definite risk to the fetus of maternal rubella reinfection in the first 16 weeks of pregnancy, there may be occasions when consideration is given to further fetal investigation by genome detection to ascertain if fetal infection has occurred. A range of possible approaches has been explored but they are all invasive (e.g. amniocentesis, fetal blood sampling) and carry a risk of adverse outcome.

The necessary virological techniques for fetal investigation are not validated and available in the UK, and it is strongly advised that management be based on risk assessment.

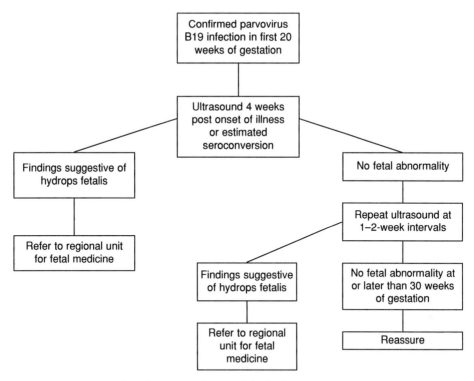

Fig. 3.5.   Management of confirmed parvovirus B19 infection in pregnancy

Parvovirus B19

The management of proven parvovirus B19 infection has become more active with the demonstration that intrauterine transfusion of the fetus improves the outcome.[28] The following management is suggested (Figure 3.5).

- On diagnosis of parvovirus B19 infection, ultrasound scanning of the fetus is started four weeks after the onset of illness or date of seroconversion and then performed at one- to two-weekly intervals until 30 weeks of gestation.
- If findings suggestive of hydrops fetalis or its development are found, the patient should be referred to a regional unit for fetal medicine for consideration of fetal blood sampling and intrauterine transfusion.

Further techniques are becoming available that may assist in fetal assessment, such as Doppler assessment of the middle cerebral artery for anaemia and parvovirus B19 genome detection in amniotic fluid.

Measles, enterovirus, infectious mononucleosis

The management of the pregnancy in these infections is expectant, although follow-up of the infant should be considered even though no congenital infection and damage would be anticipated.

The 'continuously exposed' female in the first 20 weeks of pregnancy

Exclusion is not recommended of pregnant women susceptible to rubella or varicella-zoster virus from environments that may suggest a higher rate of exposure, such as school classrooms. Rubella is now rare in children and exposure to varicella-zoster virus is as likely to occur in the wider community. Guidance on the management of pregnant women susceptible to parvovirus B19 was published in 1999.[2]

Screening for rubella antibody

Frequency of testing

It is likely that, given the low incidence of rubella in the UK, the cost benefit of the current rubella antibody screening strategy will be reviewed by the National Screening Committee.

The advice regarding frequency of testing given in *Immunisation against Infectious Disease*[3] is appropriate. This advice states that 'Women should be screened for rubella antibodies at least in the first pregnancy, irrespective of a previous positive rubella antibody result. Very occasionally, laboratory errors or errors during reporting may result in patients who are rubella antibody negative being reported as rubella antibody positive. When there are documented results available of two tests using a specific method, both confirming the presence of rubella antibody, then further screening in pregnancy is unnecessary unless contact with suspected rubella or a rubella-like rash occurs.'

PHLS guidance does update the above advice, however, in recommending that further testing is not required if contact with suspected rubella or rubella-like rash occurs.

UK health authorities and NHS trusts are recommended to review their compliance. It is appreciated, however, that a pragmatic balance has to be drawn locally on the basis of cost efficiency between screening every woman in every pregnancy against a selective screening based on documented results.

Laboratory guidance

A number of reliable and validated assays are available for rubella antibody screening, such as enzyme-linked immunosorbent assays (ELISAs), radial haemolysis and latex agglutination. The cut-off concentration of 15 iu/ml traditionally used in the UK was based on the lack of specificity of the haemagglutination inhibition test at low concentration of antibody. Many commercial ELISAs have a cut-off of approximately 10 iu/ml and such a cut-off may be accepted as valid, providing the assay is continuously monitored by the use of a second confirmatory assay, as described below. This has been endorsed in the USA.[31]

Sera giving less than 10 iu/ml in the first assay should be retested, from the clot if available, to exclude laboratory error on first testing, validate the assay run and, if an alternate assay is used, identify sera with low but detectable rubella antibody. If sera that were negative on first testing are found to be positive on further testing, the serum should be retested in the original assay. If positive on retesting, consideration should be given to retesting the batch to exclude serum transposition (i.e. another serum has been falsely identified as positive).

Given the sensitivity and specificity of ELISA, radial haemolysis and latex agglutination, if rubella-specific IgG can be detected by repeat testing in a validated assay or in two or more validated assays at whatever the concentration, the woman should be reported as 'Rubella antibody detected'. This approach would result in almost all those screened being reported as 'Rubella antibody detected', or 'Rubella antibody NOT detected' with advice being given 'Rubella immunisation advised (post delivery if pregnant)'. There may be exceptionally rare instances where further reference testing may be indicated, for example where variable results are obtained on retesting and where there is a documented history of multiple doses of vaccine yet rubella-specific IgG cannot be detected on local testing. If rubella-specific IgG is not detected, but the woman has received two or more documented doses of rubella vaccine, further doses of vaccine are unlikely to be of value and protection against primary rubella can be assumed, although such women should be advised to report any rash illness.

Parvovirus B19 antibody screening

Unselected screening of pregnant women for past infection with parvovirus B19 is not recommended as no vaccine or prophylaxis are available. This advice will need reconsideration if a licensed vaccine becomes available.

Conclusion

Although substantial progress has been made in reducing the risk of acquiring rubella in pregnancy, occasional cases, usually arising as a result of contact with an imported case, still occur. In addition, rashes in pregnancy due to the other major fetal pathogen, parvovirus B19, continue to present diagnostic problems. Investigation of pregnant women who present with a rash, or history of contact with rash, compatible with a systemic viral illness, should be investigated appropriately to confirm or exclude a diagnosis of either recent rubella or parvovirus B19 infection.

For women who present with a compatible rash, investigation for acute rubella or parvovirus B19 infection should always be undertaken, irrespective of vaccination history (rubella) or prior antibody testing (rubella or parvovirus B19). For asymptomatic women presenting with a history of contact with a rash illness compatible with a systemic viral illness, serological investigation is always recommended unless there is a documented history of rubella or parvovirus B19 immunity. The former requires two previous positive rubella antibody tests, or at least two documented doses of vaccine, or one prior positive antibody test plus one documented rubella vaccination. A single prior positive test for parvovirus B19 IgG antibody immunity should be considered evidence of immunity, unless the pregnant women develops a rash compatible with such an illness, when serological investigation for acute parvovirus B19 infection (and rubella) is indicated.

Acknowledgements

This chapter is based on a PHLS Working Group report, *Guidance on the Management of, and Exposure to, Rash Illness in Pregnancy*, which is available at the PHLS website at http://www.phls.org.uk/advice/rashillness.htm. The PHLS report also includes guidance on varicella-zoster virus infection.

References

1. Morgan-Capner P. Laboratory diagnosis of rubella. Summary of recommendations of PHLS Working Party. *PHLS Microbiol Dig* 1988;**5**:49–52.
2. Crowcroft NS, Roth CE, Cohen BJ, Miller E. Guidance for control of parvovirus B19 infection in healthcare settings and the community. *J Public Health Med* 1999;**21**:439–46.
3. Salisbury DM, Begg TM, editors. *Immunisation against Infectious Disease*. London: HMSO; 1996.
4. Miller E, Cradock-Watson JE, Pollock TM. Consequences of confirmed maternal rubella at successive stages of pregnancy. *Lancet* 1982;**ii**:781–4.
5. Anderson MJ, Kidd JM, Morgan-Capner P. Human parvovirus and rubella-like illness. *Lancet* 1985;**ii**:663.
6. Enders G, Nickerl-Pacher U, Miller E, Cradock-Watson JE. Outcome of confirmed periconceptional maternal rubella. *Lancet* 1988;**i**:1445–7.
7. Grillner L, Forsgren M, Barr B, Bottiger M, Danielsson L, De Verdier C. Outcome of rubella during pregnancy with special references to the 17th–24th weeks of gestation. *Scand J Infect Dis* 1983;**15**:321–5.
8. Best JM, Banatvala JE, Morgan-Capner P, Miller E. Fetal infection after maternal re-infection with rubella: criteria for defining re-infection. *BMJ* 1989;**299**:773–5.
9. Morgan-Capner P, Miller E, Vurdien JE, Ramsay ME. Outcome of pregnancy after maternal reinfection with rubella. *CDR (Lond Engl Rev)* 1991;**1**:R57–9.
10. Miller E, Waight P, Gay N, Ramsay M, Vurdien J, Morgan-Capner P, *et al*. The epidemiology of rubella in England and Wales before and after the 1994 measles and rubella vaccination campaign: fourth joint report from the PHLS and the National Congenital Rubella Surveillance Programme. *Commun Dis Rep CDR Rev* 1997;**7**:R26–32.
11. Tookey PA, Peckham CS. Surveillance of congenital rubella in Great Britain, 1971-96. *BMJ* 1999;**318**:769–70.
12. Tookey P, Molyneux P, Helms P. UK case of congenital rubella can be linked to Greek cases. *BMJ* 2000;**321**:766–7.
13. Pattison JR. Human parvoviruses. In: Zuckerman AJ, Banatvala JE, Pattison JR, editors. *Principles and Practice of Clinical Virology*, 4th ed. Chichester: John Wiley; 2000.
14. Miller E, Fairley CK, Cohen BJ, Seng C. Immediate and long term outcome of human parvovirus B19 infection in pregnancy. *Br J Obstet Gynaecol* 1998;**105**:174–8.
15. Donders GG, Van Lierde S, Van Elsacker-Niele AM, Moerman P, Goubau P, Vandenberghe K. Survival after intrauterine parvovirus B19 infection with persistence in early infancy: a two-year follow-up. *Pediatr Infect Dis J* 1994;**13**:234–6.
16. Anderson MJ, Higgins PG, Davis LR, Willman JS, Jones SE, Kidd IM, *et al*. Experimental parvovirus infection in man. *J Infect Dis* 1985;**152**:257–65.
17. Gay NJ, Hesketh LM, Cohen BJ, Rush M, Bates C, Morgan-Capner P, *et al*. Age specific antibody prevalence to parvovirus B19: how many women are infected in pregnancy? *Commun Dis Rep CDR Rev*

1994;**4**:R104–7.
18. Katz M. Clinical spectrum of measles. *Curr Top Microbiol Immunol* 1995;**191**:1–12.
19. Eberhart-Phillips JE, Frederick PD, Baron RC, Mascola L. Measles in pregnancy: a descriptive study of 58 cases. *Obstet Gynaecol* 1993;**82**:797–801.
20. Gay N, Ramsay N, Cohen B, Hesketh L, Morgan-Capner P, Brown D, *et al.* The epidemiology of measles in England and Wales since the 1994 vaccination campaign. *Commun Dis Rep CDR Rev* 1997;**7**:R17–21.
21. Hanratty B, Holt T, Duffell E, Patterson W, Ramsay M, White JM, *et al.* UK measles outbreak on non-immune anthroposophic communities: the implications for the elimination of measles from Europe. *Epidemiol Infect* 2000;**125**:377–83.
22. Payne D. Ireland's measles outbreak kills two. *BMJ* 2000;**321**:197.
23. Basso NG, Fonseca ME, Garcia AG, Zuardi JA, Silva MR, Outani H. Enterovirus isolation from fetal and placental tissues. *Acta Virol* 1990;**34**:49–57.
24. Nagington J, Gandy G, Walker J, Gray JJ. Use of normal immunoglobulin in an echovirus 11 outbreak in a special-care baby unit. *Lancet* 1983;**ii**:443–6.
25. Schooley RT. Epstein–Barr virus (infectious mononucleosis). In: Mandell GC, Bennett JE, Dolin R, editors. *Principles and Practice of Infectious Diseases*, 5th ed. London: Churchill Livingstone; 2000.
26. Arvin AM, Maldonado YA. Other viral infections of the fetus and newborn. In: Remington JS, Klein JO, editors. *Infectious Diseases of the Fetus and Newborn Infant*, 4th ed. Philadelphia: WB Saunders; 1995.
27. Boppana SB, Pass RF, Britt WJ, Stagno S, Alford CA. Symptomatic congenital cytomegalovirus infection: neonatal morbidity and mortality. *Pediatr Infect Dis J* 1992;**11**:93–9.
28. Fairley CK, Smoleniec JS, Caul OE, Miller E. Observational study of effect of intrauterine transfusions on outcome of fetal hydrops after parvovirus B19 infection. *Lancet* 1995;**346**:1335–7.
29. Centers for Disease Control. Measles prevention: recommendations of the Immunization Practices Advisory Committee. *MMWR Morb Mortal Wkly Rep* 1989;**38** Suppl 9:1–18.
30. Thomas JIJ, Morgan-Capner P, Enders G, *et al.* Persistence of specific IgM and low avidity specific IgG following primary rubella. *J Virol Methods* 1992;**39**:149–55.
31. Skendzel LP. Rubella immunity. Defining the level of protective antibody. *Am J Clin Pathol* 1996;**106**:170–4.

Further reading

1. Armstrong D, Cohen J. *Infectious Diseases*. London: Mosby; 1999.
2. Feigin RD, Cherry JD. *Textbook of Pediatric Infectious Diseases*, 4th ed. Philadelphia: WB Saunders; 1998.
3. Jeffries DJ, Hudson CN. *Viral Infections in Obstetrics and Gynaecology*. London: Arnold; 1999.
4. Mandell GC, Bennett JE, Dolin R, editors. *Principles and Practice of Infectious Diseases*, 5th ed. London: Churchill Livingstone; 2000.
5. Remington JS, Klein JO, editors. *Infectious Diseases of the Fetus and Newborn Infant*, 4th ed. Philadelphia: WB Saunders; 1995.
6. Zuckerman AJ, Banatvala JE, Pattison JR, editors. *Principles and Practice of Clinical Virology*, 4th ed. Chichester: John Wiley; 2000.

Chapter 4

Epidemiology of infection and pregnancy

Discussion

Discussion following Dr Newell's paper

Holliman: You stated at the end of your presentation that screening programmes needed to be introduced on the basis of scientific evidence. I am sure everybody here would agree with that but the fact of the matter is that they are probably not always done in that way. There are a number of screening programmes, in Europe particularly, which do not fulfil the World Health Organization criteria and yet they have been running for a number of years.

Newell: That is true. I have concentrated very much on the UK. The good thing about the UK is that there is a National Screening Committee, which considers all the evidence and tries to come to an informed decision. I am afraid that decision making in other countries may not be according to the same informed decision procedure.

Holliman: No, but it illustrates the importance of political influence, which must always be considered in conjunction with scientific evidence.

Newell: That is true and it also illustrates that, once you introduce something, it is much more difficult to take it out than it was to introduce it.

MacLean: There is no doubt that the Royal College has members and fellows who live outside these islands, and some of the implications of our study group go beyond these shores – whether that is Europe, or whether it extends to Africa. Obviously, all sorts of factors influence the recommendations that are relevant to our practice. The recommendations might not be applicable in other countries but it is still important to discuss them.

General discussion

MacLean: We were talking earlier about the role of the Royal College in looking at the mechanisms of surveillance. These things obviously do not happen 'on the cheap'. If rubella is less of a problem, and syphilis is not as important, will there be continuing surveillance? And who will pick up the costs?

Peckham: That is a very important question, which has been much debated as new topics are built in to the screening programme. There has been a great deal of discussion about quality assurance of some of these programmes and how they will be monitored, and ways are being discussed at the moment as to how best to co-ordinate national screening programmes.

It is more appropriate for Dr Miller to talk about what is being done through the Public Health Laboratory Service (PHLS). However, there is clearly an urgent need to improve information systems so that the laboratory data can be linked to the maternity data, together with the child health information. It is terribly crude at the moment and, as Dr Newell mentioned, during the London Implementation Group study it was found that some people were using the backs of envelopes and everyone was using different denominators, so it was very hard to find out what was going on.

Surveillance must, however, be carried on. For example, the congenital rubella surveillance is funded for the price of adding the information to the British Paediatric Surveillance Unit database and it is something we do for free because there is no funding. That is why some of these systems have collapsed. It is difficult to obtain routine funding for surveillance and this needs to be built in to discussions about new infections that are to be included in antenatal screening programmes.

Rubella surveillance is very important. I was interested in Dr Miller's figure of 1% because in some of the London hospitals the susceptibility is over 6%. I suspect that that is due to immigrants and asylum seekers, which is a different issue, and we need to question that.

Miller: That is correct. The susceptibility to rubella of women who have not been born in the UK is very much higher, as high as 9%.

On the question as to whether a woman should be screened in every pregnancy irrespective, there are practical issues about the costs in terms of identifying those who, one could say, do not need to be screened because they have had two rubella antibody positive tests in previous pregnancies, with a specific test which is documented. However, there is the cost of going through the notes and recording that information. Therefore, if you do a cost–benefit analysis, the practical issues about how to identify these women, and the cost of that, have to be borne in mind.

Surely the logic about paying for the screening programme is that if it is cost-effective in terms of the morbidity that is saved as a result of implementing it then it should save the NHS trust money and it should be paid for out of existing funds? I do not necessarily think that payment for surveillance would be covered by that.

Peckham: The quality assurance is being built into the new programmes. One hopes that this will be supported and funded. Information systems are important and we need to develop ways to bring the microbiology and clinical results together, so that this information can be obtained at low cost.

Soothill: The costs of the tests are quite easy to quantify. All the speakers have emphasised the importance of either counselling or information on patient contact. The midwifery and obstetrician time costs are almost never included in the calculations and those services are very dangerously overstretched. This is a part of the implementation of these processes that is not adequately dealt with in our thinking.

Shulman: I was quite surprised that there was such a high prevalence of parous women who were susceptible – not a much lower percentage than nulliparous women. How effective is immunisation post delivery?

Newell: We do not know, because it has not been possible to evaluate that programme. There is no documentation to say that in this hospital, or in that district, or wherever, how many pregnant women were tested, of whom how many were negative, and, of those who were negative, how many had been vaccinated. This information is desperately needed in the debate on whether the screening programme should continue.

Miller: PHLS looked at this in the mid-1980s when Princess Diana was spearheading a national rubella vaccination campaign and PHLS managed to get some money to look at exactly this. The proportion of women vaccinated postpartum varied from five percent, in susceptible women in some hospitals, to 80%. We wasted virtually all of the cost on the screening and counselling, because nothing happened as a result. We put nurses in place to establish a process whereby there would be a system for implementing, but that has not been looked at for many years.

Newell: I would like to endorse that because something similar is going to happen with hepatitis B. The antenatal screening for hepatitis B is probably easier to implement, but then no responsibility has been allocated for taking care of all the vaccinations for the children who need it. That will hinder the success of the programme, in the same way as has happened with rubella.

Ridgway: I would like to pick up Professor Soothill's throw-away remark about the costs of pathology tests being identifiable. Yes, they are, but in my experience I have almost never seen the hard cash for introducing a screening programme. It has happened by a series of subtle steps but we can no longer do that: you have to justify exactly where the costs are coming from and, until they finish up in my budget, you will not have your screening test done, because I cannot do it.

Soothill: You have expressed it very well and exactly the same argument could be applied to the clinical resources. The difficulty for us is that, if we all take your line, we will make no improvements in medicine at all. We are trying to make improvements but these are relatively underfunded. The issue about postnatal vaccination is the same one: that the postnatal midwifery resource is very seriously overstretched. We do not always have the facilities to deliver adequately those things you have described. That is a problem if we are to make progress on infection – HIV is another example.

MacLean: Before we leave Professor Peckham, one of the issues is that 14-year-old schoolgirls are vaccinated against rubella. If we are now vaccinating young children then, by the time they have grown up and become pregnant, will there be a problem with their immunity? Will we find that more and more of these women who are booking for their antenatal care are found to be rubella-susceptible because of the alteration of the time at which they are vaccinated? Will we see an alteration now in rubella susceptibility and infection?

Peckham: That is why surveillance is so critical, so that we know how many pregnant women are susceptible and can intervene where necessary. We must monitor susceptibility long-term and this monitoring should be a part of the structure. We cannot answer Professor MacLean's question, but we need to be ready to react if there is an increase in rubella susceptibility.

Regan: Could I ask about the history of consent for antenatal screening? I do not obtain written informed consent for hepatitis B or rubella screening but, in the last five years, I have been involved with introducing HIV and hepatitis C screening, which does require written consent. I am rather interested to know whether anyone else in this study group obtains consent for hepatitis B?

Peckham: Things have changed dramatically in terms of patient consent over the last few years – whether it is surveillance, or whether it is for screening. The integration of the HIV antenatal testing into the antenatal screening programmes will change what we have done in the past in relation to hepatitis B and syphilis. The information will be presented in the same sort of way with the standards of consent being brought up to those of HIV. So of course we have to obtain consent – people do not know what they are screened for at the moment, and we have just opened the box. It would be my view that written consent was probably going too far, and that is not what is usually sought. However, we have to say what we are doing and why we are doing it.

Regan: With regard to the long-term sequelae, there are, of course, long-term sequelae for hepatitis B and rubella – in the mothers, and not just the fetuses. We should perhaps think about that as a group.

I would also like to comment on the way antenatal screening is introduced. My personal experience has been that it is absolutely fundamental that the midwives, who spend most of the time doing this, are on your side. The outcome for the introduction of screening can be dramatically affected if there is a recalcitrant midwife among the ranks. It can transform to – in our hospital – 98% uptake for HIV if you have someone who is messianic about the benefits and is very proactive about it.

Newell: That is something I wanted to say. In London there are clear examples that it did not matter how well you presented the information or how good an environment you made: if you had a midwife who did not believe in testing for HIV then it did not happen. That is understandable.

MacLean: Dr Newell, could I perhaps ask you to comment on Dr Ridgway's remark? He has to save money and if he is to introduce further screening then he has to be able to recoup costs. There is therefore a great deal of benefit in dropping testing for syphilis. Is this the kind of argument that we are now having? Increasingly, you have to look at your budget and if you are going to do one thing then you have drop something else. Should we not consider dropping syphilis and perhaps selecting only those people who come from St Petersburg or Eastern Europe for testing? Or does the argument still hold that everyone should be tested for syphilis?

Newell: I very much agree that there is a problem about costing. The Department of Health issues screening recommendations but no money to go with them. The introduction of the hepatitis B screening happened, but no extra funding was available for doing it.

The deliberations that go on in the National Screening Committee are helpful in setting the relative merits of the inclusion of particular conditions. It is not only infections, but also particular conditions in the antenatal screening programmes. It therefore becomes easier for hospitals, trusts, regions or whatever to make their funding decisions.

With regard to syphilis, a syphilis test is not very expensive. It is probably more costly to sit down with a patient and ask if they have been in contact with somebody from Eastern Europe. Does Eastern Europe mean the Ukraine? It may mean Russia, it may mean Poland, and so on – and in the end it takes much more time to do that. From previous experience, that kind of selective screening does not work terribly well and so I am not sure whether, in economic terms, you save money. However, that does not mean to say that the issue of whether certain infections should or should not be part of the screening programme is not something that you should look at on a regular basis, as appropriate for the area in which you are working.

Ridgway: We have had this conversation before. I have an open chlamydia service at University College Hospital and I am now being asked where the funding came from but, to answer that question, I was not given separate funding.

As far as syphilis is concerned, this has long been one of my particular hobby horses. You are right to say that a test for syphilis is fairly cheap, but unfortunately 3500–4000 tests are not. It costs about £10 per test, in round figures, when you include laboratory and material costs, and rent, so we are looking at about £40,000. In the last few years, the only case of congenital syphilis we have had had missed antenatal screening. I therefore cannot see the justification for doing routine screening. Obviously, when you have the kinds of problems that are endemic in places such as Bristol, you have to look at it again – but that was a localised problem.

Fox: It just happens to have been replicated in Manchester.

Griffiths: Could I pick up Professor Regan's important question about consent because this is something we should discuss, and link that in with Dr Newell's comment about syphilis testing. We should be telling people openly what is being done, although I am not sure that we should necessarily give them all of the implications of every small-print answer that might come from a screening test. For example, in checking women's haemoglobin, you might find an occasional woman who has an acute leukaemia. Would it be reasonable to put that down on the consent form as an adverse event of being tested for anaemia? Most of us would probably say no, but a lawyer might take a different view and we would probably need some considered judgement on that.

As to whether it would be more cost-effective to test people for syphilis, in making those judgements you will inevitably get into value judgements of dubious validity. Is it not more efficient and better to say that the screening test is done for everybody – it is offered to everybody because there are advantages? There may come a time when it costs more to find that last remaining case within a community, but so be it: that is the cost you have to bear in running a successful programme.

Carrington: When you throw up into the air the difficulties associated with screening programmes, and therefore people fall by the wayside, we suddenly find that valuable sera – and antenatal sera are extremely valuable – get lost. Suddenly, we find that we just do not have the information that we need, not only for a particular infection but for others that subsequently become important.

We have to be very careful not to throw the baby out with the bath water here. There is a very important procedure in storing those antenatal samples, which become invaluable for a whole range of investigations subsequently, and are a valuable resource for the neonate later on when it is born. It is therefore important that we concentrate on those things which will realise an objective but we should nevertheless still maintain the view that taking blood in the antenatal period, particularly at booking, is crucial.

Brocklehurst: I would like to return to a point that Dr Newell made in her presentation, which is that the aim of most antenatal screening programmes is to prevent disease in the fetus and the newborn. I would also add that, from an obstetric point of view, subsidiary aims may be to prevent disease in the mother. For instance, one may wish to screen for group B streptococcus to prevent neonatal sepsis, but such a programme may also prevent maternal postpartum sepsis.

The very narrow focus with which many screening programmes are evaluated may actually underestimate their benefit, which is not just restricted to mother-to-child transmission.

Peckham: When the benefits are reviewed by the national screening committee, they look at the economics of it quite carefully. The secondary benefits are certainly put into screening programmes now. We have become much more sophisticated in the last five years in taking into account the benefit, for example, of treatment for the mother. There may be one prime purpose but, when you are costing it, the additional benefits that accrue are counted in as well. Health economics is a developing area and we are beginning to understand better what we should be doing.

MacLean: Dr Miller, one of the points you made concerned 'significant' contact. Is this a casual, five-minute encounter with someone at a bus station? Or is it someone who is in your house? How do you define significant? For example, what about the school teacher who has a pupil that they take for a 40-minute period of tuition – is that significant?

Miller: It is always a problem to define what 'significant' is. The bullet was bitten, so to speak, in relation to the guidelines on varicella-zoster virus, which define a significant contact as being in the same room for 15 minutes with continuous contact, with face to face exposure, as would occur during a conversation.

In these guidelines there is a definition of what constitutes 'significant' under those circumstances. When you are dealing with chickenpox, it is easier to define because the patient, generally, has a rash. When you are looking at possible exposure to parvovirus and rubella, however, there is much less certainty about the diagnosis in the index case, and there is also the possibility of asymptomatic infection. Thus, although guidelines are given as to what constitutes significant exposure, it would also have to be recognised that significant exposures outside that context may also occur because one may not be aware that the index case has the infection. Quite clearly, if you are not aware of that, you cannot instigate the whole investigations procedure.

For instance, the circumstances in a classroom, where a teacher had two or more cases of parvovirus, were considered to constitute a significant exposure, as opposed to just a single case. This is because when parvovirus is epidemic it is epidemic in the community and it was considered that there was not more of a significant exposure by having one case in the classroom than if the teacher went home on the bus or had her own children. An attempt has been made to put the clear guidelines for varicella-zoster virus into the context of rash illnesses such as rubella and parvovirus, but tempered somewhat. For varicella-zoster virus, for instance, you would take action if there was a single case in a classroom and significant exposure. In the case of parvovirus, you would not unless there were perhaps two cases in the classroom. It is incredibly difficult to be prescriptive under these circumstances but there are guidelines.

Brink: When we investigate rash illnesses in pregnancy, where at all possible we go back to the booking blood sample. Looking for an immunoglobulin G (IgG) seroconversion can be very helpful and, by the time you report back to the obstetricians, if you have an immunoglobulin M (IgM) response together with an IgG seroconversion, you are much more secure in your diagnosis. You would certainly ask for a second blood sample, but I feel much happier going back to them with indirect evidence. In pregnancy, we have this valuable resource and we should not discount it.

Miller: That is emphasised in the guidelines very strongly, for the same reason as Dr Carrington mentioned earlier. It is valuable to be able to go back to the booking blood sample in order to interpret the current antibody status.
    There is also a general recommendation – and I do not know whether the microbiologists around the table would object to this – that the booking blood sample should be stored for at least a year, so that it covers both the pregnancy and the immediate postpartum period.

MacLean: Is a year long enough? We sometimes see patients who come back several years later and we may want to go back to review previous serum.

Carrington: This is limited by the fridge space in laboratories, rather than our desire to throw this valuable resource out. It is a problem. A year at least covers the pregnancy and three months into the early infancy, and we can usually cope with that. Invariably, we do not throw it out until we have to, so that you can get one year plus in many laboratories.

Ridgway: I would agree with that – the limiting factor is the resource you have, but at least a year.

Holliman: Could I lead on from that and go into reality-based medicine? You said that these proformas relied on having accurate information on how long the rash had been present but in reality that information is not usually given to laboratories. How do you want the laboratory to proceed when they have no information available? Perhaps more importantly, how can we improve the interchange of information between the diagnostic laboratory and the clinician, to solve some of these problems before they arise?

Miller: This is why it was helpful to have an obstetrician on the working group. The kind of diagnostic conundrum that presents itself by not having accurate dates emphasises the importance of getting those dates. Sometimes, presumably, that information is available but it has just not been filled out on the form. There will be some times where that information is available but in fact the relevant rash might have been two months earlier in pregnancy, which was not reported.

This is clearly not a perfect situation but, if it is understood why the date of rash is absolutely critical for interpretation of the virological findings, then this is something for clinical colleagues. There is a table in these guidelines, indicating the information that should be provided on the request form, and it is a matter of understanding why that information is so important. Presumably, you would contact the clinician if you had an uninterpretable result, where you absolutely had to have date of rash to know whether the woman had had recent rubella or not.

Holliman: It depends on the circumstances. In some circumstances, one would. However, in other circumstances you have to send out a generic report, trying to cover the various bases. You hope that your message will get through to the relevant clinician so that they can then take the generic information that you can provide, and the specific information that they have available, and come up with the correct interpretation. The system is not perfect, however, and we need to think about improved ways of getting the right information in the right case. Throwing education at people is one way, but people are bombarded with education. We are not short of information, but we are short of knowledge these days. It is a matter of trying to make it easier for the person to provide the right information and we do not do enough of that.

MacLean: One of the recommendations that will perhaps be generated out of this is that if you are going to request a test for infection, then you have to fill in the necessary documentation. Clinicians cannot ask colleagues in the laboratory to make any sense of something unless they give the required information.

SECTION 2

NEW TECHNOLOGY FOR THE DIAGNOSIS OF
INFECTION IN PREGNANCY

Chapter 5

What obstetricians need to know about modern laboratory diagnosis

Nicola S Brink and Steven Kaye

Introduction

The rapid and accurate diagnosis of viral infections in pregnant women and fetuses forms an integral and critical part of a modern obstetric service. Increased maternal choice, together with the rapid expansion and availability of new technologies to diagnose infectious diseases, necessitates close collaboration between virologists and obstetricians. Virologists need to keep abreast of newly developed diagnostic methods. In turn, obstetricians need to be aware of the possibilities afforded by modern laboratory diagnostic methods and to collaborate with virologists in the clinical evaluation and application of these techniques.

Diagnosis of viral infections

Strategies for the diagnosis of viral infections are shown in Table 5.1. For many years, isolation of viruses in cell culture, with the generation of a cytopathic effect being used as evidence of the presence of a virus, formed the mainstay of direct virus detection. Disadvantages of this technique include the fact that virus isolation is slow and labour-intensive and that it is less sensitive than molecular amplification techniques.[1] Viral antigen detection by, for example, immunofluorescence may be used for the rapid diagnosis of infections of the respiratory tract and electron microscopy may be used for the direct visualisation of viral particles. However, these methods also often lack diagnostic sensitivity as they require the presence of high concentrations of viral antigens. Indirect evidence of a viral infection may be obtained by analysing the humoral immune response generated in response to a viral infection. Antibodies of the immunoglobulin M subclass are a good indicator of a recent infection. Serological diagnosis is often greatly assisted by the availability of an archived 'booking blood' sample from a pregnant woman where the detection of an antibody seroconversion

Table 5.1.   The diagnosis of viral infections

Direct	Indirect
Detection of virus particles, for example by electron microscopy	Detection of a viral-specific antibody response
Detection of viral antigens	
Viral culture	
Detection and quantification of viral nucleic acid (DNA or RNA)	

(when the booking blood is tested in parallel with a later blood sample) may help to time an infection in pregnancy.

In recent years, detection and quantification of viral DNA or RNA and sequence analysis of viral genomes have formed an increasingly important part of the diagnostic portfolio used for the work-up of pregnant women with viral infections. Modern obstetric services should have access to these technologies to help refine and rationalise patient care and allow for more informed maternal decision making.

Qualitative detection of viral DNA or RNA

The qualitative detection of viral genome (i.e. viral encoded DNA or RNA) has become an increasingly important technique over the last decade for the diagnosis of viral infection and disease (Table 5.2). Nucleic acid detection methods are particularly important:

- for the detection of viruses that cannot easily be cultured, for example hepatitis C virus (HCV) and human immunodeficiency virus (HIV)
- where maximum sensitivity for virus detection is required
- for the detection of viral genome at a site that is normally 'virus free', for example amniotic fluid and cerebrospinal fluid
- where antibody testing may not be clinically relevant, for example in a primary HIV infection (before antibody seroconversion) or where passively acquired maternal antibody complicates the diagnosis in infants born to HCV or HIV-infected mothers.
- for the exclusion of infectivity in, for example, blood and blood products that may be used for transfusion or treatment of the mother or baby.

The facility for detecting viral genome should be an integral part of a modern obstetric and virology service. Examples include the detection of viral nucleic acid in amniotic fluid for the prenatal diagnosis of a congenital rubella or cytomegalovirus (CMV) infection (although the infected fetus is not necessarily affected).[2,3] Close collaboration between obstetrician and virologist is essential to determine the appropriate type of sample, the timing of sample collection in relation to the fetal gestational age and time of maternal infection, as well as the most effective viral detection methods. For example, the optimal timing for the prenatal diagnosis of congenital CMV infection is at 21–22 weeks of gestation as false negative results have been obtained at earlier gestations. Such results occur as fetal diuresis is only established after 20–21 weeks of gestation and detection of CMV is dependent on fetal excretion of virus into amniotic fluid.[3] Prenatal diagnostic procedures may also form a critical part of the evaluation of pregnant women with primary rubella infection between 13 and 16 weeks of gestation. While a primary rubella infection in the first trimester of pregnancy frequently results in an infected baby with multiple defects (80–85% of cases), the risk drops dramatically to 10–17% between 13 and 16 weeks with deafness and retinopathy (that does not affect vision) usually the only clinical manifestations at this stage.[4] It is for this latter group that prenatal diagnosis may be appropriate.

Quantification of viral DNA or RNA

In addition to the qualitative detection of viral genome, methods have now been developed for the quantification of viral DNA or RNA. While initially mostly used in research, quantitative nucleic acid technology is being increasingly applied to routine diagnostic virology. Following sample preparation and nucleic acid extraction, viral DNA or RNA may be quantified by:

● target amplification techniques, for example polymerase chain reaction (PCR) based assays and nucleic acid sequence based amplification

Table 5.2. Molecular diagnosis for obstetricians

Detection of viral DNA or RNA	Clinical application
Qualitative detection of viral DNA or RNA	Prenatal diagnosis of viral infections, e.g. congenital cytomegalovirus (CMV) at 21–22 weeks of gestation and maternal primary rubella at 13–16 weeks
	Diagnosis of a current infection, e.g. hepatitis C virus (HCV) RNA detection in an HCV-antibody-positive pregnant woman and the postnatal diagnosis of HCV or HIV infection in an infant born to an HCV or HIV-infected mother
Quantitative detection of viral DNA or RNA	Association with disease severity, e.g. quantification of CMV DNA in amniotic fluid
	Prediction or staging of disease, e.g. quantification of serum HIV RNA in an HIV-infected pregnant woman Prediction of viral transmission, e.g transmission of HIV or HCV from mother to child and transmission of hepatitis B virus (HBV) from healthcare worker to patient (prediction in the HBV-infected healthcare worker)
Genotypic analysis	Useful in investigation of transmission events, e.g. in cases of suspected transmission of viruses from healthcare worker to patient
	Genotypic analysis for antiviral drug resistance, e.g. to optimise therapy in HIV-infected pregnant women

- signal amplification techniques, for example branched DNA assays or hybrid capture assays.

Target-sequence amplification relies on enzymatic reactions to increase specifically the number of target-sequence copies in a particular sample. The most widely used technique for target amplification is PCR, in which a DNA target sequence – or, in the case of an RNA virus, a DNA transcript of the viral RNA (reverse transcription or RT-PCR) – is amplified exponentially by a series of duplicating reactions. Stopping the amplification process before the reaction reaches a plateau results in a proportional relationship between the amount of virus in the sample and the amount of PCR product generated.

Viral nucleic acid quantification may be used as a prognostic marker or indicator of disease severity. The association of viral load with the clinical stage of HIV-related disease was already noted in the early 1990s using a PCR-based method to quantify plasma HIV RNA.[5] Therefore, determination of HIV viral load should form an integral part of the work-up of pregnant women infected with HIV. It has also been suggested that the amount of CMV in the urine of an infected neonate may be directly related to prognosis.[6] Data quantifying CMV DNA in amniotic fluid has shown that this may be helpful in predicting CMV disease in the fetus and newborn baby.[3] Viral genome quantification may be used to initiate and monitor antiviral therapy, the most obvious example in pregnancy being the determination of plasma HIV RNA levels to monitor the response to anti-retroviral therapy in pregnant women with HIV infection.

The use of viral genome quantification as a marker of infectivity to determine the risk of transmission from mother to child may play an important role in the future. For HCV, mother-to-child transmission is more likely if the serum HCV RNA concentration is more than 10^6–10^7 genomes per ml. One study[7] showed that only two of 30 women who transmitted infection to their infants had a viral load of less than 10^6 copies/ml. Furthermore, although a study in Italy[8] has suggested a lower rate of transmission in babies born by caesarean section (6% versus 32%), the optimal mode of delivery for the HCV-infected pregnant woman has yet to be defined. It is possible that HCV viral load may be a factor in maternal decision making in the future. The risk of transmission of HIV from mother to child is also increased with a higher viral load. However, a study[9] published in 1997 failed to demonstrate a threshold value of viral load that could discriminate between those mothers who did transmit the virus and those who did not. It also showed that transmission events occurred across the entire range of values of each of the quantification assays used, indicating the need for caution when considering viral load as a risk factor for transmission from mother to child.

Quantification of hepatitis B DNA has been introduced in the UK to determine whether healthcare workers found to be 'low infectivity' hepatitis B carriers (i.e. their serum does not contain hepatitis B antigen) can continue performing exposure-prone procedures. Those whose hepatitis B viral load exceeds 10^3 genome equivalents per ml should not perform such procedures, while those with levels below 10^3 genome per ml may continue to perform them but will need to be retested regularly at 12-monthly intervals.[10] This will clearly have an impact on a small subset of HBV-infected healthcare professionals currently working in obstetrics and gynaecology.

Genotypic analysis of viral nucleic acid may also have some relevance for obstetricians. This may be particularly important in suspected transmission events, for example the transmission of hepatitis B or C from a healthcare worker to a patient. Here the genetic relatedness of a virus in comparison with the background variation is sought. Sequence analysis has proved to be a valuable epidemiological tool in linking cases of hepatitis B infection[11] and should form an integral part in the investigation of a suspected transmission event. Nucleic acid sequencing may also be used for HIV drug-resistance testing and may help to refine and rationalise therapy in pregnant women with prior exposure to anti-retroviral drugs.

Conclusion

Diverse technologies are now available for the diagnosis and management of viral infections in pregnant women, fetuses and newborn babies. The application of these technologies depends on the clinical situation. Good communication between obstetricians and virologists and access to modern molecular diagnosis form an essential part of the management of pregnant women with viral infections.

References

1. Pillay D. Diagnostic approaches. In: Zuckerman AJ, Banatvala JE, Pattison JR, editors. *Principles and Practice of Clinical Virology*, 4th ed. Chichester: John Wiley; 2000. p. 1–18.
2. Revello M, Baldanti F, Furione M, Sarasini A, Percivalle E, Zavattoni M, *et al*. Polymerase chain reaction for prenatal diagnosis of congenital cytomegalovirus infection. *J Med Virol* 1995;**47**:462–6.
3. Guerra B, Lazzarotto T, Quarta S, Lanari M, Bovicelli L, Nicolosi A, *et al*. Prenatal diagnosis of symptomatic congenital cytomegalovirus infection. *Am J Obstet Gynecol* 2000;**183**:476–82.
4. Best JM, Banatvala JE. Rubella. In: Zuckerman AJ, Banatvala JE, Pattison JR, editors. *Principles and Practice of Clinical Virology*, 4th ed. Chichester: John Wiley; 2000. p.387–418.
5. Semple M, Loveday C, Weller I, Tedder R. Direct measurement of viraemia in patients infected with HIV-1 and its relationship to disease progression and zidovudine therapy. *J Med Virol* 1991;**35**:38–45.
6. Hodinka RL. The clinical utility of viral quantitation using molecular methods. *Clin Diagn Virol* 1998;**10**:25–47.
7. Thomas SL, Newell ML, Peckham CS, Ades AE, Hall AJ. A review of hepatitis C virus (HCV) vertical transmission: risks of transmission to infants born to mothers with and without HCV viraemia or human immunodeficiency virus infection. *Int J Epidemiol* 1998;**27**:1208–17.
8. Paccagnini S, Principi N, Massironi E, Tanzi E, Romano L, Muggiasca ML, *et al*. Perinatal transmission and manifestation of hepatitis C virus infection in a high risk population. *Pediatr Infect Dis J* 1995;**14**:195–9.
9. Cao Y, Krogstad P, Korber BT, Koup RA, Muldoon M, Macken C, *et al*. Maternal HIV-1 viral load and vertical transmission of infection: the Ariel Project for the prevention of HIV transmission from mother to infant. *Nat Med* 1997;**3**:549–52.
10. Department of Health. *Hepatitis B Infected Health Care Workers*. London: Department of Health; 23 June 2000. Health Service Circular HSC 2000/020.
11. Hawkins AE, Zuckerman MA, Briggs M, Gilson RJ, Goldstone AH, Brink NS, *et al*. Hepatitis B nucleotide sequence analysis: linking an outbreak of acute hepatitis B to contamination of a cryopreservation tank. *J Virol Methods* 1996;**60**:81–8.

Chapter 6

Prenatal diagnosis of congenital infections

Eric Jauniaux

Introduction

Gregg[1] was the first to report, in 1941, on an association between congenital cataracts in infants born to women who had contracted rubella during the first half of pregnancy. The timing of the maternal viraemia is the most important factor and it has been clearly shown that the risk of congenital defect is almost entirely confined to the first four months of pregnancy.[2,3] Congenital rubella syndrome is associated with a wide spectrum of clinical features. These mainly involve the neurological system, the heart and the eyes but defects involving virtually every organ have been reported. When considering prenatal diagnosis, it is clear that the most common fetal manifestations of rubella will only become visible during the second half of pregnancy, when termination is more difficult. The management of women with primary rubella infection before 17 weeks of gestation has thus been early termination of pregnancy, leaving little role for prenatal diagnosis. Now that the prevalence of maternal rubella has been controlled by rubella immunisation, other congenital infections, such as cytomegalovirus (CMV), *Toxoplasma gondii* and human parvovirus B19 (PVB19), have become clinically more prominent. Over the last three decades, researchers have attempted to diagnose and prevent some of the fetal complications of these congenital infections *in utero* using ultrasound information and invasive methods to detect the corresponding infectious agent inside the gestation sac. The purpose of this chapter is to critically evaluate the different ultrasound markers and invasive procedures that have been used in the management of congenital infections.

Ultrasound features in congenital infections

Prenatal diagnosis can aid the obstetrician in evaluating a mother with suspected infection that can be transmitted to her fetus(es). Ultrasonography can exclude or identify anatomical defects of the fetal heart and brain, detect thoracic or abdominal lesions, evaluate liver and spleen volume, determine the degree of haemodynamic disturbance, and even suggest anaemia. Characteristic ultrasound markers in a mother with a positive TORCH (toxoplasmosis, other agents, rubella, CMV, herpes simplex virus) screening test have high predictive value for congenital infection and may also have prognostic significance. Ultrasound techniques can be divided into three groups:

1. Single morphological marker(s), in particular, those associated with early fetal hydrops or brain anomalies

2. Multiple morphological ultrasound features viewed in combination

3. Doppler flow studies in congenital infections associated with fetal anaemia or fetal growth restriction (FGR).

Fetal Doppler evaluation may give some indication of early-stage anaemia and cardiac failure and of fetal wellbeing.

Congenital infections present with a wide spectrum of ultrasound markers and lesions, which vary with the type of pathogen involved and with the stage of gestation at which the mother contracted the infectious disease (Table 6.1). The rate of maternofetal transmission varies throughout gestation but the severity of congenital infection is greatest during the first trimester, when the fetal anatomy cannot be explored in detail by ultrasound. It is clear that viruses infect actively differentiating cells and have a profound effect on organogenesis. The risk of congenital sequelae (teratologic risk) of most viral infections is similar to the transmission rate. First-trimester viral infections often lead to miscarriage, fetal demise or major structural defects that may be identified by ultrasound, whereas late infections may lead to severe neurological defects that may not have associated sonographically detectable markers. In toxoplasmosis, the risk of the fetus being severely affected is also higher in the first trimester but there is a much lower rate of transmitted infection in this period than later in pregnancy (Table 6.1).

Early pregnancy loss

Early pregnancy loss is defined as a miscarriage occurring within the first 12 weeks of gestation.[4] Miscarriages (complete and incomplete) are the most common complication of pregnancy and chromosomal abnormalities represent at least 50% of clinically recognised early pregnancy loss. A strong correlation exists between the occurrence of a miscarriage and the following ultrasound indications: fetal bradycardia, discrepancy

Table 6.1. Timing of maternal infection, rate of mother-to-fetus transmission and risk of congenital sequelae and complications

Infectious agent	Mother-to-fetus transmission rate[a] (%)			Risk[b] (%)	
	First trimester	Second trimester	Third trimester	Early	Late
CMV primary infection	30–40	30–40	30–40	25	25
CMV secondary infection	8	8	8	5	5
Toxoplasma gondii	10	25	>80	85	10–80
PVB19	33	33	33	<10	<10
VZV	2–8	2–8	>1	<3	<1
Rubella	80–90	15–25	0	80	<1

[a] for maternal infection occurring during the specified trimester; [b] risk of congenital sequelae and complications for fetuses infected during the specified stage of pregnancy; CMV = cytomegalovirus; PVB19 = parvovirus B19; VZV = varicella-zoster virus

between the diameter of the gestation sac and the crown–rump length and discrepancy between menstrual and sonographic age of more than one week. The sonographic features of a delayed miscarriage include the presence of a gestation sac which is often collapsed, a dead fetus and no embryonic echoes within a gestation sac large enough for such structures to be visible. Provided that the equipment is technically adequate, a mean gestation sac diameter greater than 15 mm (measured using transvaginal probe) is required before diagnosis.

Infections are recognised but rare causes of early pregnancy loss. Among the many microorganisms reported to have been more frequently associated with miscarriage are listeria, PVB19, CMV and *T. gondii* (Table 6.2). Transplacental infection does occur with each of these microorganisms (Table 6.1). Sporadic losses could theoretically be caused by brucella, *Salmonella typhi*, malaria, *Mycoplasma hominis*, *Chlamydia trachomatis* and *Ureaplasma urealyticum*.[4] However, prospective epidemiological surveys suggest that the cumulative risk of these infections in first-trimester miscarriage is small.[5]

Table 6.2. Principal ultrasound features detectable in cases of congenital infection

Main clinical features		Congenital infection
General	Miscarriage	Listeria
		PVB19
		CMV
		Toxoplasmosis
	Non-immune hydrops fetalis	PVB19
		Coxsackievirus
		CMV
		Toxoplasmosis
		Rubella
		Treponema pallidum
	Fetal growth restriction	CMV
		Rubella
		VZV
		Treponema pallidum
Head	Brain tissue calcification	CMV
		Toxoplasmosis
	Hydrocephaly	CMV
		Toxoplasmosis
	Microcephaly	CMV
	Cataract	Rubella
	Chorioretinitis	Toxoplasmosis
	Microphthalmia	Rubella
Thorax	Heart defects	Rubella
	Cardiomyopathies	Coxsackievirus B
		Adenovirus
		PVB19
	Isolated pleural effusion	Adenovirus
		PVB19
Abdomen	Hyperechogenicities	CMV
		HSV
		VZV
		PVB19
	Ascites and hepatosplenomegaly	PVB19
		CMV
		Toxoplasmosis
		Treponema pallidum

CMV = cytomegalovirus; PVB19 = parvovirus B19; VZV = varicella-zoster virus

Non-immune hydrops fetalis

An increasing number of viral, bacterial and parasitic infectious agents that can cross the placenta have been reported to be present *in utero* in cases of non-immune hydrops fetalis (NIHF) (Table 6.2). Cases of hydropic fetuses due to *Treponema pallidum*, CMV, coxsackievirus B or *T. gondii* were well documented in the 1970s and 1980s.[6,7] NIHF resulting from PVB19 infection has been increasingly recognised in the last decade.[8,9] Although the association is less certain, fetal infection with trypanosomiasis, herpes simplex virus (HSV) type 1, respiratory syncytial virus (RSV) and leptospirosis have also been found with hydrops.[7] It is likely that congenital infections, which ranked as the sixth most common cause of NIHF at the end of the 1980s (Table 6.3), should now be considered as a much more frequent aetiology of NIHF. Many cases of

Table 6.3. Literature review of 600 cases of NIHF (modified from Jauniaux *et al.*[7])

Rank	NIHF Aetiologies	No.	%
1.	Chromosomal disorders	94	15.7
2.	Congenital heart disease	66	11.0
3.	α-thalassaemia	62	10.3
4.	Arrhythmia	36	6.0
5.	Twin–twin transfusion	36	6.0
6.	Congenital infections	27	4.5
7.	Skeletal dysplasia	25	4.0
8.	Placental and cord anomalies	18	3.0
9.	Genitourinary disorders	14	2.3
10.	Lung adenomatoid malformation	11	1.8
11.	Arthrogryposis multiplex syndromes	11	1.8
12.	Fetal vascular malformations	10	1.7
13.	Diaphragmatic hernia	10	1.7
14.	Multiple pterygium syndrome	9	1.5
15.	Pulmonary extralobar sequestration	9	1.5
16.	Cardiac rhabdomyoma/tumour	7	1.2
17.	Lysosomal storage disorders	6	1.0
18.	Gastrointestinal obstruction	6	1.0
19.	Congenital chylothorax	6	1.0
20.	Congenital teratoma	5	0.8
21.	Lymphatic malformations	5	0.8
22.	Fetomaternal haemorrhage	4	0.7
23.	Congenital leukaemia	4	0.7
24.	Caval or renal thrombosis	4	0.7
25.	Encephalocele/porencephaly	4	0.7
26.	Recurrent idiopathic hydrops	3	0.5
27.	Neuroblastoma	2	0.3
28.	Maternal hypertension	2	0.3
29.	Antepartum indomethacin	2	0.3
30.	Neu-Laxova syndrome	2	0.3
31.	Erythrocyte enzymopathies	1	0.2
32.	Meconium peritonitis	1	0.2
33.	Wilm's tumour	1	0.2
34.	Congenital haemophilia A	1	0.2
35.	Myotonic dystrophy	1	0.2
36.	Hydrometrocolpos	1	0.2
37.	Amniotic band syndrome	1	0.2
38.	Opitz–Frias syndrome	1	0.2
39.	Idiopathic	93	15.5

idiopathic NIHF (15.5% of all NIHF cases) reported before the 1990s were probably of an infectious origin but this was difficult to establish before the advent of modern laboratory techniques such as polymerase chain reaction (PCR) and *in situ* hybridisation.

In congenital infections, severe haemolytic or aplastic anaemia, which can precipitate cardiac failure, is often the primary cause of NIHF.[6,8,10] Fetal infections can also cause changes in the microvascular hydrostatic pressure. Plasma escapes through endothelial gaps and the basement membrane, producing NIHF.[6] Severe cardiac dysfunction with intrauterine congestive failure and high hydrostatic pressure can be secondary to severe myocarditis due to a coxsackievirus B infection or to a major cardiac structural defect secondary to a rubella infection during the first trimester. Toxoplasmosis has been reported in association with NIHF, apparently due to excessive extramedullary haematopoiesis with portal hypertension secondary to liver congestion. PVB19 is tropic to rapidly dividing cells, in particular fetal marrow red cell precursors, causing haemolysis and aplasia. The pathophysiology of NIHF in fetuses infected with CMV or *T. pallidum* is less clear and could be due to the combined effect of anaemia and hepatic dysfunction, resulting in hypoproteinaemia and portal hypertension.

The sonographic definition of intrauterine hydrops is easier than the differential diagnosis of the underlying aetiologies. Possible features are ascites, pleural or pericardial effusions, and placental and umbilical oedemas.[10] Generalised skin oedema is often the first feature of fetal hydrops revealed by ultrasound.[11,12] All fetuses presenting with hydrops between 11 and 15 weeks of gestation also have a nuchal fold thickness of more than 4 mm, suggesting that generalised skin oedema is a feature in a significant proportion of these cases in early pregnancy. The role of Doppler flow studies in detecting haemodynamic changes associated with fetal anaemia is limited because the anaemia caused by a congenital infection is acute and improves in most cases with advancing gestation. Skin oedema is most clearly observed at the level of the fetal head and in particular at the back of the neck where skin thickness can reach 15–20 mm. In severe cases, skin oedema is also prominent around the fetal thorax and abdomen, where skin thickness can reach 2–6 mm. In pregnancies with an otherwise anatomically normal fetus, the skin oedema may disappear, leaving only a small oedematous area at the back of the neck. NIHF associated with CMV or PVB19 congenital infection around mid-gestation may also resolve spontaneously before birth.[13,14]

In a survey of 426 pregnancies with an increased nuchal translucency at 10–14 weeks and 63 with unexplained second- and third-trimester fetal nuchal oedema or hydrops, Sebire *et al.*[15] found that evidence of recent maternal infection was present in only 1.4% of the early pregnancy group compared with 9.5% of the later-affected pregnancies. In one series, two mothers out of 45 (4.4%) with early fetal hydrops at 11–17 weeks had serum screening tests that suggested a recent infection by rubella and CMV, respectively.[12] Several authors[16–19] have reported that PVB19 infection can be associated with fetal hydrops from as early as the end of the first trimester of pregnancy. PVB19 may account for 10–18% of cases of NIHF[20] and 7.5% of intrauterine fetal deaths not associated with hydrops in the third trimester.[21] PVB19 immunoglobulin M (IgM) antibodies should also be measured in cases of early hydrops and unexplained intrauterine fetal death, as many PVB19 infections are subclinical in the mother. This confirms that, with the improvements in and better access to laboratory diagnostic techniques.[21,22] congenital infections are likely to be recognised as the next most common cause of NIHF after chromosomal abnormalities.

Fetal growth restriction

FGR is, like NIHF, a non-specific feature of most congenital infections. It is, however, a more prominent feature in cases of rubella, CMV and *T. pallidum* (Table 6.2).[8,23] A possible relationship also exists for malaria[24], human immunodeficiency virus (HIV)[25] and varicella-zoster virus (VZV).[26] FGR secondary to an infection is thought to arise from capillary endothelial damage during organogenesis. This induces a decrease in the number of cells having a cytoplasmic mass within the normal range and has a direct cytopathic effect.[23] If mother-to-fetus transmission occurs during the first trimester, the fetus may present with severe FGR at the beginning of the second trimester. FGR is almost always associated with reduced amniotic fluid volume and thus the fetal anatomy will be difficult to examine by ultrasound and more specific features of congenital infection may be impossible to identify *in utero*. Fetal Doppler velocimetry may reveal waveforms associated with the presence of abnormal villous development as congenital viral infections are often associated with placental damage.[23] A screen for TORCH and TORCH-like infections should, therefore, always be performed in cases of early and severe FGR with decreased fluid volume.

Lesions of the head

Cerebral calcifications, hydrocephaly or hydranencephaly and microcephaly are the most common lesions of the central nervous system detected by sonography in cases of congenital infection. These lesions are inflammatory (gliosis) and often secondary to maternal primary CMV and less often due to *T. gondii* infection or *T. pallidum*. Lesions of the fetal brain are extremely rare in other congenital infections and single cases have been reported involving VZV[26], HSV[27], lymphocytic choriomeningitis virus (LCMV)[28] and parainfluenza virus type 3.[29] Hydrocephaly secondary to CMV or toxoplasmosis is the consequence of an obstruction along the normal pathways of the cerebrospinal fluid, often at the level of the aqueduct of Sylvius.[30] In rare cases, fetal brain lesions associated with a congenital infection can be the consequence of an abscess (listeriosis), haemorrhage (CMV or VZV) or congenital malformation (rubella). Secondary abnormalities of the eyes, including microphthalmia, cataracts and chorioretinitis, are also detectable by ultrasound. Eye defects were mainly observed after congenital rubella and after congenital toxoplasmosis but are now are less common with the use of rubella vaccine in childhood and antiparasitic treatment for *T. gondii* infection during pregnancy.

Cardiothoracic lesions

Clinical features of congenital rubella syndrome include several cardiac defects, primarily pulmonary valvular stenosis and ventricular septal defect. Similar defects have occasionally been observed following first-trimester congenital CMV or toxoplasmosis infection. Congenital heart defects are believed to be multifactorial in more than 90% of cases, arising from the combined effects of a genetic predisposition and environmental factors. As a result of rubella vaccination, congenital heart defects are now more commonly associated with chromosomal abnormalities, maternal diabetes or maternal alcoholism than with rubella infection.

Cardiomyopathies such as endocardial fibroelastosis (interstitial myocarditis) have been linked to coxsackievirus B[31] and more recently to adenovirus[32] and PVB19.[33] Major congenital heart defects and severe cardiomyopathies are often complicated by NIHF. Pleural effusion may represent an early stage of NIHF and be associated with a major fetal infection usually involving the heart. Isolated pleural effusion is rarer and has only been observed in one case of adenovirus infection[34] and one case of PVB19 infection.[35]

Lesions of the gastrointestinal tract

Most congenital infections show abnormal features of the liver, spleen and bowel on ultrasound. The most common sonographically detected markers are peritoneal hyperechogenicities and/or hyperechogenic fetal bowel, which have been described mainly within the context of congenital CMV, HSV, VZV and PVB19.[27,36-41] True parenchymal liver or splenic hyperechogenicities are far less common and have occasionally been related to congenital infection.[39] The pathophysiology of these hyperechogenicities is unclear. Focal lesions are probably secondary to localised ischaemia or inflammatory reaction with calcification of the tissue. Diffuse bowel hyperechogenicity could be due to thickened meconium.[38]

Congenital infections due to PVB19, CMV, T. pallidum or toxoplasmosis may be associated with ascites and hepatosplenomegaly. These anomalies are secondary to direct infection of the fetal liver parenchyma, with secondary enlargement and progressive alteration of liver function. Liver function can also be indirectly affected if the infection involves the myocardium and leads to cardiac failure. Ascites can be detected by sonography even if there is less than 50 ml of intraperitoneal fluid and can be the first presenting sign of congenital infection. Small amounts of ascites are best visualised at the edge of the liver and may be seen to gradually outline the liver. In severe cases, ultrasound pictures of the fetal abdomen show free-floating or compressed bowel loops. Ascites is often an early manifestation of serous fluid accumulation in fetuses who later develop full-blown hydrops.

Other lesions

Although most pathogens will cross the placental barrier and may temporarily accumulate inside the placental tissue, they rarely induce placental damage that is detectable antenatally by ultrasound. Placental septic metastases from maternal haematogenous infections such as listeriosis may be observed *in utero*. Before 18 weeks, placental oedema is the feature most commonly associated with generalised skin oedema, and enlarged (thick) oedematous placentas are almost always found in NIHF.[10,11] Lesions of the urogenital tract have occasionally been reported in cases of congenital CMV or toxoplasmosis. Limb defects linked to an infectious process are exceptional and have only been observed after congenital VZV.[26]

Invasive procedures and fetal infections

Maternal TORCH and PVB19 serology cannot always be relied upon to identify or exclude an infectious cause for an ultrasound marker and/or abnormality suggesting a congenital infection. In most congenital infections, specific IgG antibodies appear early in maternal serum and may persist for several years. IgM-specific antibodies may remain for up to 16 weeks in CMV infection and for up to 18 months in toxoplasmosis. The detection of IgM in the first trimester may thus represent a maternal infection that has occurred preconceptually and it may be necessary to evaluate serial IgG and IgM titres three weeks apart. The evaluation of specific IgG-isotypes or acute-phase IgG and of IgG avidity can help. Some of the more sophisticated tests have poor reproducibility and these tests are best performed in reference laboratories.

Invasive prenatal procedures have been used to obtain placental tissue, amniotic fluid and fetal blood in order to evaluate an *in utero* infection and/or to identify the microorganism inside the gestation sac. Invasive procedures are contraindicated in women with hepatitis and HIV because the procedure may increase the risk of mother-to-fetus transmission in viruses that are mainly transmitted intra- or postpartum.

Many, but not all, viruses and protozoa can be grown in tissue culture from amniotic fluid and fetal blood. The value of using a culture is related directly to the timing of mother-to-fetus transmission. Mouse inoculation can also be used to detect toxoplasma. It appears that, when the parasite burden is small, the sensitivity of mouse inoculation is poor and tissue culture is inefficient.[42]

Depending on the agent and the gestation at the time of infection, it is possible to identify a specific fetal immunological response to infection. The value of IgG testing of the fetus is limited by the passive transfer of maternal IgG, which has been demonstrated to occur as early as the sixth week of gestation.[43] Serological evaluation has therefore focused on the IgM fraction, both total and agent-specific.[8] The normal fetal level of total IgM after 20 weeks of gestation is < 5 mg/100 ml. In infected fetuses, the IgM level will vary rapidly and may decline into normal range before delivery. Because antibody synthesis may only start after 22 weeks in the human fetus, specific IgM and IgA antibodies will not be detected in the serum of fetuses infected during the first half of pregnancy. Fetal serology *in utero* and at birth is thus insufficient as the sole method of diagnosing fetal infection (sensitivity <40%).

Electron microscopy, which can identify viral particles in fetal blood, ascites and other fluid samples and in placental tissue, has permitted antenatal diagnosis of congenital infection in the absence of serological evidence of the disease.[8] Antiviral serum may be used to immunoaggregate viral particles before they are applied to the grid so that specific serotypes can be identified. Electron microscopy techniques are expensive, time-consuming and not widely available and their use should be limited to unexplained congenital infections.

The increasing use of PCR has led to more cases of congenital abnormalities being linked to viral or protozoal infection. The PCR test is rapid (24–48 hours) and accurate with high (90–100%) sensitivity and negative predictive value. PCR has been used successfully to identify a number of infectious agents in a variety of fetal tissues and fluids in both humans and animals.[44,45]

Amniocentesis

Mid-second-trimester amniocentesis was introduced in the 1960s by Steele and Breg[46] and is still the most commonly used invasive technique for prenatal diagnosis. Its safety, when performed under ultrasound guidance, has rapidly increased its acceptance worldwide. Transabdominal amniocentesis was the first invasive procedure used to evaluate the fetus for TORCH infections.[47] The risk of pregnancy loss following a 15–18-week amniocentesis is less than 1% and is probably in the range of 1 per 200–400 when performed by experienced operators using continuous ultrasound guidance.[48] The risk of pregnancy loss and of neonatal morbidity seems to be much higher for amniocentesis performed before 14 weeks and thus early amniocentesis remains an area of continuing research. Most studies have indicated that PCR analysis of amniotic fluid is superior to fetal blood-specific IgM. Culture failure and false-negative PCR results may be related to performing amniocentesis too close to the time of initial maternal infection or too early in gestation.

Chorionic villus sampling

Placental biopsies have been used for the prenatal diagnosis of viral infection and in particular of first-trimester rubella.[49] The risk of fetal loss after chorionic villus sampling (CVS) is around 0.5% after ten weeks of gestation.[48] This method poses a theoretical risk to the fetus because it damages the placental barrier, which may result in an increased transfer of virus particles or parasites to the fetus. The only advantage of CVS is that it can be performed during the first trimester, which may be useful when there is maternal serological evidence that the infection may have occurred around conception.

Percutaneous umbilical blood sampling

Percutaneous umbilical blood sampling (PUBS) played a key role in the diagnosis of most common congenital infections in the 1980s and early 1990s. A differential white-cell count together with TORCH-specific IgM determination has been used in the assessment of an active fetal infection.[8] No fetus with a documented infection has a completely normal haematological profile.[8] Fetal liver enzymes can also be measured as they are almost always increased in congenital infection by CMV, PVB19 and enteroviruses.[8] All the above parameters can yield false-negative and false-positive results and the value of haematological and biochemical prognostic criteria has never been evaluated prospectively. The main advantage of fetal blood sampling is that it allows the evaluation of the fetal haematological profile, which is pivotal in the management of congenital PVB19.

PUBS is routinely performed from 18–20 weeks in specialist centres. The reported risk of fetal death after PUBS of 1–2% is a conservative estimate in cases of congenital infection because fetuses that are moribund at the time of the procedure are more likely to die as a result of procedure-related complications. With the development of PCR analysis on amniotic fluid, PUBS should now be used less often in the diagnosis of congenital infections. Fetal blood sampling may still be useful in the evaluation of the severity of the infection (prognosis) or in diagnostic problems such as negative prenatal amniotic fluid diagnosis in the presence of maternal symptoms and/or ultrasonographic findings that are highly suggestive of fetal infection. Like CVS, PUBS may also result in damage to the placental barrier and thus may indirectly increase the risk of fetal contamination.

Prenatal management of specific congenital infections using ultrasound markers and invasive procedures

Cytomegalovirus

CMV is thought to be the most common cause of congenital infection in the developed countries. Seroconversion occurs in approximately 1% of pregnant women in the UK[50] and more than 2% in other European countries[51] and the USA.[52]

Primary CMV carries a high mother-to-fetus transmission rate, ranging from 25% to 40% regardless of the stage of pregnancy.[44,53-59] In secondary (recurrent) infection, the transmission rate is much lower, in the region of 5%. As most pregnant women with congenital CMV but without ultrasound markers request a termination, little information is available on the timing of infection during pregnancy and on fetal outcome.[55] Overall, congenital CMV disease is asymptomatic at birth in approximately 90% of infants infected *in utero*. However, a further 15% in the primary CMV group and 5% in the secondary CMV group may develop sensorineural hearing loss and mental impairment.[54,56] In those infants who are asymptomatic at birth, such complications should not appear beyond one year of age.[56]

The classical CMV triad of blood dyscrasia (petechiae and thrombocytopenia), FGR and chorioretinitis is uncommon (<10%) *in utero* or at birth. Serial (every two weeks) ultrasound examination may identify markers such as microcephaly, FGR, discrete cerebral calcification, intestinal hyperechogenicity, mild ascites and hepatosplenomegaly (Table 6.2). Those fetuses that present with cerebral abnormality and/or severe FGR are more likely to develop neurological symptoms. The other markers are benign and are not specific to congenital CMV. PCR analysis of the amniotic fluid is highly accurate (Table 6.4) in detecting CMV, with a sensitivity ranging from 78% to 100%.[55,57-59] In congenital CMV, the sensitivity of amniotic fluid culture results is directly related to the delay between maternal seroconversion and amniocentesis.[55,59] Sensitivity increases from 45.7% for delays of ≤5 weeks to 88.6% for delays of ≥6 weeks.[59] As a result of the long-term risk (13%) of mental impairment after primary congenital CMV infection[54] in fetuses that may appear sonographically normal, PUBS may still be indicated to evaluate fetal biology. Abnormalities of fetal

Table 6.4. Sensitivity (Ss), Specificity (Sp) and Negative Predictive Value (NPV) of culture and polymerase chain reaction (PCR) on amniotic fluid in cases of primary cytomegalovirus (CMV) and *Toxoplasma gondii* congenital infection

Infectious agent	Culture			PCR		
	Ss (%)	Sp (%)	NPV (%)	Ss (%)	Sp (%)	NPV (%)
CMV[55,58,59]	56–95	100	94	78–100	97–100	93–100
Toxoplasma gondii[42,63]	15–89	100	76–99	81–97	96	94–99

haematological and biochemical parameters, primarily thrombocytopenia and high levels of γ-glutamyl transferase, are a sign of massive CMV infection.[8] These biological changes are transient and have never been evaluated prospectively.

Toxoplasmosis

In the UK, congenital toxoplasmosis affects approximately 2 per 1000 pregnancies.[60] The delay between maternal and fetal infection depends on inoculum size, virulence of the specific strain and developmental stage of the placenta.[42,61] The rate of mother-to-fetus transmission increases from approximately 10% in the first trimester and 25% in the second trimester to over 80% in the third trimester (Table 6.1). The severity of congenital infection is greatest in early pregnancy and most fetuses infected in the third trimester are asymptomatic. The overall risk of fetal infection is low but up to 85% of asymptomatic neonates from infected and untreated mothers have chorioretinitis by the age of 20 years.[62] Recurrent toxoplasmosis may occur in mothers co-infected with HIV.

The classical toxoplasmosis triad of intracerebral calcification, hydrocephaly and chorioretinitis is uncommon *in utero* or at birth. Serial ultrasound scans (every two weeks) may identify markers, mainly progressive ventricular dilatation, cerebral calcification, ascites and hepatosplenomegaly (Table 6.2). PCR analysis of the amniotic fluid is highly accurate in identifying *T. gondii* (Table 6.4), with a sensitivity of more than 80%, a specificity of 96% and a negative predictive value of almost 100%.[42,63] Variations in performance of the PCR test for *T. gondii* between different laboratories can explain sensitivity results ranging from 81% to 97%.[42,63] In a retrospective multicentre study, the combination of PCR and mouse inoculation of amniotic fluid was shown to have a sensitivity of 91%.[63]

Parvovirus B19

The incidence of congenital PVB19 is related to outbreaks of B19 virus in the general population.[64,65] Viraemia occurs six to eight days after exposure and persists for four to seven days. There is a 33% placental transmission rate following maternal seroconversion at any stage of pregnancy but the risk of fetal complication is highly variable and the teratologic risk debatable. Many cases of fetal hydrops have been reported after clinical maternal infection and, within this context, intrauterine fetal death may occur at between 1 and 21 days.[65] Overall, the risk of fetal complications following maternal PVB19 infection is less than 10%. A prospective study in 1998 has shown that 46% of infected mothers had polyarthralgia and 38% had a rash but that none of their fetuses developed NIHF and that there were no intrauterine fetal deaths attributable to PVB19.[66] No ultrasound marker other than NIHF predicts fetal demise and a survey of members of the Society of Perinatal Obstetricians has indicated that PVB19-induced NIHF resolves spontaneously in one-third of cases.[67] PCR analysis of the amniotic fluid has been used successfully to diagnose PVB19 in fetuses presenting with NIHF[68] but there are few data to support invasive modalities in non-hydropic fetuses.[67] Almost all cases of PVB19-associated NIHF have developed within eight weeks of maternal infection and therefore weekly ultrasound examinations should be performed.[67] PUBS is essential in managing NIHF with significant anaemia and more than 80% of hydropic fetuses transfused *in utero* will survive.[67,69] Thus, in congenital infection with PVB19, fetal outcome is clearly improved with intervention before the development of the hydropic state and ultrasound findings are specific enough to avoid unnecessary intervention.

Varicella-zoster virus

Varicella infection or chickenpox is rare (<2%) in adults. This mild childhood disease is much more severe in adults and, in particular, mortality is high during pregnancy.[44] The highest risk of fetal sequelae is during the first half of pregnancy and the risk of transplacental passage before 24 weeks is around 8%, with a risk of congenital varicella of 2.8%.[70] Ultrasound markers of congenital varicella include limb hypoplasia, FGR and microcalcification of the liver or spleen (Table 6.2). In primary VZV infection during pregnancy, the sensitivity of prenatal diagnosis with PCR on amniotic fluid is 100% and PUBS is not useful.[70]

Conclusions

The vast majority of congenital infections are clinically silent and a review of the maternal history may occasionally reveal prior 'flu-like illness'. Infections transmitted during the first half of pregnancy often lead to fetopathy but may be amenable to prenatal diagnosis and sometimes to therapy. Ultrasound examination and amniocentesis play a pivotal role in identifying fetuses at risk of congenital infection. The presence of ultrasound lesions of the fetal brain is a sign of severe infection and carries a worse prognosis. However, the proportion of infected fetuses going on to develop abnormalities that can be identified sonographically remains unknown. In particular, late-onset neurological damage in congenitally infected infants prevents complete reassurance in sonographically normal fetuses. Thus, in pregnancies at risk, a single ultrasound examination is not a sensitive test for fetal infection and a normal fetal anatomy cannot predict a favourable outcome.

Invasive prenatal diagnosis of most congenital infections has been revolutionised by new molecular genetic techniques involving PCR. Because of the risk of complications secondary to fetal blood sampling, amniocentesis and PCR have replaced the identification of specific IgM in fetal blood and other diagnostic tests on fetal blood. However, many technical difficulties must be addressed in order to reduce both false-negative and false-positive results and also to evaluate the risk of transmission of the pathogen to the fetus secondary to the placental damage during the invasive procedure.

In most cases of congenital infection, the timing of transmission is variable, requiring a combination of prenatal diagnostic approaches. It is important to identify mothers with *T. gondii* or PVB19 seroconversion as soon as possible because antiparasitic treatment in congenital toxoplasmosis and fetal blood transfusion in congenital PVB19 can reduce fetal mortality and neonatal morbidity. In cases of primary maternal CMV infection where there is evidence of transmission but the fetus appears sonographically normal, the options are immediate termination or follow-up and termination if fetal abnormalities are found later in pregnancy. The management of congenital infection thus requires a certain degree of fetal medicine training and laboratory expertise in PCR technology that may not be available outside specialist centres. Prospective research is needed to evaluate the impact of the combined use of ultrasound markers and amniocentesis findings on the management and outcome of congenital infection.

Recommendations

1. Fetal hydrops, brain abnormalities and hyperechogenic lesions are the most common ultrasound markers of a congenital infection and a maternal screen for TORCH and TORCH-like infections is recommended in these cases.

2. Fetal infection should also be considered when multiple organ system anomalies and/or early FGR are demonstrated on ultrasound.

3. In pregnancies at risk of congenital infection (maternal seroconversion), serial ultrasound examinations (every two weeks) should be performed until delivery.

4. Delays of more than six weeks between the serological diagnosis of maternal CMV and toxoplasmosis infection and the invasive procedure are recommended to increase the sensitivity of prenatal diagnosis.

5. Invasive procedures are contraindicated in pregnancies at risk of HIV or hepatitis.

6. Amniocentesis carries a low risk of post-procedure fetal loss and morbidity and the lowest risk of introducing a microorganism into a previously uninfected fetus and should therefore be the standard invasive procedure used for the diagnosis of congenital infection.

References

1. Gregg NM. Congenital cataract following German measles in the mother. *Trans Ophthalmol Soc Aust* 1941;**3**:35–46.
2. Miller E, Cradock-Watson JE, Pollock TM. Consequences of confirmed maternal rubella at successive stages of pregnancy. *Lancet* 1982;**ii**:781–4.
3. South MA, Sever JL. Teratogen update: the congenital rubella syndrome. *Teratology* 1985;**31**:297–307.
4. Jauniaux E, Jaffe R. Assessment of embryonic and early fetal viability. In: Jauniaux E, Barnea R, Edwards R, editors. *Embryonic Medicine and Therapy*. Oxford: Oxford University Press; 1997. p. 223–43.
5. Simpson JL, Mills JL, Kim H, Holmes LB, Lee J, Metzger B, *et al*. Infectious processes: an infrequent cause of first trimester spontaneous abortions. *Hum Reprod* 1996;**3**:668–72.
6. Keeling JW. Fetal hydrops. In: Keeling JW, editor. *Fetal and Neonatal Pathology*. London: Springer-Verlag; 1994. p. 83–93
7. Jauniaux E, Van Maldergem L, De Munter C, Moscoso G, Gillerot Y. Non-immune hydrops fetalis associated with genetic abnormalities. *Obstet Gynecol* 1990;**75**:568–72.
8. Weiner CP, Grose CF, Naides SJ. Diagnosis of fetal infection in a patient with an ultrasonographically detected abnormality but a negative clinical history. *Am J Obstet Gynecol* 1993;**168**:6–11
9. Brown KE, Green SW, Antunez de Mayolo J, Bellanti JA, Smith SD, Smith TJ, *et al*. Congenital anaemia after transplacental B19 parvovirus infection. *Lancet* 1994;**343**:895–6.
10. Jauniaux E, Kaminopetros P, Rodeck C. Hydrops fetalis. In: Brace RA, Hanson M, Rodeck C, editors. *Body Fluids and Kidney Function*. Cambridge: Cambridge University Press; 1997. p. 207–30.
11. Jauniaux E. Diagnosis and management of early non-immune hydrops fetalis. *Prenat Diagn* 1997;**17**:1261–8.

12. Iskaros J, Jauniaux E, Rodeck C. Outcome of nonimmune hydrops fetalis diagnosed during the first half of pregnancy. *Obstet Gynecol* 1997;**90**:321–5.

13. Mazeron MC, Cordovi-Voulgaropoulos L, Perol Y. Transient hydrops fetalis associated with intrauterine cytomegalovirus infection: Prenatal diagnosis. *Obstet Gynecol* 1994;**84**:692–4.

14. Bhal PS, Davies NJ, Westmoreland D, Jones A. Spontaneous resolution of non-immune hydrops fetalis secondary to transplacental parvovirus B19 infection. *Ultrasound Obstet Gynecol* 1996;**7**:55–7.

15. Sebire NJ, Bianco D, Snijders RJ, Zuckerman M, Nicolaides KH. Increased fetal nuchal translucency thickness at 10–14 weeks: is screening for maternal–fetal infection necessary? *Br J Obstet Gynaecol* 1997;**104**:212–15.

16. Petrikovsky BM, Baker D, Schneider E. Fetal hydrops secondary to human parvovirus infection in early pregnancy. *Prenat Diagn* 1996;**16**:342–4.

17. Brandenburg H, Los FJ, Cohen-Overbeek TE. A case of early intrauterine parvovirus B19 infection. *Prenat Diagn* 1996;**16**:75–7.

18. Smulian JC, Egan JF, Rodis JF. Fetal hydrops in the first trimester associated with maternal parvovirus infection. *J Clin Ultrasound* 1998;**26**:314-16.

19. Markenson G, Correia LA, Cohn G, Bayer L, Kanaan C. Parvoviral infection associated with increased nuchal translucency: a case report. *J Perinatol* 2000;**20**:129–31.

20. Jordan JA. Identification of human parvovirus B19 infection in idiopathic nonimmune hydrops fetalis. *Am J Obstet Gynecol* 1996;**174**:37–42.

21. Skjoldebrand-Sparre L, Tolfvenstam T, Papadogiannakis N, Wahren B, Broliden K, Nyman M. Parvovirus B19 infection: association with third-trimester intrauterine fetal death. *BJOG* 2000;**107**:476–80.

22. Essary LR, Vnencak-Jones CL, Manning SS, Olson SJ, Johnson JE. Frequency of parvovirus B19 infection in nonimmune hydrops fetalis and utility of three diagnositic methods. *Hum Pathol* 1998;**29**:696–701.

23. Kilby M, Hodgett S. Perinatal viral infections as a cause of intrauterine growth restriction. In: Kingdom J, Baker P, editors. *Intrauterine Growth Restriction: Aetiology and Management*. London: Springer-Verlag; 2000. p. 29–49.

24. Allen SJ, Raiko A, O'Donnell A, Alexander ND, Clegg JB. Causes of preterm delivery and intrauterine growth retardation in malaria endemic region of Papua New Guinea. *Arch Dis Child* 1998;**79**:F135–40.

25. Castetbon K, Ladner J, Leroy V, Chauliac M, Karita E, De Clercq A, *et al.* Low birthweight in infants born to African HIV-infected women: relationship with maternal body weight during pregnancy. *J Trop Pediatr* 1999;**45**:152–7.

26. Hartung J, Enders G, Chaoui R, Arents A, Tennstedt C, Bollmann R. Prenatal diagnosis of congenital varicella syndrome and detection of varicella-zoster in the fetus: a case report. *Prenat Diagn* 1999;**19**:163–6.

27. Lanouette JM, Duquette DA, Jacques SM, Qureshi F, Johnson MP, Berry SN. Prenatal diagnosis of fetal herpes simplex infection. *Fetal Diagn Ther* 1996;**11**:414–16.

28. Larsen PD, Chartrand SA, Tomashek KM, Hauser LG, Ksiazek TG. Hydrocephalus complicating lymphocytic choriomeningitis virus infection. *Pediatr Infect Dis J* 1993;**12**:528–31.

29. Seidman DS, Nass D, Mendelson E, Shehtman I, Mashiach S, Achiron R. Prenatal ultrasonographic diagnosis of fetal hydrocephalus due to infection with parainfluenza virus type 3. *Ultrasound Obstet Gynecol* 1996;**7**:52–54.

30. Johnson RT, Johnson KP, Edmonds CJ. Virus-induced hydrocephalus: development of aqueductal stenosis in hamsters after mumps infection. *Science* 1967;**157**:1066–7.

31. Burch GE, Sun SC, Chu KC, Sohal RS, Colcolough HL. Interstitial and coxsackievirus B myocarditis in infants and children. A comparative histologic and immunofluorescent study of 50 autopsied hearts. *JAMA* 1968;**203**:1–8.

32. Ranucci-Weiss D, Uerpairojkit B, Bowles N, Towbin JA, Chan L. Intrauterine adenovirus infection associated with non-immune hydrops. *Prenat Diagn* 1998;**18**:182–5.

33. Meyer K, Girgis N, McGravey V. Adenovirus associated with congenital pleural effusion. *J Pediatr* 1985;**107**:433–5.

34. Lambot MA, Noel JC, Peny MO, Rodesch F, Haot J. Fetal parvovirus B19 infection associated with myocardial necrosis. *Prenat Diagn* 1999;**19**:389–90.

35. Parilla BV, Tamura RK, Ginsberg NA. Association of parvovirus infection with isolated fetal effusions. *Am J Perinatol* 1997;**14**:357–8.

36. Forouzan I. Fetal abdominal echogenic mass: an early sign of intrauterine cytomegalovirus infection. *Obstet Gynecol* 1992;**80**:535–7.

37. Muller F, Dommergues M, Aubry MC, Simon-Bouy B, Gautier E, Oury JF, *et al.* Hyperechogenic fetal bowel: an ultrasonographic marker for adverse fetal and neonatal outcome. *Am J Obstet Gynecol*

1995;**173**:508–13.
38. MacGregor SN, Tamura R, Sabbagha R, Brenhofer JK, Kambich MP, Pergament E. Isolated hyperechoic fetal bowel: significance and implications for management. *Am J Obstet Gynecol* 1995;**173**:1254–8.
39. Achiron R, Seidman DS, Afeck A, Malinger G, Lipitz S, Mashiach S, *et al.* Prenatal ultrasonographic diagnosis of fetal hyperechogenicities: clinical significance and implications for management. *Ultrasound Obstet Gynecol* 1996;**7**:251–5.
40. Yaron Y, Hassan S, Geva E, Kupferminc MJ, Yavetz H, Evans MI. Evaluation of fetal echogenic bowel in the second trimester. *Fetal Diagn Ther* 1999;**14**:176–80.
41. Schild RL, Plath H. Thomas P, Schulte-Wissermann H, Eis-Hubinger AM, Hansmann M. Fetal parvovirus B19 infection and meconium peritonitis. *Fetal Diagn Ther* 1998;**13**:15–18.
42. Hohlfeld P, Daffos F, Costa JM, Thulliez P, Forestier F, Vidaud M. Prenatal diagnosis of congenital toxoplasmosis with polymerase-chain-reaction test on amniotic fluid. *N Engl J Med* 1994;**331**:695–9.
43. Jauniaux E, Jurkovic D, Gulbis B, Liesnard C, Lees C, Campbell S. Materno–fetal immunoglobulin transfer and passive immunity during the first trimester of human pregnancy. *Hum Reprod* 1995;**10**:3297–300.
44. Mandelbrot L. Vertical transmission of viral infections. *Curr Opin Obstet Gynecol* 1998;**10**:123–8.
45. Smith KC, McGladdery AJ, Binns MM, Mumford JA. Use of transabdominal ultrasound-guided amniocentesis for detection of equid herpesvirus 1-induced fetal infection *in utero. Am J Vet Res* 1997;**58**:997–1002.
46. Steele MW, Breg WR Jr. Chromosome analysis of human amniotic-fluid cells. *Lancet* 1966;**i**:383–5.
47. Grose C, Itani O, Weiner CP. Prenatal diagnosis of fetal infection: advances from amniocentesis to cordocentesis – congenital toxoplasmosis, rubella, cytomegalovirus, varicella virus, parvovirus and human immunodeficiency virus. *Pediatr Infect Dis J* 1989;**8**:459–68.
48. Jauniaux E. A comparison of chorionic villus sampling and amniocentesis for prenatal diagnosis in early pregnancy. In: Grudzinskas JG, Ward RHT, editors. *Screening for Down Syndrome in the First Trimester.* London: RCOG Press; 1997. p. 259–69.
49. Terry GM, Ho-Terry L, Warren RC, Rodeck CH, Cohen A, Rees KR. First trimester pre-natal diagnosis of congenital rubella: a laboratory investigation. *BMJ* 1986;**292**:930–3.
50. Timbury MC. Congenital cytomegalovirus infection: a dilemma. *BMJ* 1984;**289**:712–13.
51. Lamy ME, Mulongo KN, Gadisseux JF, Lyon G, Gaudy V, Van Lierde MV. Prenatal diagnosis of fetal cytomegalovirus infection. *Am J Obstet Gynecol* 1992;**166**:91–4.
52. Demmler GJ. Congenital cytomegalovirus infection. *Semin Pediatr Neurol* 1994;**1**:36–42.
53. Grose C, Weiner CP. Prenatal diagnosis of congenital cytomegalovirus infection: two decades later. *Am J Obstet Gynecol* 1990;**163**:447–50.
54. Fowler KB, Stagno S, Pass RF, Britt WJ, Boll TJ, Alford CA. The outcome of congenital cytomegalovirus infection in relation to maternal antibody status. *N Engl J Med* 1992;**326**:663–7.
55. Liesnar C, Donner C, Brancart F, Gosselin F, Delforge ML, Rodesch F. Prenatal diagnosis of congenital cytomegalovirus infection: prospective study of 237 pregnancies at risk. *Obstet Gynecol* 2000;**95**:881–8.
56. Ivarsson SA, Lernmark B, Svanberg L. Ten-year clinical, developmental and intellectual follow up of children with congenital cytomegalovirus infection without neurological symptoms at one year of age. *Pediatrics* 1997;**99**:800–3.
57. Lipitz S, Yagel S, Shalev E, Achiron R, Mashiach S, Schiff E. Prenatal diagnosis of fetal primary cytomegalovirus infection. *Obstet Gynecol* 1997;**89**:763–7.
58. Nigro G, Mazzocco M, Anceschi MM, La Torre R, Antonelli G, Cosmi EV. Prenatal diagnosis of fetal cytomegalovirus infection after primary or recurrent maternal infection. *Obstet Gynecol* 1999;**94**:909–14.
59. Bodeus M, Hubinont C, Bernard P, Bouckaert A, Thomas K, Goubau P. Prenatal diagnosis of human cytomegalovirus by culture and polymerase chain reaction: 98 pregnancies leading to congenital infection. *Prenat Diagn* 1999;**19**:314–17.
60. Joynson DHM, Payne R. Screening for toxoplasma in pregnancy. *Lancet* 1988;**ii**:795–6.
61. Foulon W, Villena I, Stray-Pedersen B, Decoster A, Lappalainen M, Pinon JM, *et al.* Treatment of toxoplasmosis during pregnancy: impact on fetal transmission and children's sequelae at one year of age. A multicentric study. *Am J Obstet Gynecol* 1999;**188**:410–15.
62. Koppe JG, Rothova A. Congenital toxoplasmosis. A long-term follow-up of 20 years. *Int Ophthalmol* 1989;**13**:387–90.
63. Foulon W, Pinon JM, Stray-Pedersen B, Pollak A, Lappalainen M, Decoster A, *et al.* Prenatal diagnosis of congenital toxoplasmosis: a multicenter evaluation of different diagnostic parameters. *Am J Obstet Gynecol* 1999;**181**:843–7.
64. Boley TJ, Popek E. Parvovirus infection in pregnancy. *Semin Perinatol* 1993;**17**:410–19.

65. Fairley CK, Smoleniec JS, Caul OE, Miller E. Observational study of effect of intrauterine transfusions on outcome of fetal hydrops after parvovirus B19 infection. *Lancet* 1995;**346**:1335–7.

66. Harger JH, Adler SP, Koch WC, Harger GF. Prospective evaluation of 618 pregnant women exposed to parvovirus B19: risks and symptoms. *Obstet Gynecol* 1998;**91**:413–20.

67. Rodis JF, Borgida AF, Wilson M, Eagan JF, Leo MV, Odibo AO, *et al.* Management of parvovirus infection in pregnancy and outcomes of hydrops: a survey of members of the Society of Perinatal Obstetricians. *Am J Obstet Gynecol* 1998;**179**:985–8.

68. Gentilomi G, Zerbini M, Gallinella G, Venturoli S, Manaresi E, Morandi R, *et al.* B19 parvovirus induced fetal hydrops: rapid and simple diagnosis by detection of B19 antigens in amniotic fluids. *Prenat Diagn* 1998;**18**:363–8.

69. Schild RL, Bald R, Plath H, Eis-Hubinger AM, Enders G, Hansmann M. Intrauterine management of fetal parvovirus B19 infection. *Ultrasound Obstet Gynecol* 1999;**13**:161–6.

70. Mouly F, Mirlesse V, Meritet JF, Rozenberg F, Poissonier MH, Lebon P, *et al.* Prenatal diagnosis of fetal varicella-zoster virus infection with polymerase chain reaction of amniotic fluid in 107 cases. *Am J Obstet Gynecol* 1997;**177**:894–8.

Chapter 7

New technology for the diagnosis of infection in pregnancy

Discussion

Discussion following Dr Brink's paper

Hay: Dr Brink, I suppose you did not have time to say that if someone has had past treatment with an anti-retroviral drug they can quite quickly revert back to wild type. A resistance assay is only useful to tell you about the drugs the person has been taking currently or very recently. When Dr Carrington was at St George's Hospital, London, we managed to get our purchasers to fund a deep freeze to store our viral load samples, one hopes indefinitely, so that we can always go back to a sample that is relevant to when the patient was taking those drugs.

Brink: We would obviously try to take an assay as close as possible to someone's stopping therapy. The other point is that, if someone has been on previous anti-retrovirals, and they are restarted on any drug they have been previously prescribed, if they do not have a greater than one log reduction in HIV plasma RNA viral load one month after restarting therapy we would re-test them for genotypic resistance. We would keep a very close eye on their viral load and, if there were any problem there, we would retest them for resistance.

Discussion following Dr Jauniaux's paper

Soothill: I do not think it is easy to have recommendations for all infections in one list, as proposed for this publication. In particular, there is the issue of the two weeks for scanning and the delay of six weeks before invasive procedure. That clearly does not apply to some infections, of which parvovirus is the most obvious example. It is quite hard to generalise all infections into one list of recommendations.

Jauniaux: I fully agree with you, and that is why we are here to discuss it. If you want to play the devil's advocate, and you look at American data[1,2] in the case of parvoviruses, they indirectly show that there is no need to follow these patients for 14 weeks because the vast majority will not develop fetal hydrops.

MacLean: Professor Soothill, could I ask you how you would modify the recommendation about the six week delay?

Soothill: It is quite difficult. Clearly, if you have ultrasound features in any of the conditions we are talking about, you would not want to wait that long. You are saying that, in the absence of other information on ultrasound, the earliest you would want to do your invasive procedure would be six weeks after serological diagnosis of maternal infection. Then, however, in the case of some of these conditions, you would not want to do an invasive procedure even at that time.

Dr Jauniaux has done a good job of trying to simplify this, but it would be dangerous if that list were applied to all conditions without the other information – especially ultrasound.

Griffiths: I agree with Professor Soothill. In preparing the document, we need to give a clear explanation of what is going on. The six weeks comes from the cytomegalovirus (CMV) story. The pathogenesis here is that you have fetal involvement, with fetal excretion through the fetal kidneys, with urine into the amniotic fluid, which is what you are actually sampling. It is the delay in establishing renal function of the fetus that introduces that delay, so that is specific to the CMV diagnostic side and it does not necessarily apply to some of the others. We should tabulate it according to each particular infection.

Jauniaux: I fully agree with you, but we must look at this from a practical point of view. The three main infections that we are dealing with are CMV, parvovirus B19 and toxoplasmosis. For parvovirus B19 there is no need to perform amniocentesis, which leaves CMV and toxoplasmosis for which the six-week period can apply.

If I were to summarise the recommendations, I would say that we should pay more attention to the ultrasound markers of fetal infection. Obviously, Professor Soothill and I are fetal medicine specialists, and there are only about ten of us in the UK who deal with these cases. Since I started working in this field, the emphasis that has been put on Down syndrome screening, for example, is incredible: the financial implications of Down syndrome screening are astronomical in comparison with screening for fetal infection, which is much more common and for which there is little information available in the literature to clinicians. The importance of this session is, in one aspect, to make clinicians aware of these ultrasound markers of fetal infection and to act on them when they see them.

Another aspect is that, if you discuss prenatal diagnosis of congenital infection at international meetings, many colleagues are still taking fetal blood samples in these cases. This exposes the fetus to unnecessary risk, not only of the fetus dying after the procedure, but also of transmitting the infection directly into the fetal circulation. There have been no studies aimed at trying to identify whether this is a real risk or just a hypothesis. Given the information available in the literature, amniocentesis should remain the only invasive test offered to these patients, unless there is evidence of parvovirus B19 , in which case it should be assayed with a transfusion *in utero*.

Thus, my two recommendations are: greater awareness of ultrasound markers of fetal infection, and to regard amniocentesis as being the primary invasive test in the prenatal diagnosis of the congenital infection.

MacLean: Could you elaborate on the ultrasound markers? There is no doubt that, in the UK, the majority of ultrasound scanning is performed by ultrasonographers and not by obstetricians. Following on from what Dr Miller said earlier about identifying people who may be at risk because of a rash or significant contact, would you expect an ultrasonographer to be able to see these markers? They will recognise gross hydrops, but what about the more subtle changes? Would you expect them to be able to detect those, or should these patients be referred to fetal medicine specialists who would do the scanning?

Jauniaux: They would first have to be identified, so in the UK the front line will always be the sonographer. We could also recommend that when there is high risk of fetal infection, because there is evidence that the mother has been infected and there is an ultrasound marker, the patient should be referred to regional centres that have not only fetal medicine facilities but also virology and so on. In other European countries, there are fewer or no sonographers and very often the obstetrician has limited training in carrying out ultrasound scanning.

General discussion

Soothill: I would like to follow on from what Dr Jauniaux said, i.e., that intrauterine growth restriction and hydrops may be transient markers on ultrasound. We think many of the markers must be due to viral infections, but you cannot find anything. In the new technologies that you were talking about, will there be ways of improving screening for mysterious viruses – perhaps using multiplex polymerase chain reaction (PCR), or something of that sort?

Brink: That is a relevant question. We have to be aware of the diverse viruses that could cause fetal abnormalities. A good example of that is human herpesvirus type 6, which is a beta herpesvirus, with a spectrum of disease in immunocompromised patients that is similar to that in CMV. What is its precise role in the fetus? We know it crosses to the fetus and we know it causes infection. We certainly have multiplex-based PCR for herpesviruses but the role of, for example, enteroviruses in fetal abnormalities certainly needs to be explored further. What is their role in ventriculomegaly? What is their role in unexplained myocarditis causing fetal or neonatal death? In the future, we will definitely see more viruses causing congenital abnormalities.

Griffiths: I wanted to pick up the question about multiplex PCR. The beauty of PCR is its great specificity but that means that you need to know what you are looking for before you design your primers

Soothill: One of the reasons for my question was that in the September 2000 meeting of the International Fetal Diagnosis and Therapy Society another couple of cases of adenovirus were reported. It seemed convincing that the virus was present in the fetus but they just found it by chance. As I understand it, there are a number of different types. Could you not build a system whereby there are multiple primers so that you could search?

Brink: Yes, but you have to have your detection system, so there is a limit to what we can do. Yes, the concept of 'fishing' for viruses is relevant.

Smith: This is just a point of information with respect to nucleic acid sequence based amplification (NASBA). Professor McIntyre and I were involved four years ago and we used NASBA on vaginal secretions for quantitative measurement of HIV, with respect to using it potentially as a method of measuring virucidal activity.[3] The other arena in which we have been using it is our sperm-washing programme at the Chelsea and Westminster Hospital, where the aliquots are NASBA tested prior to instillation into the negative female partner.[4]

Semprini's bank of sperm samples has been retested. Although none of the women have seroconverted, there are a couple of samples which were in fact positive on testing, which have been instilled. In fact, the first person who went through our own sperm washing programme – whose cycle had to be cancelled because the sample proved to be plasma positive – now has a baby, which was a successful outcome.

Ridgway: Dr Brink's presentation was concise and excellent – this is the sort of service we expect from her department at UCLH. Unfortunately, however, it is the exception rather than the rule throughout the country. Should your college recommend that patients who are diagnosed as having congenital infections be referred to centres of excellence, or should they struggle with a district microbiology laboratory and amateur virologists?

Brink: If you are going to make any diagnosis on a patient you have to be competent to make that diagnosis. If you cannot provide a 'top-flight' service, you should refer it on to someone who can. That is not unreasonable, because these facilities are widely available in the UK.

Carrying on from that, should all women diagnosed with a congenital infection be referred on to a fetal medicine unit? If you diagnose a parvovirus infection or varicella, for example, should these women be referred to centres for fetal medicine? I would be interested to hear the comments of the fetal medicine specialists on that question.

Soothill: I just wanted to pick up on what you said when you asked Dr Jauniaux about nonspecialised scanning for markers of infection. That is the same question, and the answer is that it is difficult to pick up the mild, but very important, markers of infection. I think patients should be referred, but only when you have identified recent definite infection in the pregnancy.

Jauniaux: There are as many fully trained fetal medicine specialists as there are virologists, and this is one of the problems. We have trained many people to become moderately competent at performing amniocentesis and basic scans but not in providing the full service. I suspect that a patient who has a massive parvovirus infection and ends up in one of these centres will have their treatment delayed for quite a long time before they reach a referral unit that can offer a transfusion *in utero* or the insertion of a chest drain.

MacLean: Presumably everyone in fetal medicine has close links with the laboratory. If they have a clinical or diagnostic challenge, and the laboratory cannot provide that service for them, then their local laboratory will facilitate transfer of specimen to somewhere where it can be provided.

Brink: Absolutely, yes. For example, Bernard Cohen at the Public Health Laboratory Service in Colindale does our parvovirus work. If we cannot do it to a satisfactory standard, we will refer it on to a laboratory that can. I see no problem with that at all.

Jauniaux: It seems to work better for you than it does for us. The main reason for this meeting is to alert clinicians about congenital infection. If I summarise my working day as a fetal medicine specialist now, it is more than 50% scanning patients and screening them for Down syndrome, whereas ten years ago this had less importance. Ten years ago, fetal medicine was mainly about treating the fetus *in utero*, detecting congenital infections and understanding the pathophysiology of fetal disease. Fetal medicine training has been transformed in this country into screening for Down syndrome. This dilutes the training and it also dilutes the working day. It is probably one of the reasons why we are missing many cases of congenital infection. If the trend continues, we will completely forget that there might be fetal conditions other than Down syndrome.

MacLean: You will certainly know that if a patient is now managed and is either not offered screening for Down syndrome or produces a false negative test then that may be an expensive mistake. Surely the same applies here. You hinted in your presentation that if you miss a parameter of infection then that may be equally costly in terms of litigation.

Jauniaux: I am not a medico-legal expert but if I were a lawyer I would have a much better case with a CMV infection that had been missed *in utero*, or toxoplasmosis, where damage can be limited by treatment, than with a Down syndrome that had been missed.

Hughes: Dr Jauniaux, what are your thoughts about non-invasive testing for anaemia associated with parvovirus, such as middle cerebral artery velocity? Do you do that?

Jauniaux: No, we do not. The hydrops seems to be quite quick – the development of this type of anaemia is a very rapid process, over a few days probably. The middle cerebral artery velocity is useful in rhesus disease, which is a slowly progressive disease and will change over weeks or sometimes months. So, no, we do not use that. We simply do a quick scan to check whether there are any markers of fetal hydrops.

Soothill: I do not quite agree with that, but I will talk about that tomorrow. Dr Jauniaux is right when he says that hydrops develops quickly but, if you are doing weekly scans for parvovirus hydrops, I certainly have had cases where the middle cerebral artery velocity was very high before development of ascites. I am convinced that it is useful to perform this test in those groups where you know that you have maternal infection and you are doing weekly scans. You might even bring that patient back before the next week if you have a very high anaemic result.

Miller: I think you advised that, ideally, women with varicella in pregnancy would be referred to a fetal medicine centre. What would be the rationale for that? What benefit would be likely to accrue as a result of that referral? The risk of fetal damage is low. Sometimes the actual defect associated with varicella may not present until late in the pregnancy, because the infection is actually intrauterine herpes zoster. Also, when the defects are present, they should be fairly obvious on ultrasound scan – although I am not sure that that is necessarily the case.

If you articulated the actual benefit you would derive from referral to a fetal medicine centre, what would that be? Remember, varicella-zoster virus is not a rare infection in pregnancy – there are probably about 2000 cases a year, so it is a common infection in pregnancy.

Soothill: The 2.5% incidence of fetal malformations is, I suspect, too high. I suspect that there may have been ascertainment bias but I do not know. I have never seen any fetal amputations in any prospective case that I have seen with chickenpox so it is probably very rare. If we could have more secure data showing that it is actually incredibly rare, then perhaps we could stop specific scanning. For the moment, however, the figure is 2.5% out on the internet sites. We would be providing reassurance that the limbs are indeed normal and that there is no cerebral lesion at that point in pregnancy. Have others seen a case in which a malformation was found on prenatal scanning?

Carrington: Basically, the answer is that it is rare, although I have certainly seen cases. It may well be that the use of hyperimmune globulin, and the intense way in which we investigate contacts and treat cases, may well have reduced the incidence – particularly in the South West, Professor Soothill, so that you have not seen it. However, it is rare, and it is difficult to know how to follow it up.

Hughes: For parvovirus, the situation is very different. Women with evidence of infection with parvovirus should definitely be referred to a fetal medicine centre because there can be a tendency for clinicians not to think of the possibility of parvovirus. They think it is a chromosomal problem, whereas parvovirus is actually a very easily treated condition, so they should definitely be referred.

References

1. Harger JH, Adler SP, Koch WC, Harger GF. Prospective evaluation of 618 pregnant women exposed to parvovirus B19: risks and symptoms. *Obstet Gynecol* 1998;**91**:413–20.
2. Rodis JF, Borgida AF, Wilson M, Eagan JF, Leo MV, Odibo AO, *et al.* Management of parvovirus infection in pregnancy and outcomes of hydrops: a survey of members of the Society of Perinatal Obstetricians. *Am J Obstet Gynecol* 1998;**179**:985–8.
3. M Stafford, personal communication.
4. Kim LU, Johnson MR, Barton S, Nelson MR, Sontag G, Smith JR, *et al.* Evaluation of sperm washing as a potential method of reducing HIV transmission in HIV-discordant couples wishing to have children. *AIDS* 1999;**13**:645–51.

SECTION 3

BACTERIAL AND OTHER INFECTIONS DURING PREGNANCY I

Chapter 8

Asymptomatic bacteriuria during pregnancy

Allan B MacLean

History

On 3 January 1906, W Anstruther Milligan[1] reported to the Obstetrical Society of London the case of Mrs Y, aged 23 years, who had been admitted two years previously to the Hospital for Women, Soho Square, in her seventh month of pregnancy. She had recently become unwell with pains in her left loin that radiated over her abdomen and into her back. Her urine was thick and had a disagreeable smell. When she was admitted, her temperature had been 101°F and she looked very ill. She had a large, dull, immobile swelling in the region of her left kidney, extending to the spinal muscles and down to the brim of the pelvis. The urine was acidic and contained a large amount of pus. The consultant surgeon had explored her retroperitoneal space and evacuated a large amount of pus from the distended renal pelvis and ureter. Drainage had been employed and the woman had gradually recovered. Her pregnancy had continued and she had delivered her child six weeks after admission.

Milligan had reviewed the literature available at that time (a bibliography of 34 references) and commented that, although the first mention of pyelonephritis in pregnancy had been made by Rayer in a French publication of 1841, its first real description was when Reblaub read a paper entitled '*Des Infections des Reins et du Bassinet Consécutives à la Compression de l'Uretère par l'Utérus Gravide*' in 1892. Reid described pyelonephritis of pregnancy in the *Philadelphia Medical Journal* of 1899 and mentioned two causative factors: ureteral compression and infection. In 1905, Opitz gave a full account, in a German publication, based on 79 cases of pyelonephritis in pregnancy. Milligan attempted to describe the mechanisms of the condition as an 'exciting cause': the entrance of pyogenic organisms that were either the colon bacillus which gained an entrance to the kidney via the blood or lymph stream, or ascending streptococcus or staphylococcus. In this case report he could not vouch for the organism as no bacteriological examination had been performed. The 'predisposing cause' was the pressure on the ureter when it was nipped between the uterus and the pelvic brim, producing dilatation of the ureter above this, and stagnation of urine. Milligan concluded his presentation, 'The point of interest lies in the question as to where and how the ureter becomes compressed, for compression seems to be an essential element, rendering the kidney and pelvis capable of being attacked by some pathogenic organism. I cannot suggest any other theory than those mentioned above, and yet at the same time we still seem to need something more definite to account for the compression.'

Professor J Whitridge Williams,[2] Professor of Obstetrics and Obstetrician-in-Chief to the Johns Hopkins Hospital in Baltimore, in his textbook of 1930 (and therefore still in the pre-antibiotic era), gives a similar description of pyelitis and pyelonephrosis in pregnancy: 'the disease usually appears in the latter half of pregnancy when the patient, who had previously been well, or had merely complained of slight vesical irritation, is suddenly seized with intense paroxysmal pains, usually in the right renal region. This is accompanied by a marked elevation of temperature and occasionally by chills, the temperature sometimes running a hectic course. Urinary examination reveals the presence of pus cells and usually of colon bacilli. If the process goes on to the development of pyelonephrosis, palpation shows that the affected kidney is definitely enlarged. In this event, the pain may disappear and the kidney become suddenly smaller after the passage of a large amount of purulent urine, the symptoms reappearing as the kidney fills again. If this condition is neglected, the patient may succumb to a septic process.'

He describes the occasional detection of an enlarged and sensitive ureter on vaginal examination, treatment by bed rest, abundant but bland diet, large quantities of water and milk and enough sodium bicarbonate to make the urine alkaline. If improvement was not rapid, premature labour was induced 'without hesitation'.

Professor R W Johnstone[3] of Edinburgh, writing in his textbook of midwifery in 1936, recommended using citrate of potash to render the urine alkaline, administering hexamine as a urinary antiseptic, and then an autogenous vaccine after the acute stage has passed.

In 1935, Dugald Baird[4-7] published a considerable experience based on six years of clinical research in the Glasgow Royal Maternity Hospital: the findings in 265 women admitted with pyelitis, the early results of a new technique for imaging (intravenous pyelography) and the findings at 102 postmortem examinations of women who had died in pregnancy or within a few days of labour. He observed that the ureter was almost always markedly dilated, due to the compression by the uterus of the ureter against the psoas muscles. Urinary tract infection was common and frequently confirmed by bacteriological culture: pyelitis was confirmed in 156 and considered probable in a further 101 in the first 1000 antenatal patients admitted for inpatient care. Treatment was bed rest, oral fluids and alkalinisation, but Baird was enthusiastic about ureteric drainage via an appropriate catheter, and acriflavine instillations.

The high prevalence of urinary tract infection among antenatal patients and the morbidity for mother and fetus reduced over the following ten years as a result of the availability of antimicrobials (sulphonamides) and antibiotics. However, pyelonephritis remained a serious complication within pregnancy, with the diagnosis increasingly supported by confirmatory bacteriology.

The pioneering work of Edward Kass,[8,9] Associate Professor of Bacteriology and Immunology at the Harvard Medical School and the Boston City Hospital, showed that 6% of women making their first antenatal visit had significant numbers of bacteria present in their urine – asymptomatic bacteriuria. A group of 48 of these patients was treated by placebo: 20 developed pyelonephritis, 24% of the infants were premature and there was a 14% perinatal mortality rate. A comparable group of 43 patients was treated with a long-acting sulphonamide until the bacteriuria cleared, or with nitrofurantoin (in the 20% of those patients with organisms that were resistant to sulphonamides). None of these patients developed pyelonephritis, the premature birth rate was 10% and there was no perinatal mortality.

Definitions

The definition of significant bacteriuria is 100 000 or more of the same pathogenic organism (or colony-forming units) per ml of urine from a clean-catch or midstream specimen. It was deemed to be asymptomatic if there were no signs or symptoms, although this ignored the urinary frequency, urgency and sometimes incontinence that occur during pregnancy. Kass[9] recognised that a single midstream urine sample had a false-positive rate of up to 20% from vulval or vaginal contamination and that the diagnosis of asymptomatic bacteriuria should therefore be based on a significant number of the same organisms in two consecutive samples. Some studies, for example Turner,[10] used a nurse to wash the vulva with liquid soap and water and to instruct the patient on the collection of a midstream urine sample into a sterile wide-mouth jar, while others confirmed the diagnosis by culture of a suprapubic aspirate of urine.[11–13] Most clinics now no longer use vulval cleansing and the patient attempts a clean catch, with or without labial separation, during voiding.[14,15]

The consequences of asymptomatic bacteriuria

Asymptomatic bacteriuria has been associated with pyelonephritis, preterm labour, intrauterine growth restriction and hypertension during pregnancy and anaemia. It is unlikely that hypertension or anaemia are direct consequences of bacteriuria and they will not be discussed further here.[15,16]

Asymptomatic bacteriuria and pyelonephritis

Kass recognised that patients with asymptomatic bacteriuria who were not treated, or who were given placebos, would develop pyelonephritis as described above. Little[17,18] studied 5000 antenatal patients at Charing Cross and Fulham Maternity Hospitals to identify those with bacteriuria. Half were not treated and, of those, 36% developed pyelonephritis, compared with only 5% of the other half who were treated. Pyelonephritis was also more likely to develop if treatment failed to clear the bacteriuria.[19] However, other reports show variation on this risk of progression. McFadyen and Eykyn[11] reported that 56% of asymptomatic bacteriuria progressed to acute pyelonephritis whereas Swapp[20] found that only 14% progressed. Accurate figures are difficult to compile as a result of the lack of confirmatory microbiology in patients with typical symptoms or the commencement of antibiotics by general practitioners who prescribe them before the patient arrives in hospital.

Acute pyelonephritis is the second most common medical problem to anaemia seen in pregnancy. The risk of ascending infection via the dilated ureter is now recognised to be due to progesterone as well as a mechanical effect. In a large study of 24 000 pregnant patients, Gilstrap et al.[21] reported in 1981 that 2% developed acute pyelonephritis. The risk is even higher following delivery and caesarean section because of intermittent or indwelling catheterisation. It is rarely seen with features as described in the pre-antibiotic days. Patients may be septicaemic and require admission, intravenous fluids and systemic antibiotics, such as cephalosporins or aminoglycosides, for example, gentamicin.[15]

Another consequence of urinary tract infection in pregnancy is the association between acute pyelonephritis and respiratory insufficiency. In 1984, Cunningham et al.,[22] of the Parkland Memorial Hospital in Dallas, Texas, described four women from among 250 seen with pyelonephritis during pregnancy who developed respiratory symptoms ranging from mild respiratory distress to overt pulmonary failure. These patients had flank pain, fever and chills, nausea and vomiting and tenderness to fist percussion in their renal angles. Pyelonephritis was confirmed by the presence of pyuria and bacteriuria and, in the four cases with respiratory complications, the causative organism was *Klebsiella pneumoniae* in two and *Escherichia coli* in the other two. These patients were between 18 and 23 years of age and gestational age was 21–36 weeks. Chest X-rays showed evidence of bilateral effusions or infiltrates. Their pyelonephritis was of significant severity to be associated with multisystem derangement including thrombocytopenia, disseminated intravascular coagulopathy and hepatic or renal dysfunction. There were no features to suggest that the lung damage was associated with left ventricular failure or fluid overload because the pulmonary capillary wedge pressures were not consistent with pulmonary oedema. The authors suggested that the pulmonary damage may have been associated with endotoxin effects from organisms reaching the circulation.

The same group[23] reviewed a total of 15 cases admitted to Parkland Memorial Hospital over a seven-year period. These patients all had acute pyelonephritis but also suffered respiratory insufficiency with dyspnoea, tachypnoea, hypoxaemia and X-ray evidence of pulmonary infiltrates. The respiratory features usually occurred 24–48 hours after admission. In three cases, respiratory failure required treatment with intubation and ventilation. The causative organisms were *E. coli* in ten cases (in four cases the organism was also found in the blood), *K. pneumoniae* in four, and *Proteus mirabilis* in one. These 15 cases occurred among approximately 750 cases of pyelonephritis (a ratio of 1 in 50) among 75 000 deliveries at the hospital. The authors again suggested that the damage may have been mediated by endotoxin-induced alveolar capillary membrane injury.

Towers et al.,[24] of the Irvine Medical Center and Long Beach Memorial Women's Hospital in California, reported 11 similar cases. Their important contribution was to recognise that the pulmonary failure may have been associated with the administration of tocolytics when there was concern about preterm labour. These drugs included magnesium sulphate (pulmonary injury occurred in four of eight women receiving magnesium sulphate in this clinical situation) and terbutaline (pulmonary injury occurred in three of eight women who received this drug). The authors also commented that the risk of pulmonary damage might be increased if the pyelonephritis was treated inadequately (there appeared to be an increased risk if ampicillin alone was used) and they recommended the prescribing of aminoglycosides in managing severe and acute pyelonephritis in pregnancy.

There is now doubt as to whether screening for and treating the 6% of pregnant women with asymptomatic bacteriuria is a useful way of preventing pyelonephritis during pregnancy, since there are likely to be more cases of pyelonephritis developing in the 94% of patients who did not have asymptomatic bacteriuria at booking. This concern is not new. Lawson and Miller[25] studied 1160 patients, 54 of whom had bacteriuria on first screening; 15 of these 54 (28%) developed symptoms suggestive of acute urinary tract infection and 9 of the 54 (17%) had bacteriologically confirmed pyelonephritis. Among the 1017 who had negative screening results, 70 (6.9%) became symptomatic and 32 (3.1%) had bacteriological confirmation. Thus, less than 20% of those patients who developed an acute urinary infection during their pregnancy had bacteriuria on initial screening. The authors concluded that 'acute pyelonephritis is unlikely to be eliminated as a disease of pregnancy by the detection and treatment of bacteriuria in early pregnancy. It seems that laboratory resources would be better used to follow closely, during and after pregnancy, those patients who develop a proven acute infection in the pregnancy rather than to screen the entire pregnant population for bacteriuria'.

Similarly, Chng and Hall[26] in Aberdeen found that urinary tract infection occurred in 25 of the 212 women who were bacteriuria-positive (12%) compared with 51 of the 1575 (3.2%) who were bacteriuria-negative, an almost four-fold increase in incidence. This also meant that 88% of the women who were bacteriuria-positive did not develop urinary tract infection at any time during their pregnancy and could be considered as false positives.

Asymptomatic bacteriuria, preterm labour and intrauterine growth restriction

Kass's experience in the Boston City Hospital was that 20–30% of bacteriuric pregnant patients failed to respond to treatment with small doses of sulphonamides or experienced recurrence or re-infection. His group[27] investigated whether a broader-spectrum antimicrobial would be more effective and tetracycline was chosen; at that time, tetracycline staining of teeth and incorporation into bone was not apparent. Tetracycline 250 mg four times a day for six weeks was given to 133 patients with asymptomatic bacteriuria and to 147 patients with sterile urine in a race-, age- and gravidity-matched control group. A placebo of identical appearance was given to 148 patients with bacteriuria, and to 132 without bacteriuria. Information was recorded from the patient's notes and about the outcome of the pregnancy. Prematurity was defined as a birthweight of 5 pounds 8 ounces (2.5 kg) or less (with no differentiation between preterm delivery and intrauterine growth restriction). Patients whose urine cleared of bacteriuria on treatment had a 10% prematurity rate, while 21% of patients whose bacteriuria did not clear with tetracycline or who had a recurrent episode were delivered of premature infants. Placebo-treated patients with bacteriuria who developed symptomatic pyelonephritis had an 18% prematurity rate, whereas if they remained asymptomatic but bacteriuric the prematurity rate was 9%. One of the interesting results from this study was that the patients in the tetracycline non-bacteriuric group had fewer premature deliveries (5%) and a longer mean length of gestation than did the placebo-treated non-bacteriuric group (15%). The authors offered no explanation. However, it is probable that tetracyclines clear organisms from the genital tract (and not just in the urinary tract), which will have a beneficial effect on preterm delivery risk.[16]

The authors also explained that, prior to 1962, when their study had been initiated, tetracyclines were widely used for the treatment of infection during pregnancy. Animal studies then suggested that bone and tooth discoloration occurred. Other studies suggested that tetracyclines could inhibit bone growth. However, follow-up of the children born in this Boston study found no increased rates of dental caries, hypoplasia of dental enamel or impairment of general growth and development. However, staining of the teeth was seen in about one-third of the children.[27]

More recent studies have used meta-analysis to evaluate larger numbers of patients and to assess the impact of bacteriuria on preterm delivery and birthweight. Romero et al.,[28] using a computer-assisted search of the English literature from 1966 to 1986, identified 31 studies of bacteriuria during pregnancy and, from these, identified 17 cohort studies where patients without bacteriuria were compared with those with untreated bacteriuria. From 13 studies analysed in depth, patients without bacteriuria had about two-thirds the risk of low birthweight (RR 0.65; 95% CI 0.56–0.74) of those with untreated bacteriuria. In four studies where there was information about preterm delivery, the relative risk was 0.50. In eight randomised studies that compared antibiotic treatment with no treatment, the relative risk of low birthweight was 0.56 (95% CI 0.43–0.73), indicating that antibiotic treatment reduced the risk of low birthweight. In a similar use of meta-analysis, Wang and Smaill[29] reported an odds ratio of 0.89 in six case-controlled studies. Their 95% confidence interval traversed unity, suggesting that treatment did not influence preterm delivery or low birthweight. It is of interest that three of the eight randomised studies included by Romero et al. were also included by Wang and Smaill but the three other studies they used included one by Gold et al.[30] that reversed the trend. In that study, two premature deliveries occurred among the 35 treated patients but none among the 30 untreated patients. The incidence of prematurity among 1216 patients without bacteriuria in that study was 13.9%. Wang and Smaill concluded that the treatment of bacteriuria with antibiotics had no significant impact on the rates of preterm delivery or low birthweight and that subsequent randomised controlled studies had not replicated the original results of Kass. More recent studies have commented on a link between acute pyelonephritis and preterm labour but, with prompt initiation of systemic antibiotics, this has not led to preterm delivery. This may explain why there is no longer a significant association.[28,31]

In a 1995 study[32] of 691 spontaneous preterm births among more than 25 000 term births in Cardiff, the spontaneous preterm births were associated with young maternal age, low maternal weight, low or high parity, previous abortion, smoking and early-pregnancy bleeding. The authors commented that there was no significant association between bacteriuria and spontaneous preterm birth and suggested that, unless subclinical urinary tract infection progressed to pyelonephritis or other renal disease, there was no association with preterm birth. The study also looked at what was called 'indicated' preterm births: ones where an induction was indicated on medical or obstetric grounds because of complications. These preterm births were associated with older age, low weight, previous stillbirth, bacteriuria and early-pregnancy bleeding. This association with bacteriuria is difficult to understand but shows that the subject cannot be totally ignored.

Screening for bacteriuria

In the past, the diagnosis of asymptomatic bacteriuria was made in the laboratory, with microscopy followed by culture, and then sensitivity patterns after positive identification of pathogens. A calibrated loop for semiquantitative counts and pour plate techniques were standard.[33] Newer methods use microscopy for pyuria, with 60 μl of urine in a 96-well tray, monitoring bacterial growth in agar, testing for sensitivity. These tests cost approximately £4 each when equipment and personnel are included. Other techniques mix urine samples and broth and monitor bacterial growth by light scattering or optical density measurements.[34]

An alternative is to use dipsticks, or multisticks, to test for the presence of nitrites and leucocyte esterase, and usually blood and protein. Nitrites are produced in urine by the breakdown (reduction) of dietary nitrates by bacteria, but group B streptococcus, enterococcus and pseudomonas species are not nitrate-reducing (and will therefore give false negatives). Leucocyte esterase is an enzyme from neutrophils and is thus a marker for pyuria. The major advantages of dipsticks are that they are inexpensive[35] (less than 15 pence per sample) and can be used in antenatal clinics, in a similar manner to tests for protein and sugar. If the result is positive, the patient should collect a clean-catch or midstream urine to go to a laboratory for culture, identification and sensitivity patterns. Robertson and Duff[36] demonstrated that if nitrite alone was used the sensitivity was 43% and specificity 99%; leucocyte esterase alone had a sensitivity of 77% and specificity of 96%. When the two tests were combined (and either test was abnormal) the sensitivity became 92% and specificity 95%. They recognised that several cases of group B streptococcal and enterococcal bacteriuria were missed. Etherington and James[37] described the use of reagent strip testing in their antenatal clinic in Bristol to examine 898 midstream urine specimens prior to formal culturing. The sensitivity for both nitrite and leucocyte esterase was 73% and specificity 86%. If these two tests were used together with blood and protein tests then the negative predictive value was 99%, and if negative urines were excluded only 242 (27%) would have been sent for culture, with significant cost savings. Tincello and Richmond[38] repeated the study in their antenatal clinic in Liverpool and found a disappointingly low sensitivity, with a maximum of 33% when all four tests were used in combination. This poor sensitivity was partly due to the pure growth of streptococci (including group B streptococci) in almost 40% of their positive cultures.

A rapid enzymatic urine screening test has been examined by Hagay et al.,[39] which is based on the detection of catalase activity, present in most bacterial species that cause urinary tract infection. A reaction after addition of urine and hydrogen peroxide is performed in a test tube as a side-room procedure. Although there was high sensitivity, there were too many false positives to make the test a practical option.

Rouse et al.[40] performed a cost-effectiveness and cost–benefit analysis of dipstick screening versus routine culture. They used an estimate of the cost of treating pyelonephritis in pregnancy on an inpatient basis, and assumed that there would be 23.2 cases of pyelonephritis per 1000 pregnancies if there was no screening, 11.2 with a routine culture strategy and 16.2 with dipstick screening. They showed that if there was a 6% or greater prevalence of asymptomatic bacteriuria, screening with either dipstick or culture and treatment of bacteriuria to prevent pyelonephritis was cost-beneficial compared with no screening. However, when the costs of routine culture are considered, it is only when the asymptomatic bacteriuria prevalence is 9% or greater that screening with culture becomes cost-beneficial. Even at low prevalence rates of 2%, screening and treatment based on dipstick screening remains cost-beneficial. The prevalence of asymptomatic bacteriuria is 4–7%, in studies from the UK, North America and Australasia. Norden and Kass[41] reported a wider range (2–13%) and there are variations according to racial and socio-economic factors. Bailey[42] reported asymptomatic bacteriuria rates as low as 2% among antenatal patients attending a private clinic and as high as 18.5% among urbanised New Zealand Maori patients. Campbell-Brown et al.[12] found a prevalence of only 2.6% in a north London population, after confirmation by suprapubic aspiration or catheterisation. Versi et al.[43] examined an east London pregnant population and found a prevalence of 6.3% among the white group and only 2.0% for Bangladeshi women.

Are there other factors that may help to direct screening towards higher risk groups? Chng and Hall[26] showed that a previous history of urinary tract infection was recorded in 20% of their antenatal patients. Screening for bacteriuria in women with a positive history would be more economical than routine testing and would give better specificity, but not sensitivity, than bacteriuria testing or history-taking alone. Twenty-eight percent of women with a past history and asymptomatic bacteriuria developed urinary tract infection during pregnancy, compared with only 2.8% among women with no past history or asymptomatic bacteriuria, a ten-fold difference. Pastore et al.[44] found among antenatal patients in North Carolina that the strongest predictors of bacteriuria were antenatal urinary tract infection prior to the booking tests and a prepregnant history of urinary tract infection.

Other risk groups include women who have previously undergone urinary tract surgery or reconstruction, women with diabetes[45] and those with sickle cell trait or disease.[44] Some of these patients will warrant bacteriuria screening at each antenatal visit.

Should we continue to screen for asymptomatic bacteriuria?

Mary Campbell-Brown and colleagues[12] at Northwick Park Hospital, London, posed a similar question in 1987. By using suprapubic aspiration or catheter specimens to confirm the diagnosis, they found that only 2.6% of their population had bacteriuria and many more cases of pyelonephritis later in pregnancy were found in patients whose urine had been sterile at booking. They noted that screening and treatment of asymptomatic bacteriuria were expensive and suggested that it was not worthwhile or cost-effective for a population if there was a low prevalence and a small proportion who progressed to overt infection.

Nevertheless, publications since the early 1990s, mainly from the USA, have continued to recommend the screening of booking patients in order to prevent preterm birth[46,47] and reduce the risk of pyelonephritis.[48–52] Pyelonephritis continues to be described as a severe infection that can result in significant maternal and fetal morbidity and mortality.[51–53] The contribution of infection to maternal mortality in the UK over the last almost 50 years is described in Chapter 32, but it is apparent that women no longer die of pyelonephritis and that the morbidity does not stand out. As described earlier, it is difficult to accept now that asymptomatic bacteriuria or even pyelonephritis contributes greatly to perinatal mortality or morbidity.

Do we continue to screen? The publication by Vause and Maresh[54] of the RCOG

Audit Unit describes 11 indicators of the quality of antenatal care in nine maternity units within 100 miles of Manchester. One of these indicators was the use of midstream urine samples to screen for asymptomatic bacteriuria. The results were expressed as the percentage of eligible patients screened, and the average over their nine units was 63%. One unit had clearly stopped screening, one had screened most patients (96%) and three units were screening less than half their patients. My own unit seems to fare little better: over a six-month period, the laboratory could identify less than half of all booking patients having urine samples sent from the clinic, although samples from the other patients may have been sent from health centres or from home by the midwife doing her booking visit. Among the 58 positive urine tests, only three patients had repeat tests that were also positive and therefore fulfilled the diagnostic criteria based on two consecutive specimens. The other patients either had subsequent negative results or were treated on the basis of the first positive result. I think our failure to screen properly for bacteriuria reflects the increasing uncertainty over its value.[55,56] Certainly among the antenatal patients admitted to hospital with abdominal pain and pyrexia, very few were proven to have pyelonephritis and those that did responded promptly to antibiotics.

If we stopped screening for asymptomatic bacteriuria, we would save £4 for every patient, as well as the costs of the patient's returning to clinic to provide repeat urine samples, and the costs of treatment. The savings for 4000 antenatal bookings would be substantial but would there be morbidity, or mortality, as a consequence? A large study, probably between nearby collaborating centres, needs to be initiated to answer the question of what harm would be done, or, if we are to continue to screen for asymptomatic bacteriuria, are dipsticks or other technologies a suitable alternative to so much laboratory work.

References

1. Milligan WA. On a case of pyelonephritis of pregnancy. *Trans Obstet Soc London* 1906;**48**:1–12.
2. Williams JW. *Obstetrics*. 6th ed. New York: Appleton; 1930.
3. Johnstone RW. *Textbook on Midwifery*. 8th ed. London: Black; 1936.
4. Baird D. The upper urinary tract in pregnancy and puerperium with special reference to pyelitis of pregnancy. *J Obstet Gynaecol Br Empire* 1935;**42**:577–95.
5. Baird D. The upper urinary tract in pregnancy and puerperium with special reference to pyelitis of pregnancy. *J Obstet Gynaecol Br Empire* 1935;**42**:733–94.
6. Baird D. The upper urinary tract in pregnancy and puerperium with special reference to pyelitis of pregnancy. *J Obstet Gynaecol Br Empire* 1935;**43**:1–59.
7. Baird D. The upper urinary tract in pregnancy and puerperium with special reference to pyelitis of pregnancy. *J Obstet Gynaecol Br Empire* 1935;**43**:435–59.
8. Kass EH. Maternal urinary tract infection. *N Y State J Med* 1962;(Part I):2822–6.
9. Kass EH. Pyelonephritis and bacteriuria. A major problem in preventive medicine. *Ann Intern Med* 1962;**56**:46–53.
10. Turner GC. Bacilluria in pregnancy. *Lancet* 1961;**ii**:1062–4.
11. McFadyen IR and Eykyn SJ. Suprapubic aspiration of urine in pregnancy. *Lancet* 1968;**i**:1112–14.
12. Campbell-Brown M, McFadyen IR, Seal DV, Stephenson ML. Is screening for bacteriuria in pregnancy worthwhile? *BMJ* 1987;**294**:1579–82.
13. Paterson L, Miller A, Henderson A. Suprapubic aspiration of urine in the diagnosis of urinary tract infection during pregnancy. *Lancet* 1970;**i**:1195–6.
14. Cattell WR. Urinary tract infection: definitions and classifications. In: Cattell WR, editor. *Infections of the Kidney and Urinary Tract*. Oxford: Oxford University Press; 1996. p. 1–7.
15. MacLean AB. Urinary tract infection and pregnancy. In: Cattell WR, editor. *Infections of the Kidney and*

Urinary Tract. Oxford: Oxford University Press; 1996. p. 206–17.

16. MacLean AB. Urinary tract infection in pregnancy. *Br J Urol* 1997;**80** Suppl 1:10–13.

17. Little PJ. Prevention of pyelonephritis of pregnancy. *Lancet* 1965;**i**:567–9.

18. Little PJ. The incidence of urinary infection in 5000 pregnant women. *Lancet* 1966;**ii**:925–8.

19. Gruneberg RN, Leigh DA, Brumfitt W. Relationship of bacteriuria in pregnancy to acute pyelonephritis, prematurity and fetal mortality. *Lancet* 1969;**ii**:1–3.

20. Swapp GH. Asymptomatic bacteriuria, birth weight and length of gestation in a defined population. In: Brumfitt W, Asscher AW, editors. *Urinary Tract Infection.* London: Oxford University Press; 1973. p. 92–102.

21. Gilstrap LC, Cunningham FG, Whalley PJ. Acute pyelonephritis in pregnancy: an anterospective study. *Obstet Gynecol* 1981;**57**:409–13.

22. Cunningham FG, Leveno KJ, Hankins GDV, Whalley PJ. Respiratory insufficiency associated with pyelonephritis during pregnancy. *Obstet Gynecol* 1984;**63**:121–5.

23. Cunningham FG, Lucas MJ, Hankins GDV. Pulmonary injury complicating antepartum pyelonephritis. *Am J Obstet Gynecol* 1987;**156**:797–807.

24. Towers CV, Kaminskas CM, Garite TJ, Nageotle MP, Dorchester W. Pulmonary injury associated with antepartum pyelonephritis: can patients at risk be identified? *Am J Obstet Gynecol* 1991;**164**:974–80.

25. Lawson DH, Miller AWF. Screening for bacteriuria in pregnancy. *Lancet* 1971;**i**:9–10.

26. Chng PK, Hall MN. Antenatal prediction of urinary tract infection in pregnancy. *Br J Obstet Gynaecol* 1982;**89**:8–11.

27. Elder HA, Santamarina BAG, Smith S, Kass EH. The natural history of asymptomatic bacteriuria during pregnancy: the effect of tetracycline on the clinical course and the outcome of pregnancy. *Am J Obstet Gynecol* 1971;**111**:441–62.

28. Romero R, Oyarzun E, Mazor M, Sirtori M. Hobbins JC, Bracken M. Meta-analysis of the relationship between asymptomatic bacteriuria and preterm delivery/low birth weight. *Obstet Gynecol* 1989;**73**:576–82.

29. Wang E, Smaill F. Infection in pregnancy. In: Chalmers I, Enkin M, Keirse MJNC, editors. *Effective Care in Pregnancy and Childbirth.* Oxford: Oxford University Press; 1990. p. 535–8.

30. Gold EM, Traub FB, Daichman I, Terris M. Asymptomatic bacteriuria during pregnancy. *Obstet Gynecol* 1966;**27**:206–9.

31. Gilstrap LC, Leveno KJ, Cunningham FG, Whalley PJ, Roark ML. Renal infection and pregnancy outcome. *Am J Obstet Gynecol* 1981;**141**:709–16.

32. Meis PJ, Michielutte R, Peters TJ, Well HB, Sands RE, Coles EC, *et al.* Factors associated with preterm birth in Cardiff, Wales. II. Indicated and spontaneous preterm birth. *Am J Obstet Gynecol* 1995;**173**:597–602.

33. Gilstrap LC, Whalley PJ. Asymptomatic bacteriuria during pregnancy. In: Brumfitt W, Hamilton-Miller JMT, Bailey RR, editors. *Urinary Tract Infections.* London: Chapman & Hall; 1998. p. 199–209.

34. Brumfitt W, Hamilton-Miller JMT. Urinary tract infection in the 1990's: the state of the art. *Infection* 1990;**18** Suppl 2:S34–9.

35. Woodward MN, Griffiths DM. Use of dipsticks for routine analysis of urine from children with acute abdominal pain. *BMJ* 1993;**306**:1512.

36. Robertson AW, Duff P. The nitrite and leucocyte esterase tests for the evaluation of asymptomatic bacteriuria in obstetric patients. *Obstet Gynecol* 1988;**71**:878–81.

37. Etherington IJ, James DK. Reagent strip testing in antenatal urine specimens for infection. *Br J Obstet Gynaecol* 1993;**100**:806–8.

38. Tincello DG, Richmond DH. Evaluation of reagent strips in detecting asymptomatic bacteriuria in early pregnancy: prospective case series. *BMJ* 1998;**316**:435–7.

39. Hagay Z, Levy R, Miskin A, Milman D, Sharabi H, Insler V. Uriscreen, a rapid enzymatic urine screening test: useful predictor of significant bacteriuria in pregnancy. *Obstet Gynecol* 1996;**87**:410–13.

40. Rouse DJ, Andrews WW, Goldenberg RL, Owen J. Screening and treatment of asymptomatic bacteriuria of pregnancy to prevent pyelonephritis: a cost-effectiveness and cost–benefit analysis. *Obstet Gynecol* 1995;**86**:119–23.

41. Norden CW, Kass EH. Bacteriuria of pregnancy – a critical appraisal. *Annu Rev Med* 1968;**19**:431–70.

42. Bailey RR. Urinary tract infection – some recent concepts. *Can Med Assoc J* 1972;**107**:316–30.

43. Versi E, Chia P, Griffiths DJ, Harlow BL. Bacteriuria in pregnancy: a comparison of Bangladeshi and Caucasian women. *Int Urogynecol J Pelvic Floor Dysfunct* 1997;**8**:8–12.

44. Pastore LM, Savitz DA, Thorpe JM. Predictors of urinary tract infection at the first prenatal visit. *Epidemiology* 1999;**10**:282–7.

45. Sobczak M, Wilczynski J, Cypryk K, Woch G. Bacterial flora in infections of the urinary system in pregnant women with pre-gestational diabetics. *Ginekol Pol* 1999;**70**:25–31.

46. Gibbs RS, Eschenbach DA. Use of antibiotics to prevent preterm birth. *Am J Obstet Gynecol* 1997;**177**:375–80.
47. Villar J, Gulmezoglu AM, de Onis M. Nutritional and antimicrobial interventions to prevent preterm birth: an overview of randomized controlled trials. *Obstet Gynecol Surv* 1998;**53**:575–85.
48. Cunningham FG, Lucas MJ. Urinary tract infections complicating pregnancy. *Baillières Clin Obstet Gynaecol* 1994;**8**:353–73.
49. Gratacos E, Torres PJ, Vila J, Alonso PL, Cararach V. Screening and treatment of asymptomatic bacteriuria in pregnancy prevent pyelonephritis. *J Infect Dis* 1994;**169**:1390–2.
50. Simon NV, Heaps KP, Chodroff CH. Improving the processes of care and outcomes in obstetrics/gynaecology. *Jt Comm J Qual Improv* 1997;**23**:485–97.
51. Millar LK, Cox SM. Urinary tract infection complicating pregnancy. *Infect Dis Clin North Am* 1997;**11**:13–26.
52. Delzell JE Jr, Lefevre ML. Urinary tract infections during pregnancy. *Am Fam Physician* 2000;**61**:713–21.
53. Patterson TF, Andriole VT. Detection, significance, and therapy of bacteriuria in pregnancy. Update in the managed health care era. *Infect Dis Clin North Am* 1997;**11**:593–608.
54. Vause S, Maresh M. Indicators of quality of antenatal care. *Br J Obstet Gynaecol* 1999;**106**:197–205.
55. MacLean AB. Pregnancy. In: Stanton S, Dwyer PL, editors. *Urinary Tract Infection in the Female*. London: Martin Dunitz; 2000. p. 145–60.
56. MacLean AB. Urinary tract infection in pregnancy. *Int J Antimicrob Agents* 2001;**17**:273–7.

Chapter 9

The group B streptococcus and pregnancy

Rhona G Hughes and A Christine McCartney

Introduction

In the last 30 years, group B streptococcal (GBS) disease has become the most common life-threatening neonatal infection in the industrialised world. This has prompted professional bodies in the USA and Australia to publish guidelines on prevention that have been widely adopted in those countries.[1,2,3] It is thought that the disease is less prevalent in the UK although this belief is based on historical data[4] and has been questioned by several authorities.[5,6] Evidence[7,8] from the USA and Australia suggests that the disease is more common in women under the age of 20 years and in ethnic minorities, both of which groups have probably been under-represented in British studies.[4,9] It is anticipated that better UK data will be provided by a 12-month nationwide study of culture-confirmed invasive GBS neonatal disease. This study commenced in February 2000 and is being conducted by the British Paediatric Surveillance Unit.

In this chapter the available evidence regarding transmission of the disease is examined and the possible strategies for preventing perinatal transmission from mother to infant discussed.

The organism

The group B streptococcus, or *Streptococcus agalactiae,* is a facultative anaerobic Gram-positive coccus. There are eight distinct serotypes, of which types Ia, Ib and III account for 70–80% of cases of invasive neonatal disease.[10,11]

Clinical spectrum

Maternal colonisation

The microorganism is a normal commensal of the female genital tract and can be recovered from 10–20% of pregnant women in the USA[1] and UK,[12] regardless of the stage of pregnancy. The gastrointestinal tract is the primary reservoir and spread is trans-perineal so that rectal and low vaginal swabs have a higher yield than high vaginal or cervical swabs.[13]

Neonatal colonisation

Between 3% and 12% of neonates are colonised with GBS during the first week of life. This figure can rise to 40–70% of the infants of colonised mothers. These infants are usually colonised with the same serotype as their mother.[14] Vertical transmission is more likely if the mother is heavily colonised, there is cervical carriage[15] or there is GBS bacteriuria.[16]

Neonatal invasive disease

The incidence of invasive neonatal disease (sepsis, meningitis or pneumonia) declined in the USA during the 1990s from 1.7 to 0.6 per 1000 live births.[17] This reduction coincided with the increased use of intrapartum ampicillin or penicillin in women considered to be at high risk of infecting their infants.[15] The UK rate is quoted as 0.5–1.15 per 1000 live births.[6,9,18]

Invasive disease can be divided into early- and late-onset disease. Early-onset disease occurs in the first week of life, with a mean age at onset of 20 hours. It accounts for 80% of cases and is due to vertical transmission. Late-onset disease occurs after the first week and is due to either vertical (approximately 50% of cases[19]) or nosocomial spread from other infants, hospital staff or other adults. As a result, the serotypes of the causative organisms in late-onset disease do not reflect those present in the mother's genital tract.

Neonatal mortality

In the 1970s, mortality was greater than 50% in neonates with invasive disease.[17] The case-fatality ratio in the USA has now fallen to less than 10%, with mortality being significantly higher in preterm infants.[20]

Epidemiology of early-onset neonatal disease

Risk factors for early-onset GBS disease during the indicated stages are as follows:

- Prepregnancy:
  - age less than 20 years[7]
  - African-American descent[21]

- Australian Aboriginal descent[8]
- previously affected baby[22]

- Antepartum:
  - GBS bacteriuria in pregnancy[16]
  - heavy GBS colonisation[2]
  - low levels of anti-GBS capsular antibodies[24]
  - prelabour rupture of membranes[25]

- Intrapartum:
  - preterm delivery[20]
  - fever greater than 38° C[26]
  - ruptured membranes for more than 18 hours.[26]

Prevention of neonatal disease

Intrapartum chemoprophylaxis

Boyer and Gotoff[27] were the first to demonstrate that intrapartum antibiotics together with postpartum antibiotics for the infant could reduce or even prevent early-onset neonatal GBS sepsis. Subsequent meta-analysis of controlled trials has confirmed their findings, with one study demonstrating a 30-fold reduction in GBS disease associated with the use of intrapartum antibiotics.[28]

In a critical appraisal of four randomised controlled trials, none of which had the power to achieve statistical significance, Ohlson and Myhr[29] concluded that intrapartum prophylaxis to reduce early-onset GBS infection was not supported by conclusive evidence from well designed and conducted randomised controlled trials. However, a more recent review of five papers, including three[30–32] not reviewed by Ohlson and Myhr, concluded that intrapartum antibiotic therapy reduces the risk of early-onset disease by 80%.[33] A systematic review[34] published by the Cochrane Pregnancy and Childbirth Group concluded that 'intrapartum antibiotic treatment of women colonised with group B streptococcus appears to reduce neonatal infection'. These studies can be criticised in terms of their failure to blind the randomisation process but their conclusion that intrapartum chemoprophylaxis is of proven benefit seems reasonable.

Penicillin is the agent of choice because its antimicrobial spectrum, narrower than that of ampicillin, reduces the likelihood of resistance developing in other organisms.[35] The recommended schedule is penicillin G 3 g (5 mU) intravenously initially and then 1.5 g (2.5 mU) at four-hourly intervals until delivery.[2] It is important that the first dose is given as soon as possible to avoid delivery of the infant prior to antibiotic treatment. It has been suggested that antibiotics should be given for at least four hours prior to delivery[1] but there is little evidence to support this.[33] Women allergic to penicillin should be given clindamycin 900 mg eight-hourly.

The question of which women should be selected for treatment is problematic and is one that clinicians in the USA have been struggling with for a number of years[1,2,5,36] They have been keen to implement intrapartum chemoprophylaxis, although there has been less enthusiasm in Europe, with some commentators suggesting that the driving factor in the USA is the fear of litigation.[5]

There are two possible strategies for selecting women for intrapartum chemoprophylaxis, both of which are endorsed by the American Academy of Pediatrics[2] and the American College of Obstetricians and Gynecologists:[36] risk-based and screening-based. A combination of the two strategies can also be used.[2]

Risk-based strategy

Using this approach, intrapartum prophylaxis is given to all women with any of the following risk factors:

1. Labour prior to 37 weeks;

2. Ruptured membranes prior to 37 weeks;

3. Fever during labour of greater than 38° C;

4. Ruptured membranes for more than 18 hours prior to delivery;

5. Previous delivery of an infant with invasive GBS disease.

This approach is similar to that recommended by the UK Public Health Laboratory Service (PHLS) Working Group on GBS (see below) and it has been estimated, based on a hypothetical population, to prevent 68.8% of cases of early-onset disease by administering prophylaxis to 18.3% of women in labour.[37] The proportion of women with clinical risk factors (who would receive intrapartum prophylaxis in practice) has been shown to be approximately 25%.[26] Studies[38-40] have demonstrated that, in fact, as few as 50% of the mothers of infants with invasive neonatal disease have identifiable risk factors. A clinical risk-based approach will thus inevitably lead to the unnecessary treatment of large numbers of women and will fail to prevent up to 50% of cases.

Screening-based strategy

With this approach, all pregnant women are offered microbiological screening at 35–37 weeks of gestation. Cultures obtained late in pregnancy (within five weeks of delivery) are much more likely to concord with intrapartum culture results. Yancey *et al.*[41] demonstrated a positive predictive value of 89% and a negative predictive value of 97% for cultures taken at 35 weeks of gestation. The rate of detection of GBS colonisation can be increased by sampling the lower vagina and rectum (27% of samples positive) rather than only the lower vagina (22% of samples positive).[42] The use of selective broth containing antibiotics to inhibit the growth of other commensal bacteria can increase the yield of GBS from swab cultures by 50%.[43]

If all women with positive cultures are treated, 25–27% of women in labour would receive intrapartum antibiotics,[26,37] resulting in the prevention of 86–90% of infant cases.[2,37] This approach is therefore more effective at preventing disease than the risk-based approach but necessitates the treatment of more women. It is also a more expensive option.[44]

Combined approach

An alternative strategy is to treat only women from whom GBS has been cultured and who also have risk factors. This approach was advocated by Boyer and Gotoff[27] and reduced the percentage of women treated to 5%, with the resulting prevention of approximately 70–75% of early-onset GBS cases. This strategy is attractive because it greatly reduces the number of women receiving antibiotic treatment. It is, however, a much more expensive option than the clinical risk-based option[44] and it will not prevent all cases that would have been prevented by treating all screen-positive women.

The UK PHLS Group B Streptococcus Working Group recommendations

In the UK, there is little consensus in the obstetric community regarding the prevention of GBS neonatal disease.[45] Because of this, a Group B Streptococcus Working Group was set up by the PHLS. This group has produced interim 'good practice' recommendations pending the results of a UK-wide British Paediatric Surveillance Unit study involving all maternity units. The recommendations suggest the following as 'good practice':

1. Do not perform routine bacteriological screening, as there is currently insufficient evidence to support this.

2. Do give intrapartum antibiotic prophylaxis specifically for GBS to the following women:
   – GBS infection in a previous baby
   – GBS found incidentally in the vagina or urine at any time during pregnancy.

3. Do give broad-spectrum antibiotics when clinically indicated and ensure that the regimen includes adequate GBS cover in the following situations:
   – chorioamnionitis diagnosed or suspected clinically
   – prolonged preterm rupture of membranes.

4. Consider giving intrapartum antibiotic prophylaxis in the following situations:
   – preterm labour
   – prolonged rupture of membranes in labour
   – fever in labour.

This approach is similar to the US risk-based strategy described above (but will result in the treatment of fewer women).

Preferences of patients and doctors

Peralta-Carcelen *et al.*[46] studied the preferences of pregnant women, obstetricians and paediatricians for two strategies for prevention of early-onset GBS disease. The two strategies were B (a combined microbiological screening at 26–28 weeks and clinical risk-factor screening strategy) and C (a purely risk-based strategy) from Table 9.1. Interestingly, 81% of women (and 65% of paediatricians) opted for strategy B despite being advised that the risk of neonatal infection with this strategy would be 1.5 per 1000 live births versus 1.0 per 1000 for strategy C and that the chance of the baby requiring extra diagnostic tests would be 132 per 1000 live births. Strategy C would

Table 9.1.   Estimated impact of several strategies for the use of intrapartum antimicrobial prophylaxis (IAP) against early-onset group B streptococcal (GBS) disease in a *hypothetical* population (from Rouse *et al.*[37])

Prevention strategy	Proportion of deliveries receiving IAP (%)	Proportion of early-onset GBS disease prevented (%)
A Prenatal culture at 35–37 weeks of gestation; IAP for preterm deliveries and all GBS carriers	26.7	86.0
B Prenatal culture at 26–28 weeks of gestation; IAP for GBS carriers who develop intrapartum risk factors[b, 27]	3.4[a]	50.7
C No routine prenatal cultures; IAP for all women with intrapartum risk factors[b]	18.3[c]	68.8[d]

[a] the percentage was estimated for a hypothetical population[37] – the actual proportion of deliveries among women who were screen-positive for GBS and who developed intrapartum risk factors was 4.6%[26]; [b] e.g. fever, prolonged rupture of membranes, preterm labour; [c] the percentage was estimated for a hypothetical population[37] – the actual proportion of deliveries among women who had intrapartum risk factors was 24.7%[26]; [d] later studies report a figure around 50%[38–40]

require additional tests for 107 per 1000 live births. Women preferred strategy B because they ranked knowledge of maternal GBS status highly and as more important than did paediatricians and obstetricians. Eighty-five percent of obstetricians preferred strategy C. At the time of the study, strategy B was endorsed by the American Academy of Pediatrics[47] and strategy C was endorsed by the American College of Obstetricians and Gynecologists[48] so that the preferences of the clinicians may possibly be explained by loyalty to their respective professional bodies.

Disadvantages of intrapartum chemoprophylaxis

POTENTIAL SEVERE ADVERSE REACTIONS TO PENICILLIN
The rate of fatal anaphylaxis to penicillin is quoted as 1 in 100 000, with less severe reactions affecting 1 in 10 000.[26] Maternal anaphylaxis can cause serious fetal compromise.[49] It is important to bear these potentially disastrous consequences in mind when considering administration of antibiotics to 18–27% of healthy pregnant women.

EMERGENCE OF ANTIBIOTIC RESISTANCE
Clinically significant resistance to penicillin in GBS is rare but has been described.[50] Resistance to erythromycin and clindamycin has been reported in 7.4% and 3.4% of invasive GBS isolates, respectively.[51] This has some clinical relevance as clindamycin is recommended for intrapartum prophylaxis in women with a history of penicillin allergy.

The use of ampicillin rather than penicillin for intrapartum GBS prophylaxis has been reported to be associated with an increase in the incidence of ampicillin-resistant Gram-negative neonatal sepsis, with a resultant increased mortality rate.[52–54]

FINANCIAL COST

Mohle-Boetani et al.[44] compared the cost of three strategies, one based on a combined bacteriological screening and clinical risk-based approach as described by Boyer and Gotoff,[27] one a purely risk-based approach and one based on a hypothetical vaccine. The vaccine was least expensive while the combined approach cost US$28,800 and the risk-based approach US$12,200 per case prevented. These estimates are based on 1993 figures. The cost of introducing the risk-based approach was greater than the calculated cost of the disease until the incidence of early-onset GBS disease exceeded 0.6 per 1000 live births. The cost of introducing the combined approach was greater than the cost of the disease until the incidence of the infection exceeded 1.2 per 1000 live births. On this basis and on the basis of limited UK data demonstrating an incidence of 0.5–1.15 per 1000 live births,[6,9,18,55] a risk-based screening approach could be justified in the UK but not a microbiological screening-based approach.

MEDICALISATION OF LABOUR

Normal labour is a physiological not a pathological process and this remains true for the majority of women colonised with GBS. The introduction of four-hourly intravenous antibiotics can medicalise an otherwise normal labour. It may mean that the woman is no longer eligible to deliver in a midwife-run unit and may thus have a less positive birth experience.[56,57] It is recognised that interventions during labour reduce maternal satisfaction with labour.[58] This may seem a trivial concern compared with the risk of neonatal disease. However, this risk is relatively low (approximately 1 in 200 in women known to be colonised[26]) and, after counselling, some women will decline administration of intrapartum antibiotics.[1]

INCREASED DEMAND FOR PRENATAL COUNSELLING AND INCREASED MATERNAL ANXIETY

If approximately 20–25% of women in labour were to be given intrapartum antibiotics (if a screening- or risk-based strategy was adopted), it would be necessary to inform all women at booking of this possibility. Women attending booking clinics already receive a large quantity of information regarding screening for HIV, hepatitis B, rubella and syphilis infections, chromosomal disorders, neural tube defects and other fetal structural abnormalities. It has been demonstrated that 'low-risk' women retain little of this information[59,60] and that prenatal screening tests cause 'significant negative psychosocial effects'.[61] It is likely that women would respond in a similar manner if a policy of universal screening for GBS carriage were to be adopted.

MEDICALISATION OF THE NEONATAL PERIOD

An increasing use of intrapartum antimicrobial agents may have a substantial impact on the clinical management of the healthy neonate.[30,62] Some paediatricians advise a 48-hour inpatient observation period or routine additional diagnostic tests for the asymptomatic infant of a mother who has received intrapartum antibiotics.[62] There is currently no conclusive evidence to support this practice. If a mother has received 'inadequate' prophylaxis (i.e. if she delivers within four hours of the first dose of antibiotic or receives no chemoprophylaxis contrary to local guidelines), many neonatologists feel uneasy about sanctioning an early discharge from hospital. Again, there is no current evidence to support the use of extra interventions for these infants.[63,64]

FAILURE TO PREVENT DISEASE

Intrapartum antimicrobial prophylaxis does not prevent all cases of early-onset disease,[33] probably because of failure to eradicate an established fetal infection. More than 80% of treatment failures are associated with chorioamnionitis or maternal fever.[63] Intrapartum prophylaxis causes only a temporary reduction in neonatal colonisation[49] and therefore has no influence on the incidence of late-onset GBS disease, which is an important cause of neonatal mortality and serious morbidity.[35]

Other strategies

Vaginal disinfectants

Vaginal disinfectants have been used in research trials in Sweden[65] and Malawi[66] and are less invasive than intrapartum antibiotics. The Malawi study demonstrated a significantly reduced rate of admission for neonatal sepsis associated with disinfectant use but an effect on GBS disease was not demonstrated.

Postnatal antibiotic prophylaxis

In some centres, postnatal penicillin is given to all infants[67] or to the infants of colonised mothers without intrapartum risk factors.[68] The strategy does reduce the incidence of early-onset disease in term infants but has no effect on the disease in low-birthweight infants or on late-onset disease.[35] Universal postpartum prophylaxis has been shown to increase overall mortality rates due to mortality attributable to penicillin-resistant pathogens[33] and has not, therefore, been widely adopted.

Vaccines

Studies in the 1970s established a relationship between low levels of maternal antibodies to GBS capsular polysaccharides and susceptibility of the infant to invasive GBS infection.[24] This finding prompted research on GBS polysaccharide antigens and resulted in production of purified polysaccharides and, more recently, conjugated vaccines against the major serotypes causing the disease.[35] A vaccine specific for serotype III has been produced and has been shown to cause a four-fold or greater rise in antibody levels in 90% of volunteers.[69] The antibody crossed the mouse placenta and protected neonatal mice from lethal challenge with type III organisms.[69] A vaccine specific for serotypes Ia and Ib has also been produced, with encouraging results.[70]

For statistical validation purposes, sample sizes for trials to measure the clinical protective efficacy of vaccines against invasive GBS disease would be prohibitively large given the low incidence of the disease. In view of this, research has focused on surrogates for clinical protection through a variety of immunological assays. GBS colonisation may also be a useful surrogate. At present the optimum timing for vaccination has not been established.

In addition to the above considerations, there has been a shift in the serotypes of strains causing disease, which creates a challenge for vaccine development.[35] Serotype V was first recognised in the USA in 1993 and is now responsible for approximately 10% of neonatal disease.[35]

Rapid detection techniques

If a rapid detection test was available which matched culture in selective broth in terms of sensitivity and specificity, the use of intrapartum prophylaxis could be refined, with some women avoiding unnecessary exposure to antibiotics. To date, the available rapid detection tests (Gram stain, latex particle agglutination, enzyme immunoassay) have not proved sufficiently reliable.[14] Bergeron *et al.*[71] have recently described the use of two polymerase chain reaction techniques for the rapid detection of GBS in anal and vaginal specimens in labour. The tests were compared with culture using a selective broth medium and were shown to have a sensitivity of 97% and a specificity of 100%. If these tests perform as well in routine practice as reported, they have the potential to make a significant impact on the intrapartum management of women at risk of GBS colonisation.

Maternal disease

Preterm delivery

The relationship between GBS and preterm delivery is complex and it is difficult to establish causality. Preterm prelabour rupture of the fetal membranes is strongly associated with early-onset GBS disease.[35] This may be due to the fact that antibody transport across the placenta is reduced in early pregnancy so that infants born prematurely have less protection from maternal antibodies.[35] It is postulated that group B streptococci, in common with several other bacteria, cause preterm prelabour rupture of the membranes by a variety of mechanisms, including secretion of proteases that degrade collagen and weaken fetal membranes.[72] A Cochrane review[73] demonstrated that antibiotic treatment of women with preterm prelabour rupture of the membranes does prolong pregnancy to a significant extent, suggesting that infection may be an important factor in the aetiology of labour under these circumstances.

Thomsen *et al.*[74] reported a significant reduction in the risk of preterm labour and preterm rupture of membranes among women with asymptomatic GBS bacteriuria that was treated with penicillin. Regan *et al.*[75] confirmed the association between heavy GBS colonisation at 23–26 weeks and an increased risk of delivering a preterm, low-birthweight infant. However, long-term erythromycin treatment of the women with heavy GBS colonisation failed to reduce the risk of preterm labour.[76]

In summary, no firm conclusions can be drawn, at present, with regard to the role of GBS in the aetiology of preterm labour.

Maternal infectious morbidity

Chorioamnionitis and endometritis are often associated with GBS carriage. The rates of both can be significantly lowered by a policy of universal screening and intrapartum antibiotic treatment of colonised women.[77] Puerperal septicaemia due to GBS occurs at a rate of approximately 1–2 per 1000 deliveries and can account for up to 15% of positive blood cultures from postpartum patients.[78]

Conclusions

It is generally accepted that the incidence of neonatal GBS disease can be reduced by intrapartum chemoprophylaxis. However, there is insufficient evidence at present to recommend either a microbiological screening-based strategy, a clinical risk-based screening strategy or a combined approach for the UK. The introduction of universal antenatal microbiological screening of pregnant women in the UK would have enormous financial implications and would be hard to justify given the current evidence. If a rapid detection technique or a vaccine was available this could potentially revolutionise the management of perinatal GBS disease.

Women with a previously affected infant[22] or with preterm rupture of the membranes[25] should be offered intrapartum chemoprophylaxis. Women with GBS bacteriuria[16] or vaginal colonisation[23] should also be offered prophylaxis. Their risk of disease will be low (approximately 1 in 200[26]) but from a medico-legal perspective it would be difficult to defend a decision not to offer treatment at present. The possibility of GBS disease should always be considered in women with intrapartum risk factors.

There is still considerable uncertainty surrounding this condition and there is an urgent need for UK-based research. The results of the British Paediatric Surveillance Unit study are awaited with interest.

References

1. Centers for Disease Control and Prevention. Prevention of perinatal group B streptococcal disease: a public health perspective. *MMWR Morb Mortal Wkly Rep* 1996;**45**(RR-7):1–24.
2. American Academy of Pediatrics Committee on Infectious Diseases and Committee on Fetus and Newborn. Revised guidelines for prevention of early-onset group B streptococcal (GBS) infection. *Pediatrics* 1997;**99**:489–96.
3. Jeffery HE, Moses LM. Eight year outcome of universal screening and intrapartum antibiotics for maternal group B carriers. *Pediatrics* 1998;**101**:96–7.
4. Mayon-White RT. The incidence of GBS disease in neonates in different countries. *Antibiot Chemother* 1985;**35**:17–27.
5. Isaacs D. Prevention of early onset group B streptococcal infection: screen, treat or observe? *Arch Dis Child Fetal Neonatal Ed* 1998;**79**:F81–2.
6. Embleton N, Wariyar U, Hey E. Mortality from early onset group B streptococcal infection in the United Kingdom. *Arch Dis Child Fetal Neonatal Ed* 1999;**80**:F139–41.
7. Schuchat A, Deaver-Robinson K, Plikaytis BD, *et al.* Multistate case control study of maternal risk factors for neonatal group B streptococcal disease. *Pediatr Infect Dis J* 1994;**13**:623–9.
8. Australasian Study Group for Neonatal Infections. Early-onset group B streptococcal infections in Aboriginal and non-Aboriginal infants. *Med J Aust* 1995;**163**:302–6.
9. Moses LM, Heath PT, Wilkinson AR, Jeffery HE, Isaacs D. Early onset group B streptococcal neonatal infection in Oxford 1985–96. *Arch Dis Child Fetal Neonatal Ed* 1998;**79**:F148–50.
10. Lin FY, Clemens JD, Azimi PH, *et al.* Capsular polysaccharide types of group B streptococcal isolates from neonates with early-onset systemic infection. *J Infect Dis* 1998;**177**:790–2.
11. Harrison LH, Elliot JA, Dwyer DM, *et al.* Serotype distribution of invasive group B streptococcal isolates in Maryland: implications for vaccine formulation. Maryland Emerging Infections Program. *J Infect Dis* 1998;**177**:998–1002.
12. Easmon CSF. The carrier state: group B streptococcus. *J Antimicrob Chemother* 1986;**18** Suppl A:59–65.
13. Dillon HC, Gray E, Pass MA, Gray BM. Anorectal and vaginal carriage of group B streptococci during pregnancy. *J Infect Dis* 1982;**145**:794–9.

14. Sampson JE, Gravett MG. Other infectious conditions in pregnancy. In: James DK, Steer PJ, Weiner CP, Gonik B, editors. *High Risk Pregnancy: Management Options*, 2nd ed. London: WB Saunders; 1999. p. 559–98.

15. Hoogkamp-Korstanje JAA, Gerards LJ, Cats BP. Maternal carriage and neonatal acquisition of group B streptococci. *J Infect Dis* 1982;**145**:800–5.

16. Wood EG, Dillon HC. A prospective study of group B streptococcal bacteriuria in pregnancy. *Am J Obstet Gynecol* 1981;**140**:515–20.

17. Schrag SJ, Zywicki S, Farley MM, *et al*. Group B streptococcal disease in the era of intrapartum antibiotic prophylaxis. *N Engl J Med* 2000;**342**:15–20.

18. Beardsall K, Thompson MH, Mulla RJ. Neonatal group B streptococcal infection in South Bedfordshire, 1993–1998. *Arch Dis Child Fetal Neonatal Ed* 2000;**82**:F205–7.

19. Dillon HC, Khare S, Gray BM. Group B streptococcal carriage and disease: a 6-year prospective study. *J Pediatr* 1987;**110**:31–6.

20. Schuchat A. Neonatal group B streptococcal disease – screening and prevention. *N Engl J Med* 2000;**343**:209–10.

21. Zangwill KM, Schuchat A, Wenger JD. Group B streptococcal disease in the United States, 1990: report from a multistate active surveillance system. *Mor Mortal Wkly Rep CDC Surveill Summ* 1992;**41**:25–32.

22. Carstensen H, Christensen KK, Grennert L, Persson K, Polberger S. Early-onset neonatal group B streptococcal septicaemia in siblings. *J Infect* 1988;**17**:201–4.

23. Pass MA, Gray BM, Khare S, Dillon HC. Prospective studies of group B streptococcal infection in infants. *J Pediatr* 1979;**95**:437–43.

24. Baker CJ, Kasper DL. Correlation of maternal antibody deficiency with susceptibility to neonatal group B streptococcal infection. *N Engl J Med* 1976;**294**:753–6.

25. Regan JA, Chao S, James LS. Premature rupture of membranes, preterm delivery and group B streptococcal colonisation of mothers. *Am J Obstet Gynecol* 1981;**141**:184–6.

26. Boyer KM, Gotoff SP. Strategies for chemoprophylaxis of GBS early-onset infections. *Antibiot Chemother* 1985;**35**:267–80.

27. Boyer KM, Gotoff SP. Prevention of early-onset group B streptococcal disease with selective intrapartum chemoprophylaxis. *N Engl J Med* 1986;**314**:1665–9.

28. Allen UD, Navas L, King S. Effectiveness of intrapartum penicillin prophylaxis in preventing early onset group B streptococcal infection: results of a meta-analysis. *Can Med Assoc J* 1993;**149**:1659–65.

29. Ohlsson A, Myhr TL. Intrapartum chemoprophylaxis of perinatal group B streptococcal infections: a critical review of randomized controlled trials. *Am J Obstet Gynecol* 1994;**170**:910–17.

30. Pylipow M, Gaddis M, Kinney JS. Selective intrapartum prophylaxis for group B streptococcus colonization; management and outcome of newborns. *Pediatrics* 1994;**93**:631–5.

31. Allardice JG, Baskett TF, Seshia MM, Bowman N, Malazdrewicz R. Perinatal group B streptococcal colonization and infection. *Am J Obstet Gynecol* 1982;**142**:617–20.

32. Morales WJ, Lim D. Reduction of group B streptococcal and neonatal infections in preterm pregnancies with premature rupture of membranes through a rapid identification test. *Am J Obstet Gynecol* 1987;**157**:13–16.

33. Benitz WE, Gould JB, Druzin ML. Antimicrobial prevention of early-onset group B streptococcal sepsis: estimates of risk reduction based on a critical literature review. *Pediatrics* 1999;**103**:e78–98.

34. Smaill F. Intrapartum antibiotics for group B streptococcal colonisation. *Cochrane Database Syst Rev* 2000;(2):CD000115.

35. Schuchat A. Group B streptococcus. *Lancet* 1999;**353**:51–6.

36. American College of Obstetricians and Gynecologists Committee on Obstetric Practice. *Prevention of Early-Onset Group B Streptococcal Disease in Newborns*. Washington DC: ACOG; June 1996. ACOG Committee Opinion No. 173.

37. Rouse DJ, Goldenberg RL, Cliver SP, Cutter GR, Mennemeyer ST, Fargason CA. Strategies for the prevention of early-onset neonatal group B streptococcal sepsis: a decision analysis. *Obstet Gynecol* 1994;**83**:483–94.

38. McLaren RA, Chauhan SP, Gross TL. Intrapartum factors in early-onset group B streptococcal sepsis in term neonates: a case-control study. *Am J Obstet Gynecol* 1996;**174**:1934–40.

39. Philipson EH, Herson VC. Intrapartum chemoprophylaxis for group B streptococcus infection to prevent neonatal disease: who should be treated? *Am J Perinatol* 1996;**13**:487–90.

40. Rosenstein NE, Schuchat A. Opportunities for prevention of perinatal group B streptococcal disease: a multistate surveillance analysis. *Obstet Gynecol* 1997;**90**:901–6.

41. Yancey MK, Schuchat A, Brown LK, Ventura VL, Markenson GR. The accuracy of late antenatal screening cultures in predicting genital group B streptococcal colonization at delivery. *Obstet Gynecol* 1996;**88**:51–5.

42. Badri MS, Zawaneh S, Cruz AC, *et al.* Rectal colonization with group B streptococcus: relation to vaginal colonization of pregnant women. *J Infect Dis* 1977;**135**:308–12.
43. Baker CJ, Goroff DK, Alpert S, *et al.* Vaginal colonization with group B streptococcus: a study of college women. *J Infect Dis* 1977;**135**:392–7.
44. Mohle-Boetani JC, Schuchat A, Plikaytis BD, Smith JD, Broome CV. Comparison of prevention strategies for neonatal group B streptococcal infection. A population-based economic analysis. *JAMA* 1993;**270**:1442–8.
45. Brocklehurst P. UK national survey of maternity units to determine their policies for managing Group B Strep infection in pregnancy. Unpublished data.
46. Peralta-Carcelen M, Fargason CA, Coston D, Dolan JG. Preferences of pregnant women and physicians for 2 strategies for prevention of early-onset group B streptococcal sepsis in neonates. *Arch Pediatr Adolesc Med* 1997;**151**:712–18.
47. American Academy of Pediatrics Committee on Infectious Diseases and Committee on Fetus and Newborn. Guidelines for prevention of group B streptococcal (GBS) infection by chemoprophylaxis. *Pediatrics* 1992;**90**:775–8.
48. Hankins GV, Chalas E. Group B streptococcal infection in pregnancy: ACOG's recommendations. *ACOG Newslett* 1993;**37**:2
49. Heim K, Alge A, Marth C. Anaphylactic reaction to ampicillin and severe complication in the fetus. *Lancet* 1991;**337**:859–60.
50. Easmon CSF, Hastings MJG, Deeley J, Bloxham B, Rivers RPA, Marwood R. The effect of intrapartum chemoprophylaxis on the vertical transmission of group B streptococci. *Br J Obstet Gynaecol* 1983;**90**:633–5.
51. Fernandez M, Hickman ME, Baker CJ. Antimicrobial susceptibilities of group B streptococci isolated between 1992 and 1996 from patients with bacteremia or meningitis. *Antimicrob Agents Chemother* 1998;**42**:1517–19.
52. Levine EM, Ghai V, Barton JJ, Strom CM. Intrapartum antibiotic prophylaxis increases the incidence of Gram-negative neonatal sepsis. *Infect Dis Obstet Gynecol* 1999;**7**:210–13.
53. McDuffie RS, McGregor JA, Gibbs RS. Adverse perinatal outcome and resistant Enterobacteriaceae after antibiotic usage for premature rupture of the membranes and group B streptococcus carriage. *Obstet Gynecol* 1993;**82**:487–9.
54. Joseph TA, Pyatt SP, Jacobs N. Neonatal early-onset *Escherichia coli* disease. The effect of intrapartum ampicillin. *Arch Pediatr Adolesc Med* 1998;**152**:35–40.
55. Nicoll A, Heath P. Commentary. *Arch Dis Child Fetal Neonatal Ed* 2000;**82**:F207.
56. Waldenstrom U, Nilsson CA. Experience of birth in birth center care. A randomized controlled study. *Acta Obstet Gynecol Scand* 1994;**73**:547–54.
57. Shields N, Turnbull D, Reid M, Holmes A, McGinley M, Smith LN. Satisfaction with midwife-managed care in different time periods: a randomised controlled trial of 1299 women. *Midwifery* 1998;**14**:85–93.
58. Waldenstrom U. Experience of labour and birth in 1111 women. *J Psychosom Res* 1999;**47**:471–82.
59. Marteau T, Johnston M, Plenicar M, Shaw RW, Slack J. Development of a self-administered questionnaire to measure women's knowledge of prenatal screening and diagnostic tests. *J Psychosom Res* 1988;**32**:403–8.
60. Browner CH, Preloran M, Press NA. The effects of ethnicity, education and an informational video on pregnant women's knowledge and decisions about a prenatal diagnostic screening test. *Patient Educ Couns* 1996;**27**:135–46.
61. Santalaahti P, Latikka AM, Ryynanen M, Hemminki E. Women's experiences of prenatal serum screening. *Birth* 1996;**23**:101–7.
62. Wiswell TE, Stoll BJ, Tuggle JM. Management of asymptomatic, term gestation neonates born to mothers treated with intrapartum antibiotics. *Pediatr Infect Dis J* 1990;**9**:826–31.
63. Mecredy RL, Wiswell TE, Hume RF. Outcome of term gestation neonates whose mothers received intrapartum antibiotics for suspected chorioamnionitis. *Am J Perinatol* 1993;**10**:365–8.
64. Gotoff SP. Chemoprophylaxis of early-onset group B streptococcal disease in 1999. *Curr Opin Pediatr* 2000;**12**:105–10.
65. Burman LG, Christensen P, Christensen K, *et al.* Prevention of excess neonatal morbidity associated with group B streptococci by vaginal chlorhexidine disinfection during labour. *Lancet* 1992;**340**:65–9.
66. Taha TE, Biggar RJ, Broadhead RL, *et al.* Effect of cleansing the birth canal with antiseptic solution on maternal and newborn morbidity and mortality in Malawi: clinical trial. *BMJ* 1997;**315**:216–19.
67. Siegel JD, Cushion NB. Prevention of early-onset group B streptococcal disease: another look at single-dose penicillin at birth. *Obstet Gynecol* 1996;**87**:692–8.
68. Gotoff SP, Boyer KM. Prevention of early-onset neonatal group B streptococcal disease. *Pediatrics* 1997;**99**:86–9.

69. Kasper DL, Paoletti LC, Wessels MR, *et al.* Immune response to type III group B streptococcal polysaccharide-tetanus toxoid conjugate vaccine. *J Clin Invest* 1996;**98**:2308–14.
70. Baker CJ, Paoletti LC, Wessels MR, *et al.* Safety and immunogenicity of capsular polysaccharide-tetanus toxoid conjugate vaccines for group B streptococcal types Ia and Ib. *J Infect Dis* 1999;**179**:142–50.
71. Bergeron MG, Ke D, Menard C, Picard FJ, Gagnon M, Bernier M, *et al.* Rapid detection of group B streptococci in pregnant women at delivery. *N Engl J Med* 2000;343:175–9.
72. Parry S, Strauss JF. Premature rupture of the fetal membranes. *N Engl J Med* 1998;**338**:63–70.
73. Kenyon S, Boulvain M. Antibiotics for preterm premature rupture of membranes. *Cochrane Database Syst Rev* 2000;(2):CD001058.
74. Thomsen AC, Morup L, Brogaard-Hansen K. Antibiotic elimination of group B streptococci in urine in prevention of preterm labour. *Lancet* 1987;**i**:591–3.
75. Regan JA, Klebanoff MA, Nugent RP, *et al.* Colonization with group B streptococci in pregnancy and adverse outcome. *Am J Obstet Gynecol* 1996;**174**:1354–60.
76. Klebanoff MA, Regan JA, Rao AV, *et al.* Outcome of the Vaginal Infections and Prematurity Study: results of a clinical trial of erythromycin among pregnant women colonized with group B streptococci. *Am J Obstet Gynecol* 1995;**172**:1540–5.
77. Locksmith GJ, Clark P, Duff P. Maternal and neonatal infection rates with three different protocols for prevention of group B streptococcal disease. *Am J Obstet Gynecol* 1999;**180**:416–22.
78. Blanco JD, Gibbs RS, Castaneda YS. Bacteremia in obstetrics: clinical course. *Obstet Gynecol* 1981;**58**:621–6.

Chapter 10

Tuberculosis in pregnancy

Geoff M Scott

Summary

Tuberculosis in pregnancy is now rare in the UK and is most likely to be seen in recent immigrants. Occasionally, genital tuberculosis may render a patient infertile and the diagnosis should become clear as investigations are undertaken. Reactivation of tuberculosis is no more common in pregnancy than in matched controls and probably does not significantly affect the outcome of pregnancy if the mother receives timely therapy. The diagnosis of tuberculosis, especially extrapulmonary forms of the disease, may be extremely difficult and requires radiological and invasive procedures on which obstetricians may be reluctant to embark. Failure to identify a case in pregnancy threatens the mother's health, the success of the pregnancy and the health of all those around her, including other antenatal patients. The treatment of tuberculosis in pregnancy is the same as in nonpregnant individuals: first-line drugs carry negligible risk to the fetus and results are excellent. Congenital tuberculosis is exceptionally rare and babies may be more at risk after they have been born to a mother with the disease. The diagnosis is difficult to make in newborns. Serious problems may arise in individuals with resistant isolates and in those co-infected with HIV. Obstetric outcomes for all reasons in low-income countries where tuberculosis is common are not as favourable as in high-income countries.

Epidemiology

In the UK, the incidence of tuberculosis fell progressively until the mid-1980s, when the rate of decline decreased. The number of elderly white people with reactivation tuberculosis in the indigenous population has continued to fall and most new cases are seen in immigrants, some with HIV.

The risk of transmission of tuberculosis to HIV-infected individuals appears to be high because they are susceptible before the CD4 lymphocyte count has fallen to low levels. However, patients with tuberculosis and HIV may, paradoxically, be less infectious than non-AIDS patients.

In the UK, people with HIV are predisposed to tuberculosis and there have been some outbreaks, especially in hospitals, because these patients are particularly susceptible. Nevertheless, at present, incidents of HIV and tuberculosis in the heterosexual population remain relatively infrequent. Some tuberculosis is seen in the socially deprived, where it is often associated with excessive alcohol consumption and illicit drug use.

Tuberculosis in pregnancy is therefore most likely to present in immigrants from areas of high endemicity and in those who are socially deprived.

In New Orleans, LA, immigration rather than HIV status has been shown to be a more potent risk factor for skin-test positivity.[1] Elsewhere in the USA, however, there has been a major increase in tuberculosis in general, in pregnant women[2] and in the HIV-infected population.[3] As HIV becomes more prevalent in the heterosexual population in the UK, occasional patients may be expected to present with both infections.

For a number of years, control measures seemed to be having substantial effects on the incidence of tuberculosis in many local areas in low-income countries. Unfortunately, all this advantage has now been lost with the emergence of the HIV pandemic. In Cote D'Ivoire, the rate of HIV seropositivity in newly diagnosed tuberculosis between 1989 and 1996 was stable in men at around 45%, but increased in women from 33% to 42%.[4] The commonest cause of death in Sub-Saharan Africa in HIV-infected individuals is tuberculosis; HIV-1 and HIV-2 seropositivity in themselves carry a profound risk to the outcome of pregnancy.[5] Elsewhere in Africa, the incidence and mortality from tuberculosis is now rising again[6] and, because the most common age group coincides with the reproductive age, there is an inevitable rise in perinatal tuberculosis.[7] Connolly and Nunn[8] have summarised the profound impact of tuberculosis in women, highlighting poverty, poor access to health care, cultural suppression, stigmatisation and social deprivation as important considerations in their high mortality. Worldwide, tuberculosis is a more important cause of mortality than childbearing.

In countries with a low background prevalence of tuberculosis, disease is most common in conurbations with a high population of immigrants and will be seen in clusters in particular subpopulations. It is here that there should be a high index of clinical suspicion in those with classical symptoms or those who are deprived economically, appear malnourished and whose pregnancy does not develop normally. Tuberculosis is most common in immigrants around two years after arrival. The strategy of screening immigrants on arrival may therefore not be effective at identifying those who are likely to have a problem with tuberculosis. The longer an immigrant group has been established in the UK, the lower the incidence of tuberculosis in that group.

The influence of pregnancy on tuberculosis

In the second half of the 19th century, it was felt that cyesis was of benefit, purportedly because the enlarging uterus splinted the lungs and encouraged healing. Women with tuberculosis were actively encouraged to become pregnant. Following a study showing that the disease actually worsened when they got pregnant, there was a move in the first half of the 20th century towards termination of pregnancy.[9] Perceptions have now changed completely, with the benefit of chemotherapy being so profound that the influence of pregnancy is generally undetectable. Termination is not considered at all now unless a patient has multi-drug-resistant tuberculosis that indicates the use of drugs that may affect the fetus.

It was long held that the immunosuppression of pregnancy would encourage reactivation of dormant tuberculosis. The observations by Warner et al.[10] of three women in whom tuberculous lymphadenitis appeared to reactivate, and occasional cases of tuberculous meningitis in pregnancy,[11] seemed to reinforce this concept. However, proper epidemiological studies have shown that tuberculosis is no more common in pregnancy or in the puerperium than in matched controls.[12–14] There is also no evidence that the outcome of treated tuberculosis is worse.[15] Before treatment was available, it was shown that the condition of 84% of pregnant patients with active disease remained stable, while the rest deteriorated or improved in equal measure.[16] More (15%) deteriorated in the puerperium, however. Of 486 pregnant patients with dormant tuberculosis studied between 1933 and 1956, only 3.7% developed active disease.[17] However, there are now relatively few cases for study in the West and all those diagnosed are treated unless there are exceptional reasons for delaying antibiotic treatment (e.g. primary disease with spontaneous resolution and intolerance of chemotherapy).

Resistance to antibiotics is an additional source of anxiety when treating pregnant women.[18] Some of the drugs used in second-line regimens are recognised as causing damage to the fetus *in utero*. At present, resistance is still unusual enough for it to be a rare problem in pregnancy. Advances are being made to speed up the identification of important resistance (e.g. to rifampicin) although these are not widely applied to all fresh isolates in the laboratory and the technology is expensive. The number of new isolates per year and their resistance patterns at University College London Hospitals are shown in Table 10.1. Only a few of these cases were in pregnant women. The resistance patterns reflect the patterns seen countrywide in the current Mycobnet survey.[19] An outbreak of isoniazid-resistant tuberculosis, for instance, can markedly skew local data.

The influence of tuberculosis on pregnancy

Before chemotherapy was available, active tuberculosis was inevitably associated with significant mortality in pregnancy and an increased risk of complications, including miscarriage and difficult labour. In these days of improved antibiotic treatment and obstetric practice in the West, suitable data about outcomes in large cohorts of patients are not available. Patients diagnosed and treated before or early in pregnancy have similar outcomes to matched controls but those diagnosed in the second and third trimester have a worse prognosis.[20] The danger is probably greatest in those who book late and who are not recognised as having the disease. This is classically illustrated by disastrous cases where tuberculosis in a mother is diagnosed by postmortem of an infant.[21] One study in India in 1994[22] found that, in pregnancies complicated by pulmonary tuberculosis, babies are premature, small for dates and have low birthweights. Perinatal mortality is also much

Table 10.1.   Isolates of *Mycobacterium tuberculosis* at University College London Hospitals

Year	Total number of isolates (n)	H	S	Z	E	SH	Other
						Multiple	
1989	59						1 (SHR), 1 (HEZ)
1990	62	1				1	
1991	70	2	1			1	
1992	73	4					
1993	59	1	3	1			1 (HRE), 1 (HREClo)
1994	65	3	2	1			
1995	47	3	3	1[a]			
1996	59	2	2	1		2	1 (HRZ), 1 (HR)
1997	52	3	1	1[a]		1	1 (HR), 1 (SHRZRib)
1998	60	2	4			3	1 (SHRZCycCapAmi), 1 (HRCla)
1999	66	2	3		1		
Total	672	23	19	5	1	8	10
% resistant	(3)	(3)	(<1)	(0.1)	(1)	(1.5)	

[a]*M. bovis*; Ami = amikacin; Cap = capreomycin; Cla = clarithromycin Clo = clofazimine; Cyc = cycloserine; E = ethambutol; H = isoniazid; R = rifampicin; Rib = rifabutin; S = streptomycin; Z = pyrazinamide

higher than in matched controls. A more recent study[23] from the same group found that outcomes in women with extra-nodal extrapulmonary disease, such as intestinal, skeletal, renal and meningeal, were worse than those in women with pulmonary or nodal disease, where there were no differences in obstetric outcomes from non-infected patients. In small groups in the UK, the outcome of tuberculosis and the pregnancy is currently excellent.[24] By contrast, in Zambia, tuberculosis has emerged as the cause of 25% of non-obstetric mortality and is closely linked to HIV-seropositivity.[25] Patients with life-threatening forms of tuberculosis, such as miliary and meningeal, are likely to do badly whether pregnant or not.[26]

Management

Diagnosis

It is important for those caring for antenatal patients to be aware of the risks of tuberculosis in certain sectors of the population and to screen those patients appropriately. A good history, if necessary taken with the aid of an interpreter, should be sufficient. At high risk would be immigrants from a high-risk area who have entered the UK within the last two years or have had any known contact with tuberculosis. Referral of contacts to the tuberculosis clinic may reveal someone in the family with active tuberculosis. Language difficulties and shyness may preclude obtaining a good history and the symptoms are often so subtle that the patient does not recognise that she is ill. The median interval from the first symptom to the diagnosis of tuberculosis is three months, with a very wide range. In those perceived to be at risk, a symptom complex including any one of anorexia, weight loss, fevers, night sweats, headaches, cough, sputum, haemoptysis or enlarged lymph nodes or any focal symptoms (e.g. backache) may indicate active tuberculosis. Although classical tuberculosis is pulmonary, more than one-third of patients from the Asian subcontinent have extrapulmonary disease, often in lymph nodes, but possibly in any organ. The presenting features are protean but activity of tuberculosis in pregnancy is usually associated with mild to moderate non-specific features of chronic inflammation.[27] In Rhode Island, Carter and Mates[28] showed that pregnant patients were more likely to be discovered to have tuberculosis through routine screening and were likely to be asymptomatic. If a suspicion is raised but not confirmed during pregnancy, the patient should be sent to a tuberculosis clinic postpartum for further assessment.

Investigations

Tuberculin reactivity

This test may not be of much value when considering a difficult case. Most people in the UK have been immunised with bCG, including nearly all the immigrants seen. Thus low-grade reactivity is normal and cannot, as in the USA, be used as a basis for instituting treatment. In a prospective study of Mantoux reactions to 5TU tuberculin in pregnant women in New Orleans, only Hispanic race was a significant risk factor for positivity, this being the most recent group of immigrants to the city.[29] In Houston, TX, there were no differences in the population skin-test reactivity to tuberculin and other skin-test antigens between pregnant and nonpregnant women with HIV.[30]

Interestingly, about one-third of patients with active tuberculosis have no reactivity to low dose (1TU) intradermal tuberculin.[31] Those with low reactivity become positive within two weeks of starting treatment, so this can be used as an important sign that a presumptive diagnosis was correct. Others have a strong reaction and often have significant swelling at the injection site at 6 hours. The important feature here is that the test has to be carried out carefully as any tendency to inject subcutaneously renders the test invalid. Mantoux tests must be read at 6 and 48 hours and the results clearly recorded as the diameters of swelling in millimetres. The Heaf multipuncture test is less valuable in the acute diagnostic setting and is used for convenience in chest clinics because the test is standardised to be read at one week. A rather high dose of tuberculin is inoculated intradermally and may give rise to large necrotic reactions in those who have active disease without anergy.

Surrogate markers

Of these, C-reactive protein and serum albumin are the most useful subtle indicators of inflammation and its chronicity. Patients often have normochromic, normocytic anaemia (unless they are also iron deficient, which is not unusual), raised erythrocyte sedimentation rate and serum ferritin. Severely ill patients will, in addition to the above, have abnormal liver enzymes, high or low platelet counts and low blood urea. However, all of these tests may be completely normal in a patient with active tuberculosis.

Imaging

A chest X-ray is an important prerequisite for diagnosing and assessing the extent of pulmonary tuberculosis. A decision to request an X-ray is made with the interests of the developing fetus in mind.[32] Chest X-rays must not be used routinely in pregnant women to exclude tuberculosis because the yield is too low to justify the potential harm of even low-dose radiation.[33,34] For Example, Bonebrake *et al.*[34] showed that only 48 out of 12 109 chest radiographs were abnormal and that all 48 were from patients with symptoms. One in twenty patients with active pulmonary tuberculosis has a completely normal chest radiograph.[35] For sites of disease other than pulmonary, other imaging techniques that are safe in pregnancy should be able to illustrate any pathological abnormality. Magnetic resonance imaging is useful for lesions of bone and intracranial disease.

Specific tests

The diagnosis of tuberculosis is best made by seeing acid/alcohol-fast bacilli (AAFB) in appropriate specimens. Three consecutive early-morning sputum specimens are better than occasional random specimens. Gastric washings, bronchoscopy and broncho-alveolar lavage or induced sputum may be necessary for those showing a change on chest X-ray but no sputum. The latter two procedures should be performed in properly ventilated facilities, away from susceptible patients. Lymph nodes should be aspirated for cytology and a specimen sent to the microbiology laboratory. Biopsy and removal of nodes give more precise histology and it is more likely that AAFB will be seen. If the lymph nodes are intrapulmonary, endoscopic mediastinoscopy with biopsy is valuable. Any abnormal tissue can be biopsied using minimally invasive techniques, although intense radiation will have to be avoided. Miliary disease is more difficult to diagnose but liver and bone-marrow biopsies are helpful. It is those with miliary disease who are particularly likely to infect the placenta (and the diagnosis can be made rapidly by examining the placenta histologically)[36] and fetus by the blood-borne route.

If AAFB are not visible, cultures are established and continued for two or three months. Rapid broth cultures are used by some laboratories and halve the time to positivity but are more likely to become contaminated than Lowenstein–Jensen slopes. After identification of a positive culture, the reference laboratory takes about four weeks to provide speciation and antibiotic sensitivities of an isolate. It may be necessary to embark on treatment without positive microbiology or histology and with mere hints as to the diagnosis.

Treatment

Decisions about treatment should always be made as a partnership between patient, obstetrician and specialist tuberculosis physician. The diagnosis is always presumptive until data are received from the reference laboratory, which will not be until 5–16 weeks after taking specimens. Treatment is sometimes undertaken on subtle grounds and such decisions must be clearly documented in the patient's notes. Occasionally, the diagnosis will not be confirmed but, in general, unless an alternative diagnosis to explain the patient's syndrome is made positively, it is wise to complete a full course of treatment.

The minimum course of treatment is six months. Any less than this and the relapse rate is unacceptably high. For a minimum of two months, rifampicin, isoniazid and pyrazinamide are given and, when the sensitivity test results are received, pyrazinamide is discontinued. If no isolate is forthcoming, at University College London Hospitals the three drugs are continued for six months. Although it is recommended that ethambutol be added at the start of therapy in case of a possible resistant isolate, this is a controversial recommendation and has proved to be unnecessary in our group. Although ethambutol appears to be safe in pregnancy, it adds nothing to the efficacy of a regimen and the fewer the drugs that are used, the better. An alternative strategy of an initial phase of rifampicin, isoniazid and ethambutol for a minimum of two months with a continuation of rifampicin and isoniazid to a total of nine months is favoured in the USA. Ethambutol is probably better tolerated than pyrazinamide in terms of simple toxicity, and the knowledge of lack of adverse effects on the fetus is greater for ethambutol than for pyrazinamide.[37]

For lone isoniazid resistance, a longer continuation phase of rifampicin and ethambutol is used. When multiple drug resistance occurs (defined by an isolate with resistance at least to isoniazid and rifampicin), serious problems arise because two of the important second-line antibiotics (streptomycin[38] and ethionamide[37]) cause fetal abnormalities and others (such as the fluoroquinolones) are considered risky. A range of other drugs that are all weak antituberculosis agents with adverse effects must be used until delivery, at which stage these latter drugs may be introduced, taking in to account the risks of transference in the breast milk.[39] By the time it is known that an isolate is multi-drug-resistant, the pregnancy has usually advanced to a stage where abortion is not an option, although this might be offered to a patient who becomes pregnant during a course of treatment involving teratogenic drugs.

Drugs used and their adverse effects

Rifampicin

Together with isoniazid, rifampicin forms the mainstay of modern treatment of tuberculosis. This is a red dye that appears in the urine, sweat and tears and may stain soft contact lenses. Absorption is affected by food and it is preferable, although not essential, to give the drug on an empty stomach half an hour before food. Powerful induction of cytochrome P-450 results in accelerated degradation of hormones, with the effect that women who rely solely on the contraceptive pill may fall pregnant as a result of this treatment.[40] Among a host of relatively unusual adverse effects, rifampicin is hepatotoxic. Rifampicin has a broad spectrum of antimicrobial activity and is one of the most potent agents against staphylococci, although, when used alone, resistance is rapidly selected.

Isoniazid

Although generally well tolerated, adverse effects of isoniazid include hepatotoxicity and neurological abnormalities, in part caused by interference with pyridoxine metabolism. Whereas peripheral neuritis is rare, minor psychotropic effects, including insomnia, are more common. Fits may occur particularly in children who are pyridoxine deficient. Supplemental pyridoxine must be given to pregnant women and children on isoniazid. Of considerable concern is the excessive mortality in women given isoniazid in pregnancy and the puerperium.[41,42] Close observation and monitoring are necessary. The symptoms of hepatitis must be explained and patients must be able to gain immediate access to their physician for advice. Although there has been some anxiety in the past, there is no evidence that isoniazid is associated with a higher risk of fetal abnormalities than would be expected in the general population.[43]

Pyrazinamide

Pyrazinamide will often cause nausea and itching. The nausea can be reduced by dividing the dose through the day but this is not encouraged because of difficulties with compliance. Hyperuricaemia also occurs, and serum uric acid can be a useful guide to compliance. Rarely, pyrazinamide can cause idiosyncratic hepatic necrosis. The tablets are large and hard to swallow but may be crushed and mixed with milk or yoghurt.

Ethambutol

High doses of ethambutol given for a prolonged period and normal doses in renal failure may cause optic neuritis with scotomata and, eventually, distortion of colour vision. Patients must be warned of this effect and referred for a vision and fundal review near the start of treatment, to allow a baseline set of data to be collected for reference, should the vision deteriorate. It seems that the fetus is not likely to develop this complication. Ethambutol may occasionally cause hepatitis. Ethambutol causes neural tube defects in rodents but this has not been reported in humans.

Streptomycin

Streptomycin, which used to be given during the induction phase, has the usual adverse effects of the aminoglycosides but with deafness predominating over renal damage. It may damage the VIIIth cranial nerve of the fetus. Alternative aminoglycosides, such as amikacin, carry a similar risk. Streptomycin is useful with ethambutol in patients who have developed such hepatitis on the induction phase of treatment and require continuing treatment because they are ill.

Ethionamide

Ethionamide and its congener prothionamide are second-line drugs that may cause teratogenic damage in animals and must not be used in pregnant women. They would only rarely be considered.

Fluoroquinolones

Ciprofloxacin, ofloxacin and sparfloxacin have moderately antituberculosis activity but are contraindicated in pregnancy and in young children because this class of antibiotics causes developmental abnormalities of the growing ends of long bones in beagle puppies.

Other drugs

If the patient has multi-drug-resistant tuberculosis, it may be necessary to use some or all of the drugs mentioned above. Other drugs that can be obtained include para-aminosalicylic acid, thiacetazone, capreomycin, amikacin and cycloserine. A regimen of these drugs alone would be relatively ineffective at gaining control over the infection compared with regimens including isoniazid, rifampicin or streptomycin (or another aminoglycoside) and would be less well tolerated.

Management of toxicity

Most commonly, patients will develop anorexia and mild nausea. This can be ameliorated by dividing the pyrazinamide through the day although this may lead to problems with compliance. These symptoms tend to wear off as patients get used to taking the drugs. Severe nausea and vomiting presage hepatitis and the transaminases will then generally be found to be high, when all drugs must be stopped. It is common to admit the patient to hospital under these circumstances. If ill, the patient is started on streptomycin and ethambutol, with appropriate regular monitoring of streptomycin levels and renal function. The trough level of streptomycin should be < 5 mg/l and dose or dose intervals adjusted accordingly. When the transaminases settle to near normal, which usually takes a week, rifampicin is introduced at full dosage and liver-function tests are repeated every day. If there is no worsening, isoniazid is added at full dose and again the liver function is watched. If these two drugs are well tolerated, then it is preferable not to reintroduce pyrazinamide but to stop the streptomycin and continue with rifampicin, isoniazid and ethambutol. Assuming the isolate is sensitive, the ethambutol will be discontinued after two months and the rifampicin and isoniazid continued until a total of nine months of therapy (measured from the time of reintroduction of the full regimen) have been given.

Itching often accompanies pyrazinamide therapy and, if severe, can be relieved by antihistamines, although it normally becomes more tolerable after a week or two of therapy. More severe manifestations of allergy to any of the drugs include fever and influenza-like symptoms, and rash, which can be suppressed by corticosteroids. Because of the effects of rifampicin on corticosteroid metabolism, the effective dose is about one half of that administered. It is conventional to start prednisolone at 30 mg/day and to reduce the dose progressively to the minimum needed to keep the symptoms suppressed.[44]

Compliance

There has been much emphasis in recent guidelines on directly observed (supervised) therapy for tuberculosis, as failure to take the drugs is the main reason for failure of a treatment regimen, and intermittent therapy is a major cause for the selection of resistance. For an intransigent patient who wilfully refuses to take the drugs, admission to hospital may be the only solution. It is usually sufficient to spend some time discussing the need for drugs with the patient and requesting someone at home, usually the partner, to help the patient to remember. The regimen is made easier by still being effective if taken once per day all together on awakening. It is preferable but not essential to take rifampicin on an empty stomach 30 minutes before food. It may be preferable to take pyrazinamide with breakfast rather than on an empty stomach.

Compliance can be assessed by questioning the patient and by monitoring the symptom response to therapy, weight gain and reduction of an elevated C-reactive protein. Tablets should be brought to the clinic and counted and the urine should be tested for isoniazid and rifampicin at every clinic visit. The serum urate is elevated on pyrazinamide and this is also a useful marker. None of these indications is a foolproof measure of complete adherence to treatment but clinicians soon get a feeling if the treatment is not being taken and the simplest strategy is then to admit the patient for a period of monitoring. Directly observed therapy can be arranged by any agency but it is essential that the patient is watched swallowing the drugs rather than simply handed them to take later. A thrice-weekly regimen of antituberculosis therapy is available to make it easier to arrange directly observed therapy.

Congenital tuberculosis

Infection of a fetus is extremely rare, even in mothers who develop primary tuberculosis in pregnancy.[17,45,46] Only around 30 cases were reported between 1980 and 1994.[47] In order for the diagnosis to be made, proven tuberculosis must be demonstrated in the first two weeks of life, with a primary focus on the liver or caseating hepatic granulomas or tuberculosis of the placenta or the genital tract and exclusion of the possibility of postnatal transmission. Blood-borne spread through the umbilical vein will result in infection, first of the liver and lymph nodes and then potentially of all the developing organs of the fetus. Hepatomegaly is present in more than one-half of infected babies.[48] A liver biopsy is rarely performed, yet this is the most direct way of making the diagnosis. Infection of the placenta and rupture of a tubercle into the amniotic fluid will result in the fetus inhaling and swallowing bacilli and will cause local tissue infection.[49] Babies present at a mean of 24 days (range 1–84) with hepatosplenomegaly (76%), respiratory distress (48%), fever (48%) and lymphadenopathy (38%).[47] Failure to thrive is unusual.

Macroscopic areas of abnormality in the placenta should be examined histologically and microbiologically. Gastric washings, specimens from the middle ear and bone marrow are useful.[48] If the diagnosis is made in life, the treatment is more or less conventional[50] but delay in diagnosis is common and in several series the diagnosis was only made post mortem.[51]

Perinatally acquired tuberculosis

A baby born to a mother with infectious tuberculosis is at higher risk of acquiring the infection in the puerperium. The later a baby presents with disease, the more difficult it is to know when the infection was acquired, *in utero* or postpartum. Each case must be judged on its own merits.

Prophylaxis

Chemoprophylaxis should be offered to infants who are contacts of patients with infectious tuberculosis and appears to be effective at preventing disease.[52] bCG also appears to offer protection[53-55] but immunisation may cause a change in skin-test reactivity so that a skin-test conversion is not available to confirm the diagnosis. It is therefore recommended that chemoprophylaxis is given first and then bCG after two to six months if the child contact remains skin-test negative. bCG is not contraindicated in infants born to HIV-seropositive mothers.[56]

The puerperium

Snider and Powell[57] calculated that 6–20% of an infant's required therapeutic dose of isoniazid would be transferred in the breast milk. Rifampicin achieves peak concentrations of 10–30 mg/l in breast milk after a single dose.[58] It is not advised that mothers should discontinue breastfeeding. However, it would be a disadvantage to an infected infant to be given subtherapeutic concentrations of drugs for fear of selecting resistance. Potential overdosing should also be taken into consideration when deciding on the doses of antibiotics to give the child.

Tuberculous mastitis

Tuberculosis of the breast is a rare finding today.[59] Although mostly reported during lactation,[60] at University College London Hospitals two cases in postmenopausal women were seen in the period 1995–99 associated with tuberculosis of the thoracic spine. It will generally come to light when a lump is found and appropriate specimens are taken and sent for histological examination. Further specimens will then need to be taken for microbiology. Although *Staphylococcus aureus* is the most common isolate in postpartum breast abscesses, it is important to bear tuberculosis in mind and request examination for AAFB when sending specimens from patients at high risk of tuberculosis, especially when preliminary cultures are sterile.

Genital tuberculosis

Tuberculosis of the female genital tract is presumed to be a manifestation of reactivation disease. It has become increasingly rare in the developed world but remains an important cause of infertility (or ectopic pregnancy) in countries where tuberculosis is common.[61] Classically, patients have amenorrhoea (50%) or menorrhagia and dysmenorrhoea. One-half of the patients will have a normal examination; the rest may have only an adnexal mass. The diagnosis is commonly made at hysterosalpingography or laparoscopy. The uterine cavity is often normal. In countries with a low incidence, it is often diagnosed postmenopausally.[62] *In vitro* fertilisation may be indicated for the occasional patient who presents in the West.[63]

Contact tracing

The family and household contacts of patients should be referred to the tuberculosis clinic. The chest-clinic health visitor may visit the household to make sure that everyone attends for screening. This will essentially consist of clinical evaluation with tuberculin skin test (usually a Heaf multipuncture test) and chest X-ray. The nurse practitioners will additionally have a low threshold for performing blood screening and for referring anyone with symptoms for medical review. This is less easy since the dissolution of the open-access chest clinics in the early 1980s but most hospitals in areas where tuberculosis is common are again moving towards having special tuberculosis clinics.

Infection control

Although pulmonary tuberculosis is a disease of relatively low infectivity, patients known to have open disease should be kept separate from other patients during the early phase of treatment. There are clear dangers in failing to make the diagnosis.[21] Known infectious patients should not wait with other patients in antenatal clinics but should be seen separately and without any delay. If in hospital, it is generally recommended that patients should be kept isolated for two weeks into active chemotherapy (or, preferably, sent home before this time). It is not so much that the patient will be guaranteed not to be excreting viable bacilli by that time, but rather that the infective load will have been significantly reduced. One problem with this strategy is that the bacillary load will remain much the same in those with resistant tuberculosis and it is transmission of such a strain that is of great concern in hospital infection control. Some patients are exceptionally infectious.[64] Patients with extensive cavitating lung lesions, multibacillary disease and laryngeal disease should be kept in a side room for longer and preferably sent home rather than being put in an open ward with other antenatal patients. Optimally, the patient's room should be properly ventilated, although few hospitals have proper facilities for this. Alternatively, keeping the window open in a nonventilated room can reduce the concentration of infectious aerosol particles. Nurses and doctors can protect themselves by using special dust-mist masks. Children should not visit tuberculous patients in hospital.

Conclusion

The management of tuberculosis is difficult in so far as making a diagnosis, gaining patients' confidence and persuading them to take long courses of antibiotics are concerned. Some patients, such as those with problems of antibiotic intolerance and compliance and those with antibiotic-resistant isolates, require a disproportionately large amount of extra time spent on their medical care. Adding the extra dimension of pregnancy should create no more significant problems. The results of chemotherapy are excellent and the outcome of the pregnancy is likely to be favourable.

References

1. Nolan TE, Espinosa TL, Pastorek JG II. Tuberculosis skin testing in pregnancy: trends in a population. *J Perinatol* 1997;**17**:199–201.
2. Anonymous. Tuberculosis among pregnant women – New York City, 1985–1992. *MMWR Morb Mortal Wkly Rep* 1993;**42**:611–12.
3. Margona F, Mroueh J, Garely A, White D, Duerr A, Minkoff HL. Resurgence of active tuberculosis among pregnant women. *Obstet Gynecol* 1994;**83**:911–14.
4. Abouya L, Coulibaly IM, Wiktor SZ, Coulibaly D, N'kragbo M, N'gbo A, *et al*. The Cote d'Ivoire national HIV counseling and testing program for tuberculosis patients: implementation and analysis of epidemiologic data. *AIDS* 1998;**12**:505–12.
5. De Cock KM, Zadi F, Adjorlolo G, Diallo MO, Sassan-Morokro M, Ekpini E, *et al*. Retrospective study of maternal HIV-1 and HIV-2 infections and child survival in Abidjan, Cote d'Ivoire. *BMJ* 1994;**308**:441–3.
6. Harries AD, Parry C, Nyongonya Mbewe L, Graham SM, Daley HM, Maher D, *et al*. The pattern of tuberculosis in Queen Elizabeth Central Hospital, Blantyre, Malawi: 1986–1995. *Int J Tuberc Lung Dis* 1997;**1**:346–51.
7. Adhikari M, Pillay T, Pillay DG. Tuberculosis in the newborn: an emerging disease. *Pediatr Infect Dis J* 1997;**16**:1108–12.
8. Connolly M, Nunn P. Women and tuberculosis. *World Health Stat Q* 1996;**49**:115–19.
9. Lerner BH. Constructing medical indications: the sterilization of women with heart disease or tuberculosis, 1905–1935. *J Hist Med Allied Sci* 1994;**49**:362–79.
10 . Warner TT, Khoo SH, Wilkins EG. Reactivation of tuberculous lymphadenitis during pregnancy. *J Infect* 1992;**24**:181–4.
11. Ogawa SK, Smith MA, Brennessel DJ, Lowy FD. Tuberculous meningitis in an urban medical center. *Medicine (Baltimore)* 1987;**66**:317–26.
12. Espinal MA, Reingold AL, Lavandera M. Effect of pregnancy on the risk of developing active tuberculosis. *J Infect Dis* 1996;**173**:488–91.
13. Edge JR. Pulmonary tuberculosis and pregnancy. *BMJ* 1952;**i**:845–7.
14. Bjerkedal T, Bahna S, Lehman EH. Course and outcome of pregnancy in women with pulmonary tuberculosis. *Scand J Resp Dis* 1975;**56**:245–50.
15. Pridie R, Stradling P. Management of pulmonary tuberculosis during pregnancy. *BMJ* 1961;**ii**:78–9.
16. Hedvall E. Pregnancy and tuberculosis. *Acta Med Scand* 1953;**147** Suppl 1:1–101.
17. Schaefer G, Zervoudakis IA, Fuchs FF, Sami D. Pregnancy and pulmonary tuberculosis. *Obstet Gynecol* 1975;**46**:706–15.
18. Good JT, Iseman MD, Davidson PT, Lakshminarayan S, Sahn SA. Tuberculosis in association with pregnancy. *Am J Obstet Gynecol* 1981;**140**:492–8.
19. Drobniewski FA, Magee JG, Smith EG, Williams R. PHLS mycobacteriology reference services in England and Wales. *Commun Dis Rep CDR Rev* 1997;**7**:R106–9.
20. Figueroa-Damian R, Arrendo-Garcia JL. Pregnancy and tuberculosis: influence of treatment on perinatal outcome. *Am J Perinatol* 1998;**15**:303–6.
21. Spark RP, Pock NA, Pedron SL, Fox C, Opulski A. Perinatal tuberculosis and its public health impact: a case report. *Tex Med* 1996;**92**:50–53.
22. Jana N, Vasishta K, Jindal SK, Khunnu B, Ghosh K. Perinatal outcome in pregnancies complicated by pulmonary tuberculosis. *Int J Gynaecol Obstet* 1994;**44**:119–24.
23. Jana N, Vasishta K, Saha SC, Ghosh K. Obstetrical outcomes among women with extrapulmonary tuberculosis *N Engl J Med* 1999;**341**:645–9.
24. Llewellyn M, Cropley I, Wilkinson RJ, Davidson RN. Tuberculosis diagnosed during pregnancy: a prospective study from London. *Thorax* 2000;**55**:129–32.

25. Ahmed Y, Mwaba P, Chintu C, Grange JM, Ustianowski A, Zumla A. A study of maternal mortality at the University Teaching Hospital, Lusaka, Zambia: the emergence of tuberculosis as a major non-obstetric cause of maternal death. *Int J Tuberc Lung Dis* 1999;**3**:675–80.
26. Prevost MR, Fung Kee Fung KM. Tuberculous meningitis in pregnancy – implications for mother and fetus: case report and literature review. *J Matern Fetal Med* 1999;**8**:289–94.
27. Doveren RF, Block R. Tuberculosis and pregnancy – a provincial study (1990–1996). *Neth J Med* 1998;**52**:100–6.
28. Carter EJ, Mates S. Tuberculosis during pregnancy. The Rhode Island experience, 1987 to 1991. *Chest* 1994;**106**:1466–70.
29. Nolan TE, Espinosa TL, Pastorek JG II. Tuberculosis skin testing in pregnancy: trends in a population. *J Perinatol* 1997;**17**:199–201.
30. Eriksen NL, Helfgott AW. Cutaneous anergy in pregnant and nonpregnant women with human immunodeficiency virus. *Infect Dis Obstet Gynecol* 1998;**6**:13–17.
31. Onwubalili JK, Scott GM. Immune status in tuberculosis and response to treatment. *Tubercle* 1988;**69**:81–94.
32. Swartz HM, Reichling BA. Hazards of radiation exposure for pregnant women. *JAMA* 1978;**239**:1907–8.
33. Hadlock FP, Park SK, Wallace R. Routine radiographic screening of the chest in pregnant women: is it indicated? *Obstet Gynecol* 1979;**54**:433–6.
34. Bonebrake CR, Noller KL, Loehnen CP, Muhm JR, Fish JR. Routine chest roentgenography in pregnancy. *JAMA* 1978;**240**:2747–8.
35. Marciniuk DD, McNab BD, Martin WT, Hoeppner VH. Detection of pulmonary tuberculosis in patients with a normal chest radiograph. *Chest* 1999;**115**:445–52.
36. Henderson CE, Turk R, Dobkin J, Comfort C, Divon MY. Miliary tuberculosis in pregnancy. *J Natl Med Assoc* 1993;**85**:685–7.
37. Holdiness MR. Teratology of the antituberculosis drugs. *Early Hum Dev* 1987;**15**:61–74.
38. Donald PR, Doherty E, Van Zyl FJ. Hearing loss in the child following streptomycin administration in pregnancy. *Cent Afr J Med* 1991;**37**:268–71.
39. Nitta AT, Milligan D. Management of four pregnant women with multidrug-resistant tuberculosis. *Clin Infect Dis* 1999;**28**:1298–1304.
40. Szoke PR, Edgren RA. Drug interactions with oral contraceptives: compilation and analysis of an adverse experience report database. *Fertil Steril* 1988;**49**:31S–38S.
41. Snider DE Jr, Caras GJ. Isoniazid-associated hepatitis deaths: a review of available information. *Am Rev Respir Dis* 1992;**145**:494–7.
42. Franks AL, Binkin NJ, Snider DE Jr, Rokaw WM, Becker S. Isoniazid hepatitis among pregnant and post-partum Hispanic patients. *Public Health Rep* 1989;**104**:151–5.
43. Snider DE Jr. Pyridoxine supplementation during isoniazid therapy *Tubercle* 1980;**62**:191–6.
44. Morris H, Muckerjee J, Akhtar S, Abdullahi L, Harrison M, Scott GM. Use of corticosteroids to suppress drug toxicity in complicated tuberculosis. *J Infect* 2000;**40**:237–40.
45. Grenville-Mathers R. Tuberculous primary infection in pregnancy and its relation to congenital tuberculosis. *Tubercle* 1960;**41**:181–5.
46. Snider DE Jr, Block AB. Congenital tuberculosis. *Tubercle* 1994;**65**:81–2.
47. Cantwell MF, Shehab ZM, Costello AM, Sands L, Green WF, Ewing EP, *et al.* Brief report: congenital tuberculosis. *N Engl J Med* 1994;**330**:1051–4.
48. Hageman J, Shulman S, Schrieber M, Luck S, Yogev R. Congenital tuberculosis: critical reappraisal of clinical findings and diagnostic procedures. *Pediatrics* 1980;**66**:980–4.
49. Narabhai RC, Mathiassen W, Malan AF. Congenital tuberculosis localised to the ear. *Arch Dis Child* 1989;**64**:738–40.
50. Steinhoff MC, Lionel J. Treatment of tuberculosis in newborn infants and their mothers. *Indian J Pediatr* 1988;**55**:240–5.
51. Machin GA, Honore LH, Fanning EA, Molesky M. Perinatally acquired neonatal tuberculosis: report of two cases. *Pediatr Pathol* 1992;**12**:707–16.
52. Dormer BA, Swart JA, Harrison I, Vidor SR. Prophylactic isoniazid protection of infants in a tuberculosis hospital. *Lancet* 1959;**ii**:902–3.
53. Kendig EL Jr. The place of BCG vaccine in the management of infants born of tuberculous mothers. *N Engl J Med* 1969;**281**:520–3.
54. Curtis H, Leck I, Bamford F. Incidence of childhood tuberculosis after neonatal BCG vaccination. *Lancet* 1984;**i**:145–8.
55. Young T, Hershfield E. A case-control study to evaluate the effectiveness of mass neonatal BCG vaccination among Canadian Indians. *Am J Public Health* 1986;**76**:783–6.

56. Lallemont-Le Coeur S, Lallemant M, Cheynier D, Nzingoula S, Drucker J, Larouze B. Bacillus Calmette-Guerin immunization in infants born to HIV-1-seropositive mothers. *AIDS* 1991;**5**:195–9.
57. Snider DE Jr, Powell K. Should women taking antituberculosis drugs breast-feed? *Arch Intern Med* 1984;**144**:589–90.
58. Vorherr H. Drug excretion in breast milk. *Postgrad Med J* 1974;**56**:97–104.
59. Goldman KP. Tuberculosis of the breast. *Tubercle* 1978;**59**:41–5.
60. Muckerjee P, George M, Maheswasi HB, Rao CP. Tuberculosis of the breast. *J Indian Med Assoc* 1974;**62**:410–12.
61. Parikh FR, Nadkarni SG, Kamat SA, Naik N, Soonawala SB, Parikh RM. Genital tuberculosis – a major pelvic factor causing infertility in Indian women. *Fertil Steril* 1997;**67**:497–500.
62 . Falk V, Ludviksson K, Agren G. Genital tuberculosis in women: analysis of 187 newly diagnosed cases from 47 Swedish hospitals during the ten-year period from 1968–1977. *Am J Obstet Gynecol* 1980;**138**:974–7.
63. Soussis I, Trew G, Matalliotakis I, Margara R, Winston RM. *In vitro* fertilization treatment in genital tuberculosis. *J Assist Reprod Genet* 1998;**15**:378–80.
64. Braden CR. Infectiousness of a university student with laryngeal and cavitatory tuberculosis. *Clin Infect Dis* 1995;**21**:565–70.

Chapter 11

Malaria in pregnancy

Caroline Shulman, Edgar Dorman and Bernard Brabin

Historical background and global burden

The effects of malaria in pregnancy are quite well understood for *Plasmodium falciparum* infection in several tropical settings. This has enabled a rational approach to control and therapy to be developed. Many of the initial studies in the 1950s and 1960s, which described the pattern of *P. falciparum* infection in pregnancy and its effects on maternal anaemia and low birthweight, were carried out in Nigeria. These included the first reports of the high prevalence of malaria in primigravidae and the effects of this on low birthweight and maternal anaemia.[1-4] The first trial of antimalarial prophylaxis in pregnancy was also undertaken in Nigeria.[5] The global burden of malaria in pregnancy has since become recognised as a major public health problem. This is because, in endemic areas, pregnant women are the main groups of adults at risk for malaria. On a global basis, 40% of pregnant women are exposed to malaria infections. The disease has been evaluated mostly in sub-Saharan Africa, where it is associated with significant numbers of maternal and neonatal deaths.[6] The annual death toll from malaria in pregnancy is unknown and difficult to calculate because malaria is frequently overlooked as a cause of death, tending to be asymptomatic but contributing to deaths from severe anaemia. Recent estimates would indicate that malaria may account for as many as 5–10% of all maternal deaths, due to severe anaemia alone.[7] Recognition of its impact is important, as there is widespread concern that the malaria problem will be magnified in the near future due to the quickening pace of antimalarial drug resistance.

Epidemiology of falciparum malaria

The clinical features of falciparum malaria in pregnancy depend to a large extent on the immune status of the woman, which in turn is determined by her previous and continued exposure to malaria.

Low- or unstable-transmission areas

In areas with low or unstable transmission of malaria, exposure is not constant enough to result in effective immunity in the population. People of all ages are at risk of severe disease if exposed to infection. In these settings, pregnant women of all parities are at two to three times greater risk of developing severe disease than nonpregnant women and at approximately three times greater risk of dying if they do develop severe disease.[8,9] Severe disease in pregnant women has been associated with 20–30% maternal mortality and a high risk of miscarriage, premature delivery and neonatal death.[10] Particular dangers of malaria in pregnancy in women with absent or low levels of immunity are hyperpyrexia, hypoglycaemia, severe haemolytic anaemia, cerebral malaria and pulmonary oedema. Women of all parities are affected. Maternal and fetal complications are also significant during malaria epidemics.

Moderate- or high-transmission areas

In most of sub-Saharan Africa and many parts of Asia, malaria transmission is moderate or high. Malaria is present every year, commonly with seasonal peaks. Immunity to malarial disease takes a number of years to develop so, in these settings, children under five years are at particular risk of severe disease and death. With continued exposure, older children and adults still become infected with malaria and may have a low-grade fever in association with infection but rarely develop severe disease.

During pregnancy, this immunity to malaria is altered. Pregnant women have higher rates of parasitaemia and a higher density of parasitaemia than nonpregnant women. Primigravidae are affected most, with the risk of malaria decreasing with each successive pregnancy. Severe disease is uncommon, although placental parasitisation is frequent. The main clinical problems of malaria in pregnancy in these settings are the development of maternal anaemia, which is often severe, and low-birthweight babies. Infection is frequently asymptomatic and thus malaria may remain unsuspected and undetected.

Clinical features of falciparum malaria

Table 11.1 summarises the clinical features and consequences of malaria in pregnancy in low-transmission settings or during epidemics, compared with moderate- and high-transmission settings.

The pattern of falciparum malaria in pregnancy may vary between the two extremes described in the table. Outlined below are features that are of particular relevance to pregnant women.[11]

Table 11.1. Features of and risks associated with falciparum malaria in pregnancy in areas of different transmission

	Low transmission or epidemic malaria (little or no immunity)	Moderate or high transmission (pre-existing immunity)
Mother		
Groups at risk	All parities	Mainly primigravidae
High fever	Yes	Often asymptomatic
Maternal death	Yes	Yes, secondary to severe anaemia or postpartum haemorrhage
Cerebral malaria	Yes	Rare
Pulmonary oedema	Yes	Rare
Hypoglycaemia	Yes	Inconclusive
Severe anaemia	Yes	Yes, may develop slowly
Fetus		
Miscarriage	Yes	Uncommon
Stillbirth	Yes	Inconclusive
Low birthweight	Yes	Yes
Prematurity	Yes	Yes
Intrauterine growth restriction	Inconclusive	Yes

Effects on the mother

Fever

Fever, particularly in non-immune women with malaria, is associated with miscarriage and preterm labour.

Severe anaemia

Severe anaemia in pregnancy is defined by the World Health Organization (WHO) as blood haemoglobin concentration less than 7 g/dl and very severe anaemia as haemoglobin less than 5 g/dl. Haemolytic anaemia due to malaria may develop rapidly, in which case it is usually highly symptomatic. In women with pre-existing immunity, it may be more insidious in onset and may therefore be overlooked until very severe. In the latter group, peripheral parasitaemia may be absent although placental parasitaemia is present. Malaria may then be overlooked as the cause of the anaemia.

Hypoglycaemia

Hypoglycaemia (blood sugar less than 2.2 mmol/l) is a recognised complication of severe malaria,[12] with pregnant and recently delivered non-immune women being at particularly high risk. It may be present prior to commencement of treatment but is particularly common in patients treated with quinine, due to quinine-induced hyperinsulinism. It is associated with fetal heart-rate abnormalities. Hypoglycaemia in pregnancy may be asymptomatic, although it usually presents as an alteration in the woman's level of consciousness or as abnormal behaviour, often with sweating and an increased respiratory rate or dyspnoea. In uncomplicated malaria, a classical presentation would be of someone recovering from falciparum malaria and then suddenly losing consciousness.

Coma

Any impairment of consciousness should be regarded as a sign of possible cerebral involvement. Patients with cerebral malaria may have signs of upper motor neurone lesion and may present with unrousable coma or seizures.[13]

Pulmonary oedema

Pregnant or recently delivered non-immune women with malaria are at particular risk of pulmonary oedema.[14,15] The condition carries a high mortality, of around 50%. This is a serious complication and is usually due to abnormal capillary permeability. It may occur as a consequence of over-hydration but can occur without positive fluid balance, as adult respiratory distress syndrome. Tachypnoea or dyspnoea are usually the first clinical features and should alert staff to the possibility of pulmonary oedema. Ventilatory support of these patients in late pregnancy may be difficult due to diaphragmatic splinting, so delivery may be indicated.

Other effects on the mother

Non-immune pregnant women may also present with any other features of severe malaria, including jaundice, renal failure, coagulopathy, acidosis and shock.

Effects on the fetus

Fetal heart-rate abnormalities, premature delivery and fetal distress

The patient with symptomatic malaria in pregnancy may present with fetal heart-rate abnormalities suggestive of fetal distress (e.g. tachycardia, loss of baseline variability and decelerations). Hypoglycaemia may also produce similar effects. Immediate delivery is not usually indicated and assessment, resuscitation and treatment of the pregnant woman should be instituted before consideration is given to delivery. Fetal heart-rate abnormalities often resolve with control of fever, correction of hypoglycaemia and initiation of antimalarial treatment.[8]

Malaria may trigger premature labour and careful examination, including vaginal examination, should be part of the initial assessment. If labour is established, continuous fetal heart-rate monitoring should be employed and delivery should be expedited if there is good evidence of fetal distress in labour.

Uteroplacental bloodflow

In the antenatal patient with acute malaria, there may be Doppler ultrasound evidence of uteroplacental insufficiency with bilateral uterine artery notching, oligohydramnios and evidence of fetal arterial redistribution.[16,17] These findings may be accompanied by other features suggestive of pre-eclampsia, such as thrombocytopenia, raised serum urate and significant proteinuria. All these abnormalities may resolve during the course of treatment and the pregnancy may be allowed to continue. However, regular assessment of fetal growth and wellbeing should be continued for the rest of the affected pregnancy, as growth restriction may remain a problem.

Low birthweight

Malaria is an important cause of low birthweight (less than 2500 g) in women from endemic areas. The increased low-birthweight prevalence in primiparae is substantial, ranging from below 10% in low transmission areas to over 50% in moderate- and high-transmission areas. Anaemia independent of malaria is possibly a less important contributor. In The Gambia, reduction of low birthweight by chemoprophylaxis was estimated to reduce the neonatal death rate by 42% and infant mortality by 18% among children of primigravidae, and by 6% and 4% respectively among children of multigravidae.[18]

Congenital malaria

Cord-blood parasitaemia may be present where placental malaria has been active at the time of delivery. It is not clear how commonly parasites cross the placenta in the antenatal period or whether cord parasitaemia represents peripartum transfer of parasites.

In babies born to immune women, cord parasite prevalence may be as high as 10% in some settings. Clinically significant disease in the neonate is rare, although cord parasitaemia has been associated with preterm delivery. Parasites are rapidly cleared in most cases, presumably as a result of passively acquired immunity, which continues to protect these infants for some months. However, recent anecdotal reports from both East and West Africa suggest that clinical congenital malaria may be an increasing problem. This may be associated with the rising prevalence of HIV infection. Research into this phenomenon is needed urgently.

Babies born to non-immune women with untreated or incompletely treated malaria may suffer overwhelming congenital infection. Hepatosplenomegaly is a common feature and the mortality is high.

Impact of HIV on malaria in pregnancy

The emergence of HIV in malaria-infected pregnant women creates a new situation. A number of studies from Malawi and Kenya have shown that *P. falciparum* parasitaemia occurs more frequently in HIV-infected pregnant women.[19–21] This effect is apparent in primigravidae and multigravidae and may be independent of maternal age. HIV infection appears to impair malarial immunity from early in pregnancy, such that HIV-infected multigravidae may show higher malaria prevalence than primigravidae not infected with HIV. Further studies are necessary to determine the consequences of higher parasite prevalence in HIV-infected women. The interaction may be synergistic in increasing the risk of maternal anaemia and low birthweight and consequently reducing child survival. It is also possible that placental malaria increases the risk of mother-to-child HIV transmission.

Pathophysiology of falciparum malaria in pregnancy

A unique feature of *P. falciparum* is its ability to sequester in deep capillary beds during the asexual stages of parasite replication, thereby avoiding host immune surveillance and splenic clearance. Infected erythrocytes adhere to a variety of ligands on vascular endothelium.[22] It is this feature that is thought to result in *P. falciparum* being responsible for most of the severe disease and almost all of the mortality associated with malaria worldwide.

What makes malaria in pregnancy unique is that parasites sequester in the placenta, where infection is often extremely heavy. Parasites are seen in maternal erythrocytes in the intervillous space in active/acute infection. If there is longer-standing infection, haemozoin (malaria pigment) is seen in perivillous fibrin deposits in the placenta (Figures 11.1 and 11.2). Thickening of the syncytiotrophoblast basement membrane in association with placental malaria infection is a consistent feature and an intervillous inflammation usually occurs with infiltration of mononuclear inflammatory cells.[23,24]

Until recently, the mechanism through which placental parasite sequestration occurs had been unclear. Studies in Malawi and Kenya, however, have identified strains of parasite that are pregnancy-specific and may be selected by their ability to adhere to chondroitin sulphate A on the syncytiotrophoblast.[25–27]

The maternal anaemia that develops in association with falciparum malaria infection is mediated through haemolysis of both infected and uninfected red cells. It is thought that the haemolysis of uninfected cells is immune-complex mediated. Dyserythropoiesis may also contribute to the development of anaemia during and after malaria infection. In addition, folate deficiency may develop secondary to haemolysis and the already increased demands for folate in pregnancy.[28]

The low birthweight that commonly occurs in pregnancies affected by malaria results from a combination of intrauterine growth restriction and prematurity. The mechanisms through which it occurs may include an effect of maternal anaemia: haemodynamic disturbance of uteroplacental circulation, placental damage leading to impaired nutrient supply and/or possibly an association with pre-eclampsia or a similar process.[29]

Management of falciparum malaria in pregnancy

Non-immune pregnant women with malaria infection are more ill, more anaemic, more hypoglycaemic and deteriorate faster than nonpregnant women. They must thus be

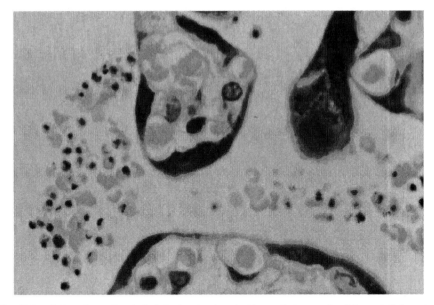

Fig. 11.1. Active placental malaria infection; section showing malaria parasites (pigmented) in maternal erythrocytes in the intervillous space; note the absence of parasites in fetal capillaries in the terminal villi (Giemsa × 1000)

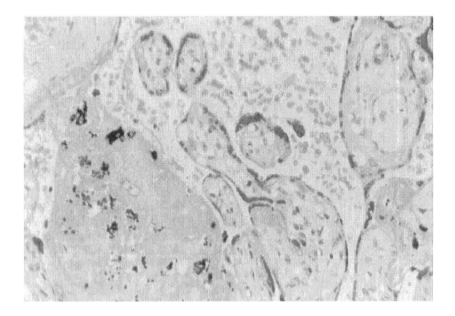

Fig. 11.2. Past/old placental malaria infection; section showing perivillous fibrin deposits, containing haemozoin (H&E × 450)

treated more aggressively and transfused earlier than nonpregnant women. Those with severe disease should be transferred to an intensive care facility, if available.[30] In a non-malarious area, a travel history should be taken from all pregnant women with a fever.

In areas of moderate or high transmission, urgent treatment of symptomatic disease is also vital. However, malaria in pregnancy is often asymptomatic. Peripheral films may be negative despite placental parasitisation, so malaria during pregnancy cannot easily be diagnosed. The mainstay of management in areas of moderate or high transmission is prevention of infection and presumptive treatment, based on the knowledge that many pregnant women will be parasitaemic although asymptomatic. In addition, effective antimalarial treatment should be part of the management of any febrile or severely anaemic pregnant women.

Antimalarial therapy in pregnancy

The most appropriate antimalarial therapy will depend on local antimalarial drug resistance, the severity of the malaria and the degree of pre-existing immunity. The drugs used will often depend on what is locally available. Prompt treatment of symptomatic malaria with appropriate effective antimalarials is essential. Concerns about possible adverse drug effects will be outweighed by the danger of malaria to the mother and fetus.

In the first trimester, quinine is usually the drug of choice. Chloroquine was widely used in the past but widespread resistance has rendered it useless in most parts of the world. There is less experience with most other antimalarials in the first trimester but data suggest that it is reasonable to use sulfadoxine-pyrimethamine (assuming sensitivity to it) for symptomatic disease.

In the second or third trimesters, quinine, sulfadoxine-pyrimethamine, artemesinin derivatives or amodiaquine can be used. Mefloquine should be used only if no other drug is available, as it carries a higher risk of neuropsychiatric effects.

In many parts of South-East Asia, there is multi-drug-resistance. The following schedule is used in such an area on the Thai–Burmese border: uncomplicated malaria is treated with oral quinine sulphate for seven days. A second infection is treated with either quinine for seven days if first trimester or artesunate if second or third trimester. Third infections are treated with artesunate irrespective of trimester. Severe malaria is treated with either intramuscular artemether or intravenous quinine.[31]

In areas of Africa where there is sensitivity to sulfadoxine-pyrimethamine, it can be used for non-severe disease. However, quinine should be used if there is sulfadoxine-pyrimethamine resistance or severe malaria.

New combinations of drugs that may be of use for resistant strains of parasite include atovaquone-proguanil and chlorproguanil-dapsone. These preparations require evaluation for use in pregnancy.

Prevention of falciparum malaria

Antenatal screening and case management

In areas of low or unstable transmission, regular screening and prompt treatment of women with parasitaemia or symptomatic disease may be an effective option. In Thailand, in an area of low, seasonal transmission and a high proportion of non-immune pregnant women, weekly antenatal screening has resulted in a huge reduction in maternal and perinatal morbidity and mortality.[31]

In areas of moderate or high transmission, examining for peripheral parasitaemia is not a sensitive way of screening for malaria infection. In some studies, only half of the women with placental infection at delivery were found to have concurrent peripheral parasitaemia. Screening women and treating only those with a positive peripheral slide will therefore miss women with placental infection alone. Furthermore, infection is asymptomatic in the majority of women, so if treatment is only given to women who present with clinical illness, many women with malaria infection will be missed.

Chemoprophylaxis or intermittent treatment

In areas of moderate or high transmission, the prevention of malaria in pregnancy with effective antimalarial prophylaxis or intermittent treatment has been shown to increase haemoglobin levels and birthweight.

Most countries in malaria-endemic areas of sub-Saharan Africa have had policies for the prevention of malaria in pregnancy. Historically, the mainstay of this prevention has been with chloroquine but, with increasing levels of resistance, this is now inadequate in the majority of countries. In parts of West Africa, weekly pyrimethamine prophylaxis has been used for many years but high levels of parasite resistance have rendered this approach ineffective. Proguanil is safe in pregnancy but needs to be given daily and must be preceded by effective parasite clearance. Fortnightly pyrimethamine-dapsone has been shown to be effective in increasing birthweight and reducing anaemia in primigravidae in The Gambia. In South-East Asia and in Malawi, weekly prophylaxis with mefloquine has been effectively used.[33,34] The initial large study in Malawi found that mefloquine was not associated with an increased risk of stillbirths or miscarriages.[35] However, another study conducted on the Thai–Burmese border found a higher stillbirth rate among women treated for malaria with mefloquine compared with women treated with quinine. However, most of the stillbirths were explained by obstetric factors unlikely to be related to malaria or its treatment.[36]

With a requirement for regular daily or weekly prophylaxis, there is often a problem of low effectiveness due to poor adherence. To try to overcome these problems, trials of intermittent treatment with sulfadoxine-pyrimethamine have been undertaken. Full treatment doses are given to all women (irrespective of peripheral parasite status) at specified intervals during the second and third trimesters of their pregnancies. In a research setting, sulfadoxine-pyrimethamine taken two or three times during pregnancy has been shown to be effective in reducing placental parasitaemia, improving birthweight[21] and reducing severe maternal anaemia[37] in primigravid women. This is an operationally feasible regimen that can be given when women attend antenatal clinics, as it does not rely on medication being taken regularly at home. HIV-positive women appear to respond less well to intermittent treatment than HIV-negative women and they may require more doses.[21]

The WHO recommends that intermittent treatment with an effective, preferably one-dose, antimalarial drug should be provided as part of antenatal care and be made available in highly endemic areas to women in their first and second pregnancies. Such intermittent treatment should be started from the second trimester onwards and be given at intervals of not less than one month.[38] In most countries in sub-Saharan Africa, policy for the management of malaria in pregnancy has been the domain of malaria control programmes. However, for the strategy to be successful, the providers of reproductive health services need to drive implementation as part of an antenatal anaemia control strategy.[39]

Parasite resistance to sulfadoxine-pyrimethamine is increasing in many areas. While there is good evidence that appropriate implementation of this policy should occur in areas with poor weekly compliance and chloroquine resistance, there is also an urgent need for alternative regimens to be identified and tested.

Insecticide-treated bed nets

In areas of moderate or high transmission, it is unlikely that insecticide-treated bed nets, when used without additional preventive measures, offer sufficient protection to pregnant women. In Kenya and Ghana, they had no impact on maternal anaemia or parasitaemia.[40,41] However, in an area of low transmission in Thailand[42] and an area of highly seasonal transmission in The Gambia,[43] their use was associated with a reduction in maternal anaemia, but the effect was not marked. Nevertheless, pregnant women should be a target group for insecticide-treated bed nets as an addition to other preventive measures, particularly in areas of highly seasonal or low transmission.

Non-falciparum malaria

The other species of malaria are *P. vivax, P. ovale* and *P. malariae*. These are not associated with severe disease and usually present with fever. There is also evidence that infection with *P. vivax* during pregnancy is associated with mild anaemia and low-birthweight babies.[44] In *P. vivax* and *P. ovale* infections, there is a stage of the parasite that can lie dormant in the liver (as hypnozoites). Relapses can occur many months or years after the original infection due to reactivation of these liver-stage parasites.

Non-falciparum malaria can be treated with chloroquine sulphate with relapses due to *P. vivax* and *P. ovale* being prevented by chloroquine 600 mg base weekly for the remainder of the pregnancy and during breastfeeding. After cessation of breastfeeding, the liver stage parasites of these species may be cleared with primaquine 15 mg twice daily for two weeks, provided that the patient is not glucose-6-phosphate dehydrogenase-deficient.

Advice to travellers

Pregnant women should be advised against travel to a malaria-endemic area and should be warned that pregnancy is an added risk factor for severe disease. If travel is unavoidable, advice should be given regarding personal protection and chemoprophylaxis.

Avoidance of bites is of paramount importance. Women should sleep under insecticide-treated bed nets or in a closed, air-conditioned room. Long-sleeved garments should be worn after dark and exposed skin should be well covered in insect repellent. Advice should always be sought from a specialist travel clinic regarding up-to-date chemoprophylactic recommendations for the areas to be visited. Currently, for travel to areas of chloroquine sensitivity, women can take proguanil 200 mg daily and chloroquine base 300 mg weekly. However, for travel to areas with chloroquine resistance, the Centres for Disease Control, Atlanta, and the Hospital for Tropical Diseases travel clinic, London, are recommending mefloquine prophylaxis in the second and third trimesters. Though travelling in the first trimester is not recommended, where mefloquine has been taken in the first trimester it has not been associated with any significant increase in miscarriages or congenital abnormalities. Prophylaxis should be continued for six weeks after leaving the malaria-endemic area. All of these measures are safe in pregnancy when weighed against even a small potential risk of contracting malaria. Any febrile illness during or after travel should be promptly investigated and treated, with treatment for falciparum malaria being instituted where there is any doubt about the diagnosis. Any traveller who becomes unwell after returning home should ensure that their travel history is known and the possibility of malaria considered even several months after return.

An important high-risk group, many of whom fail to take prophylaxis, is immigrants from malarious areas who settle in non-endemic areas but return to visit family during their pregnancy. This group of patients may be unaware that their immunity to malaria will have significantly declined since leaving their home and that they are at serious risk.

Research challenges

1. New strategies for preventing malaria in pregnancy in areas of low- and moderate- or high-transmission areas need to be identified and tested.

2. Information is required to establish more clearly the risk of malaria-attributable maternal mortality in areas of low, moderate and high transmission.

3. A co-ordinated international effort is needed, to increase knowledge and awareness of the scale and consequences of malaria in pregnancy for both mothers and babies.

4. The risks and consequences of malaria in the postpartum period should be studied.

5. The influence of placental malaria on mother-to-child transmission of HIV and on maternal HIV progression needs further investigation.

6. The influence of HIV on congenital infection needs exploration.

Conclusion

Plasmodium falciparum malaria in pregnancy is a potentially life-threatening condition demanding urgent treatment. The clinical features of falciparum malaria depend on the immune status of the woman, which is a consequence of her exposure to malaria over the previous 5–10 years.

Non-immune pregnant patients with malaria are more prone to acquiring and to dying from severe disease than nonpregnant women. Particular dangers are hyperpyrexia, hypoglycaemia, severe haemolytic anaemia, cerebral malaria and pulmonary oedema.

Women from a malaria-endemic area may not present with a high fever but are at high risk of severe anaemia and of delivering a low-birthweight baby. Any severely anaemic woman from a malarious area should be treated for malaria irrespective of whether or not she has a fever or positive blood slide. The mainstay for preventing the complications of malaria in pregnancy in areas of moderate or high transmission is antimalarial chemoprophylaxis or intermittent treatment. A regimen that has been shown to be safe and effective in East Africa is intermittent treatment with sulfadoxine-pyrimethamine.

References

1. Bruce-Chwatt LJ. Malaria in African infants and chidren in Southern Nigeria. *Ann Trop Med Parasitol* 1952;**46**:173–200.
2. Archibold HM. The influence of maternal malaria on newborn infants. *BMJ* 1958; **ii**: 1512–4.
3. Spitz AJW. Malaria infection of the placenta and its influence on prematurity in Eastern Nigeria. *Bull World Health Organ* 1959;**21**:242–4.
4. Gilles HM, Lawson JB, Sibelas M, Voller A, Allan N. Malaria, anaemia and pregnancy. *Ann Trop Med Parasitol* 1969;**63**:245–63.
5. Morley D, Woodland M, Cuthbertson WFJ. Controlled trial of pyrimethamine in pregnant women in an African village. *BMJ* 1964;**i**:667–8.
6. Brabin BJ, Rogerson S. The epidemiology and outcome of maternal malaria. In: Duffy P, Fried M, editors. *Malaria in Pregnancy: Deadly Parasite, Susceptible Host*. London: Harwood Academic; 2001.
7. Brabin BJ, Hakimi M, Pelletier D. An analysis of anemia and pregnancy-related maternal mortality. *J Nutr* 2001;**131**:604–15S.
8. Looareesuwan S, White NJ, Silamut K, Phillips RE, Warrell DA. Quinine and severe falciparum malaria in late pregnancy. *Lancet* 1985;**ii**:4–8.
9. Luxemburger C, Ricci F, Nosten F, Raimond D, Bathet S, White NJ. The epidemiology of severe malaria in an area of low transmission in Thailand. *Trans R Soc Trop Med Hyg* 1997;**91**:256–62.
10. Meek SR. Epidemiology of malaria in displaced Khmers on the Thai–Kampuchean border. *Southeast Asian J Trop Med Public Health* 1988;**19**:243–52.
11. Shulman CE, Dorman EK. Clinical features of malaria in pregnancy. In: Warrell DA, Gilles HM, editors. *Bruce-Chwatt's Essential Malariology*, 4th ed. London: Edward Arnold; 2002.
12. White NJ, Warrell DA, Chanthavanich P, Looareesuwan S, Warrell MJ, Krishna S, *et al*. Severe hypoglycemia and hyperinsulinemia in falciparum malaria. *N Engl J Med* 1983;**309**:61–6.
13. Granja AC, Machungo F, Gomes A, Bergstrom S, Brabin B. Malaria-related maternal mortality in urban Mozambique. *Ann Trop Med Parasitol* 1998;**92**:257–63.
14. Gilles H. *Management of Severe and Complicated Malaria. A Practical Handbook*. Geneva: World Health Organization; 1991.
15. Warrell D, Molyneux M, Beales P. Severe and complicated malaria. *Trans R Soc Trop Med Hyg* 1990;**84** Suppl 2:43–4.
16. Arbeille P, Carles G, Bousquet F, Body G, Lansac J. Fetal cerebral and umbilical artery blood flow changes during pregnancy complicated by malaria. *J Ultrasound Med* 1998;**17**:223–9.
17. Dorman EK, Shulman CE, Kingdom J, Marsh K. Impaired uteroplacental blood flow in pregnancies complicated by falciparum malaria [abstract]. *J Obstet Gynaecol* 2000;**20** Suppl 1:S15.
18. Greenwood AM, Armstrong JR, Byass P, Snow RW, Greenwood BM. Malaria chemoprophylaxis, birth weight and child survival. *Trans R Soc Trop Med Hyg* 1992;**86**:483–5.
19. Steketee RW, Wirima JJ, Bloland PB, Chilima B, Mermin JH, Chitsulo L, *et al*. Impairment of a pregnant woman's acquired ability to limit *Plasmodium falciparum* by infection with human immunodeficiency virus type-1. *Am J Trop Med Hyg* 1996;**55** Suppl 1:42–9.

20. Verhoeff FH, Brabin BJ, Hart CA, Chimsuku L, Kazembe P, Broadhead R. Increased prevalence of malaria in HIV-infected pregnant women and its implications for malaria control. *Trop Med Int Health* 1999;**4**:5–12.
21. Parise ME, Ayisi JG, Nahlen BL, Schultz LJ, Roberts JM, Misore A, *et al.* Efficacy of sulfadoxine-pyrimethamine for prevention of placental malaria in an area of Kenya with a high prevalence of malaria and human immunodeficiency virus infection. *Am J Trop Med Hyg* 1998;**59**:813–22.
22. Roberts DJ, Craig AG, Berendt AR, Pinches R, Nash G, Marsh K, *et al.* Rapid switching to multiple antigenic and adhesive phenotypes in malaria. *Nature* 1992;**357**:689–92.
23. Galbraith RM, Fox H, Hsi B, Galbraith GM, Bray RS, Faulk WP. The human materno-foetal relationship in malaria. II. Histological, ultrastructural and immunopathological studies of the placenta. *Trans R Soc Trop Med Hyg* 1980;**74**:61–72.
24. Ismail MR, Ordi J, Menendez C, Ventura PJ, Aponte JJ, Kahigwa E, *et al.* Placental pathology in malaria: an histological, immunohistochemical and quantitative study. *Hum Pathol* 2000;**31**:85–92.
25. Rogerson SJ, Chaiyaroj SC, Ng K, Reeder JC, Brown GV. Chondroitin sulphate A is a cell surface receptor for *Plasmodium falciparum*-infected erythrocytes. *J Exp Med* 1995;**182**:15–20.
26. Fried M, Duffy PE. Adherence of *Plasmodium falciparum* to chondroitin sulfate A in the human placenta. *Science* 1996;**272**:1502–4.
27. Maubert B, Fievert N, Tami G, Cot M, Boudin C, Deloron P. Development of antibodies against chondroitin sulfate A-adherent *Plasmodium falciparum* in pregnant women. *Infect Immun* 1999;**67**:5367–71.
28. Fleming AF. Tropical obstetrics and gynaecology. 1. Anaemia in pregnancy in tropical Africa. *Trans R Soc Trop Med Hyg* 1989;**83**:441–8.
29. Sartelet J, Rogier C, Milko-Sartelet I, Angel G, Michel G. Malaria associated pre-eclampsia in Senegal [letter]. *Lancet* 1996;**347**:1121.
30. World Health Organizaiton. Severe falciparum malaria. *Trans R Soc Trop Med Hyg* 2000;**94** Suppl 1:S1–90.
31. F Nosten, personal communication.
32. Nosten F, ter Kuile F, Maelankirri L, Decludt B, White NJ. Malaria during pregnancy in an area of unstable endemicity. *Trans R Soc Trop Med Hyg* 1991;**85**:424–9.
33. Nosten F, ter Kuile F, Maelankiri L, Chongsuphajaisiddhi T, Nopdonrattakoon L, Tangkitchot S, *et al.* Mefloquine prophylaxis prevents malaria during pregnancy: a double-blind, placebo-controlled study. *J Infect Dis* 1994;**169**:595–603.
34. Steketee RW, Wirima JJ, Hightower AW, Slutsker L, Heymann DL, Breman JG. The effect of malaria and malaria prevention in pregnancy on offspring birthweight, prematurity, and intrauterine growth retardation in rural Malawi. *Am J Trop Med Hyg* 1996;**55**:33–41.
35. Steketee RW, Wirima JJ, Slutsker L, Khoromana CO, Heymann DL, Breman JG. Malaria treatment and prevention in pregnancy: indications for use and adverse events associated with use of chloroquine or mefloquine. *Am J Trop Med Hyg* 1996;**55** Suppl 1:50–6.
36. Nosten F, Vincenti M, Simpson J, Yei P, Thwai KL, de Vries A, *et al.* The effects of mefloquine treatment in pregnancy. *Clin Infect Dis* 1999;**28**:808–15.
37. Shulman CE, Dorman EK, Cutts F, Kawuondo K, Bulmer JN, Peshu N, *et al.* Intermittent sulphadoxine-pyrimethamine to prevent severe anaemia secondary to malaria in pregnancy: a randomised placebo-controlled trial. *Lancet* 1999;**353**:632–6.
38. World Health Organization. *WHO Expert Committee on Malaria 20th Report.* Geneva; 2000.
39. Shulman CE. Malaria in pregnancy: its relevance to safe-motherhood programmes. *Ann Trop Med Parasitol* 1999;**93** Suppl 1:S59–66.
40. Browne ENL. Insecticide-treated nets for malaria in control in pregnancy in rural Ghana. 18th African Health Sciences Congress, 1997, Cape Town, South Africa.
41. Shulman CE, Dorman EK, Talisuna AO, Lowe BS, Nevill C, Snow RW, *et al.* A community randomized controlled trial of insecticide-treated bednets for the prevention of malaria and anaemia among primigravid women on the Kenyan coast. *Trop Med Int Health* 1998;**3**:197–204.
42. Dolan G, ter Kuile FO, Jacoutot V, White NJ, Luxemburger C, Malankirii L, *et al.* Bed nets for the prevention of malaria and anaemia in pregnancy. *Trans R Soc Trop Med Hyg* 1993;**87**:620–6.
43. D'Alessandro U, Langerock P, Bennett S, Francis N, Cham K, Greenwood BM. The impact of a national impregnated bed net programme on the outcome of pregnancy in primigravidae in The Gambia. *Trans R Soc Trop Med Hyg* 1996;**90**:487–92.
44. Nosten F, McGready R, Simpson JA, Thwai KL, Balkan S, Cho T, *et al.* Effects of *Plasmodium vivax* malaria in pregnancy. *Lancet* 1999;**354**:546–9.

Chapter 12

Bacterial and other infections during pregnancy I

Discussion

Discussion following Professor MacLean's paper

MacLean: Has anyone seen a serious case of pyelonephritis during pregnancy? From what I can ascertain, there have been no maternal deaths from pyelonephritis in the last 20 years.

Soothill: There was a woman who became very sick at about 28 weeks and developed disseminated intravascular coagulation (DIC) and became ill – but she recovered completely and the baby was all right.

Ridgway: I was Professor Brumfitt's research technician in the sixties, and we collected a series of cases.

MacLean: And of the patients you saw who were sick, was that because you did not treat them properly?

Ridgway: I was only a laboratory technician in those days. The treatment, as you have implied, was a sulphonamide or, later, ampicillin. We had cases – I was aware of them because I was doing the bacteriology on them but I did not actually see them.

MacLean: In the past, pyelonephritis must have been a dramatic illness but I am not sure that it is the same now. In renal units, maybe it is, but I am not sure that we see serious pyelonephritis in pregnancy and therefore some of the implications have changed.

Smith: I saw one case when I was working for Dr John Grant in Bellshill Maternity Hospital. This was a woman who came in at 28 weeks and developed septic shock, the cause of which was pyelonephritis. We managed her shock as if it had been hypovolaemic – in other words, we did not manage it particularly well, because we did not have much experience of pyelonephritis. That was the only time I have ever seen it.

MacLean: Was there a delay in making the diagnosis and therefore in treating her appropriately?

Smith: There was not a long delay. She came in and, during the initial assessment by the senior house officer, she became shocked. The thinking during the initial management was that she was having an intra-abdominal bleed. It was over the course of the next half hour that it became clear that this was not what was happening but, by that time, she had had a great deal of fluid poured into her. She narrowly missed going off to theatre for a caesarean.

Brocklehurst: One reason why we might be seeing less pyelonephritis is that, when most people think about screening, they think about screening of midstream urine at booking. However, we do a great deal more opportunistic screening than that. We screen for proteinuria all the way through pregnancy, at every antenatal visit. The first thing you do when you get a positive proteinuria screen is to send the specimen off for a midstream urine test and, if bacteriuria is present, you treat it. We are probably using many more antibiotics for that indication during pregnancy than was the case with the earlier studies you presented.

You may be aware that the Health Technology Assessment exercise specifically prioritised this question of whether routine screening for asymptomatic bacteriuria should happen. Unfortunately, they have not funded anything and everything was turned down, so routine screening will not be going ahead. We were one of the applicants and we reviewed the literature, which revealed that almost all the randomised trials of treatment for asymptomatic bacteriuria had been carried out before the use of routine proteinuria tests in pregnancy. I am much too young to remember, but it involved using a test tube and a Bunsen burner to look for protein. That may be why part of the natural history of pyelonephritis has changed, in that we look for it all the way through pregnancy.

MacLean: Is there an enthusiasm among microbiologists to drop this? You would save a great deal of money if you stopped screening urines?

Ridgway: We would not actually save all that much money because it is quite cheap to do, provided you do not have to do the microscopy – which I certainly have not been doing for many years.

I prefer to target my screening. I would much rather that we picked up patients with abnormal proteinuria tests. One point that worries me about the nitrite dipstick, for example, is that not all organisms reduce nitrates to nitrites, which is why you have a lower sensitivity. Like all these things, you need to think about what you are doing.

MacLean: I accept that you will not pick up the Gram-positive cocci and the enterococci but, if you use a dipstick, you will get the majority.

Ridgway: Yes. But going back to your original comment, if I understood you properly, you are actually not convinced that asymptomatic bacteriuria in itself is a major risk factor for problems now. We are really looking for the symptomatic, are we not?

MacLean: With the patients who were seen originally, I suspect the reason why they had organisms present in their urine was because they had organisms in their genital tract as well – although several studies looked at that and showed that it did not necessarily correlate.[1,2] I am sure there are reasons why these patients get organisms within the vagina that are more important in causing preterm labour than the organisms present in the urine.

Ridgway: I like the idea of you doing suprapubic aspirates – a nice clean specimen.

MacLean: But we are very reluctant to do that now. Paediatricians still do it in some units in babies, but they now have fancy devices for collecting urine from children. There seems to be a general move away from sticking needles into mothers and babies.

Regan: You posed the question whether these women from the 1960s and 1970s were unusual. Do you not think that the question is rather different and that in the 1960s and 1970s we had a much poorer understanding of renal disease? There were underlying renal tract disorders, which actually then presented when they were compromised in pregnancy.

I say that because I look after all the renal transplants and renal failures in our catchment area. I will have six or eight women a year who come in with pyelonephritis, but none of them are very sick and the urine is always sterile because they are on multiple antibiosis for all sorts of other things. It is picked up very quickly because they were collecting urine for creatinine clearance throughout their pregnancy.

The answer to your question is probably that it is the other branches of medicine that have improved and caught up.

Hughes: That relates to something Professor Soothill said. Another way women are screened in pregnancy is that they are scanned. If a woman comes in with a pain of any sort, she is quite likely to have someone looking at her kidneys. Gross hydronephrosis is detected. These may be women who, if they were not picked up in that way, would present later with severe pyelonephritis.

Holliman: I would like to go back to a point you made, Professor MacLean. If you are going to screen – whether it is by culture, microscopy or dipstick – you have to have a midstream urine. That really has slipped out of medical attention now, and the number of samples that are badly contaminated and frankly misleading is rising all the time. That needs to be looked at.

MacLean: Is that because the size of the pottle now means that it is acrobatically impossible to collect a specimen? It is all right if you are a male but not a pregnant woman.

Holliman: Taking a midstream urine sample is not a natural human activity. If you just give a pot to a woman and ask her to micturate in it, you will not get one: you have to instruct her how to do it. I do not think the staffing, the resources and the time are available any more.

Discussion following Dr Hughes' paper

Ridgway: I have two questions of fact. First, did you have any data on the sensitivity of a single swab for detecting group B streptococcus (GBS)? Second, are there any data on the intermittent carriage? These are obviously both relevant to the guidelines one makes.

Hughes: There is good evidence that carriage is intermittent. If you swab women at different times in pregnancy, they will be positive and then negative. Do you mean sensitivity for a single swab at the time of labour?

Ridgway: At any time – just sending a mere swab for group B streptococcus. If I fail to isolate it, how sensitive is that?

Hughes: As I understand it, it depends on how it is cultured. Taking a swab from the lower vagina or the rectum and culturing it in enriched broth seems to be the gold standard, but I do not know whether anyone else can comment. I am not sure.

Ridgway: My understanding is that the sensitivity on a single swab is 60–80%.

Hughes: The polymerase chain reaction (PCR) study[3] compared PCR with a culture. It was discussing sensitivity in relation to that. I will let the bacteriologists answer.

Ridgway: The point I am making is that diagnostic sensitivity is not very good.

Scott: The disease is associated with heavy bacterial load.

Hughes: Yes.

Scott: And we probably would detect that on a single swab. The studies in the USA were about trying to detect a high load in the vagina during labour. Then, if the test became positive – it might have been a colour change test – the midwife could detect that and then give antibiotics. That was quite an interesting and valuable strategy.

Discussion following Dr Scott's paper

Holliman: Yesterday we heard about the advantages and disadvantages of molecular techniques for virological diagnosis. What is your feeling for the place of tests such as PCR in suspected tuberculosis patients – particularly women with negative smear tests?

Scott: For just over a year, we did ligase chain reaction (LCR) tests on all our specimens.[4] This is a DNA amplification method that lends itself to routine laboratory work. There was a small group of patients in which that was the first specimen that was positive before a smear. That test being positive implied that the patient had tuberculosis and not *Mycobacterium avium intracellulare* (MAI) infection. There are therefore several areas in which that approach is valuable.

In practice, clinical acumen in deciding on whether a patient has tuberculosis is probably slightly more important. Anything that can bring down the length of time it takes to make a diagnosis, and make a specific diagnosis, must be a good thing, but it is at an enormous cost. It cost us about £42,000 for a year's work. In fact, we have discontinued doing it simply because of the expense. I am sad about that, because it is a good and valuable additional thing to do. It was particularly good at confirming a positive culture – but in fact our technician can look at the culture and say that it is tuberculosis, or she can look at an MAI and say it is MAI.[4]

Holliman: I agree with that. My experience is that when the patient is smear-negative, molecular techniques seem, in practice, to add very little, and they are most valuable for speciation and occasionally for resistance testing.

Scott: Yes, absolutely.

Discussion following Dr Shulman's paper

MacLean: As obstetricians, we need your guidance. I am always amazed by the number of women who come to a booking clinic and then announce that they have a holiday planned and they are going to the middle of Africa. It might be a holiday they had paid for some months previously, and they are concerned that they might have to take toxic antimalarials, and therefore they will not take them – they will just take the risk. It appears to me that, as you defined it, these are the very people who, if they contract malaria, have significant morbidity if not mortality. I am not sure that we have patients returning and dying of malaria in the UK but it must be a risk.

Shulman: My first recommendation to anyone who is pregnant is that, if they can avoid it, they should not travel to a malarious area, although clearly, if they have paid £4,000 for their African safari, that is very difficult. If travel is unavoidable, then women need to take regular chemoprophylaxis and to reduce the risk of being bitten.

The main antimalarials that have been used in pregnancy for prophylaxis are daily proguanil and chloroquine. However, the efficacy of these is not high enough to offer sufficient protection in many areas, due to high rates of drug resistance. In areas of chloroquine resistance, the Hospital for Tropical Diseases in London and the Centres for Disease Control in Atlanta are recommending mefloquine prophylaxis in the second and third trimesters, as the risks of infection are much greater than the potential risks of the drug. Data also suggest that where mefloquine has been used inadvertently in any trimester it is not associated with any increased risk of congenital abnormalities. However, in one study from the Thai–Burmese border women treated with mefloquine for symptomatic disease had a higher stillbirth rate than women who were treated with quinine. However, when you looked at the reasons for stillbirth, most of them were explained causes, unlikely to be related to malaria or the treatment.[5]

Preventive strategies, such as wearing long-sleeved clothing after dusk, using a diethyltoluamide-containing repellent and sleeping under an insecticide-treated bed net, are also important.

Sulfadoxine/pyrimethamine, given as intermittent presumptive treatment (i.e. treatment to all women assuming that they are infected), is primarily used for women in endemic areas who have, or are likely to have, placental parasitaemia. Intermittent presumptive treatment is not appropriate for a non-immune person travelling to an area where they would develop symptomatic disease if they contracted malaria. There are newer drugs, such as Malarone® (GlaxoSmithKline), which are yet to be tested in pregnancy.

MacLean: What do you think about making the recommendation that patients should be discouraged from travelling to such areas?

Shulman: I would make that recommendation.

Jauniaux: As an obstetrician, I am asked the opposite question. I have people who have been travelling, perhaps on their honeymoon, and they have discovered that they are pregnant when they come back, after they have been taking antimalarial drugs for a while. That is the most common question I hear related to malaria. It is very difficult to give them any information on the safety of these drugs. Is there any new information? And what information is available on the new drugs?

Shulman: There has been a good deal of data collected from the often inadvertent use of antimalarials in the first trimester, including sulfadoxine-pyrimethamine or Fansidar® (Roche, Welwyn Garden City), mefloquine, quinine and artemesinin derivatives, and currently none have been shown to be associated with congenital abnormalities.[6] There are currently no data available for the new drug Malarone®.

McIntyre: On your recommendations on intermittent treatment, would you stratify that by gravidity? Some of the World Health Organization (WHO) recommendations are doing that.[7]

Shulman: I contributed to the WHO recommendations, which say that priority should be given to primigravidae and secundigravidae. Policy in Kenya is for all pregnant women to receive this treatment. The reason that it became a recommendation – and again, I was on the working groups looking at that – was because it was very difficult to say to people working in the field that they should only give this treatment to primigravidae and secundigravidae.

I was initially quite anxious at the thought of this drug being given to many multigravidae, because most trial data are based on primigravidae and secundigravidae only. However, subsequent analysis of other data shows that, in Kilifi, infected multigravidae are likely to benefit as much as primigravidae from intermittent treatment with antimalarials. As there are more pregnancies to multigravidae than to primigravidae, the number of low-birthweight deliveries that are prevented will actually be greater amongst multigravidae. With the increasing risk of HIV, we know that HIV-positive multigravidae are probably at as high a risk as primigravidae who are HIV-negative. That, again, makes it easier to suggest that all pregnant women from malarious areas should be receiving intermittent treatment.

If there is limited availability of drugs, priority should be given to primigravidae because, on an individual level, they are at a higher risk. However, on a population level, probably all women from malarious areas should receive chemoprophylaxis or intermittent presumptive treatment.

General discussion

Soothill: From an international perspective, we in the UK are somewhat out of line. The Americans and the Australians are screening for GBS. The main problem seems to be the large percentage of our population who would be on antibiotics if we did that. However, we have a problem if we are going to say that if, by chance, someone does a swab and finds GBS, we should treat. It is therefore not really logical not to look for it. I understand why your group has taken that line but it will be quite hard to sustain in the population.

Brocklehurst: I take an alternative viewpoint. Although the Americans, Australians and New Zealanders now screen routinely for GBS – and it is difficult to stop a screening programme once it has been initiated – the potential adverse effects of screening, which have not been very well quantified in the USA and are now emerging, are very distressing. It is estimated that a maternal death will be caused to one in every 100 000 women given intrapartum penicillin.[8] In the UK that represents over three maternal deaths every two years. This is based on giving 20% of women intrapartum antibiotics and, as Dr Hughes described, 20% is the minimum we could expect, using any of the screening programmes being suggested.

Although most of the studies in the USA[9] have looked at neonatal GBS disease, researchers are now beginning to look at severe neonatal sepsis as a whole, and not just that due to GBS. There is a suggestion[10] that severe neonatal sepsis incidence is not being affected by intrapartum antibiotic prophylaxis, even though the proportion of neonatal sepsis due to GBS is reducing. There are real concerns that, although this screening programme may be preventing babies from dying of GBS, these babies may be dying from other causes of neonatal sepsis. All-cause mortality may not be affected by giving 25% of women intrapartum antibiotic prophylaxis.

The other point to mention is that the UK's Health Technology Assessment (HTA) exercise has prioritised this as a specific question that it wants to have addressed in the UK. There is currently a proposal for a large randomised controlled trial of risk-based screening versus current policy in the UK with the HTA, to look at the impact on neonatal sepsis, neonatal all-cause mortality and maternal morbidity.

Soothill: I understand that. However, if you take that line then we should be asking our laboratories not to report GBS in asymptomatic women. We are doing something halfway between those two lines.

Ridgway: I would like to clarify that. When we are talking about 'screen and treat if positive', we are talking about 'screen and treat intrapartum if positive'. Many of my colleagues, particularly in the private sector, will treat at the time they receive the positive result back from us, and that to me is entirely wrong.

Regan: On that point, could I ask Dr Hughes what a PCR test costs? My understanding is that the advantage is that it seemed to be accurate – both sensitive and specific – whether the woman had ruptured membranes or not, and you had an answer within an hour. Would that not be a potential way of resolving many of these problems?

Hughes: I do not know what the cost is.

MacLean:　I suspect that, if you include the cost of someone being available after midnight, when the patient comes in, to give an answer at 2 a.m. so that you can make a decision, it will not be the kind of side-room test that the obstetric senior house officer does.

Ridgway:　You have to bear in mind that you cannot just do one-off PCR tests. These tests have to be properly controlled and the fewer tests you do at any one time, and the more controls you do, the higher the unit cost. In the case of LCR, which is the technique we use in our laboratory for an entirely different reason, the cost is £12 a test when you do 40–50 at a time.

Holliman:　We touched on antimicrobial resistance, both in tuberculosis and in malaria. Perhaps, taking a worldwide view, we should appreciate that counterfeit drugs are probably a more significant problem than resistance. I have had the good fortune to work in Ghana over the last few years and there, if somebody does not respond to chloroquine, the first thought is that you have a bad batch of chloroquine, and not that the malaria is actually resistant. The WHO believes that most antimicrobials given worldwide are actually counterfeit and therefore likely to be of suboptimal dosage, or indeed to have no active agent in them at all. Treatment is all very well but you have to be sure that your drug supply is safe.

Regan:　Dr Shulman, you mentioned that there was a high risk of fetal loss. What do you mean by fetal loss? I took on board the stillbirth issue, and the low transmission and the high transmission, but what does fetal loss mean? Specifically, patients will ask whether they are going to lose their pregnancy in the first trimester because they are unwell, or because the malaria has attacked the pregnancy.

Shulman:　It is not absolutely clear what causes the fetal loss. The group working in the area of low transmission, at the Thai–Burmese border, believe that the fetal loss is due to inadequate treatment and is a result of the high fever.[11] They say that they can achieve good pregnancy outcome by their regular screening for parasitaemia and rigorous treatment of infection.

Fetal loss is probably due to a mixture of things, including the high fever causing uterine contractions, cytokines such as tumour necrosis factors, etc. Abnormalities of the fetal heart rate have been found in association with active infection, with the hypoglycaemia contributing to this. Congenital infection may be a contributing factor in low-transmission settings, but most of the data on congenital infection in stillbirths come from the 1930s in women at much later gestation, rather than in the first trimester.

Fox:　There is a high incidence of intrauterine growth restriction. In fact, worldwide, malaria is the most common cause of intrauterine growth restriction. I have always naively thought that this is due to the rather massive collection of inflammatory cells in the intervillous space in the placenta. Whatever else that does, it is bound to alter the haemodynamics in the intervillous space and interfere with maternofetal transfer of nutrients and oxygen. That is almost certainly not the whole story, but I wonder how much you thought it was actually a contributory factor.

I would further add that all the placentas that have ever been looked at in cases of malaria come from Africa. We have not seen any from the Thai–Burmese border, to the best of my knowledge.

Shulman: That is right. There are some placentas from the Thai–Burmese border. However, there is believed to be much less placental infection – they have a large number of placentas, which they have been trying to have examined.

In terms of haemodynamic disturbances, while we were in Kenya, Dr Ed Dorman was looking at uterine artery bloodflow Dopplers and found an association between active malaria (as diagnosed by peripheral parasitaemias) and abnormal uterine artery bloodflow and increased notching. That suggests that there is some haemodynamic disturbance, as well as probable nutrient and oxygen problems in terms of transfer.

Smith: Dr Mike Haxton published a paper in the *Scottish Medical Journal* 12 to 15 years ago, looking at tuberculosis in women in Glasgow, who were presenting with primary infertility. There was a 1% positive Ziehl–Neelsen culture rate on curettings taken at that time. This is not directly pregnancy but rather prepregnancy, and I just wondered whether any other work had been done around that subject, because I have never seen any.

Scott: I did not see the paper. The endometrium tends not to become infected, because it tends to shed every month – that was my reading of the subject – so that you tend to get higher tubercle problems and so on. Was it tuberculosis that they found?

Fox: The endometrium is in fact infected but it does not reach the stage of forming tuberculous granulomas, because it takes longer than a month to develop a granuloma, by which time the endometrium has been shed. It is, nevertheless, infected.

References

1. Thomsen AC, Morup L, Hansen KB. Antibiotic elimination of group-B streptococci in urine in prevention of preterm labour. *Lancet* 1987;**i**:591–3.
2. Schultz R, Read AW, Straton JA, Stanley FJ, Morich P. Genitourinary tract infections in pregnancy and low birth weight: case-control study in Australian Aboriginal women. *BMJ* 1991;**303**:1369–73.
3. Bergeron MG, Ke D, Menard C, Picard FJ, Gagnon M, Bernier M, *et al.* Rapid detection of group B streptococci in pregnant women at delivery. *N Engl J Med* 2000;**343**:175–9.
4. Shetty N, Shemko M, Holton J, Scott GM. Is the detection of *Mycobacterium tuberculosis* DNA by ligase chain reaction worth the cost: experiences from an inner London teaching hospital. *J Clin Pathol* 2000;**53**:924–8.
5. Nosten F, Vincenti M, Simpson J, Yei P, Thwai KL, de Vries A, *et al.* The effects of mefloquine treatment in pregnancy. *Clin Infect Dis* 1999;**28**:808–15.
6. Phillips-Howard PA, Steffen R, Kerr L, Vanhauwere B, Schildknecht J, Fuchs E, *et al.* Safety of mefloquine and other antimalarial agents in the first trimester of pregnancy. *J Travel Med* 1998;**5**:121–6.
7. World Health Organization. *WHO Expert Committee on Malaria 20th Report*. Geneva; 2000.
8. Isaacs D. Prevention of early onset group B streptococcal infection: screen, treat, or observe? *Arch Dis Child Fetal Neonatal Ed* 1998;**79**:F81–2.
9. Schrag SJ, Zywicki S, Farley MM, Reingold AL, Harrison LH, Lefkowitz LB, *et al.* Group B streptococcal disease in the era of intrapartum antibiotic prophylaxis. *N Engl J Med* 2000;**342**:15–20.
10. Towers CV, Carr MH, Padilla G, Asrat T. *et al.* Potential consequences of widespread antepartal use of ampicillin. *Am J Obstet Gynecol* 1998;**179**:879–83.
11. F Nosten, personal communication.

SECTION 4

BACTERIAL AND OTHER INFECTIONS
DURING PREGNANCY II

Chapter 13

Chlamydia and pregnancy

Geoffrey L Ridgway

Introduction

Chlamydia trachomatis is an obligate intracellular bacterium with a unique life history characterised by an infectious extracellular phase, the elementary body, and an intracellular reproductive phase, the reticulate body. The organism is the most common cause of sexually transmitted bacterial infection. Cervical and urethral infection occurs in women, and sequelae in nonpregnant women include ascending infection leading to endometritis, salpingitis and pelvic abscess. Extension of infection into the peritoneal cavity leads to the signs of perihepatitis (Curtis and Fitz-Hugh syndrome), characterised by fibrin deposition between the diaphragm and the liver capsule. The long-term consequences include secondary infertility in 10% of women with one known episode of pelvic inflammatory disease (PID), rising to over 50% in cases of recurrent PID, making *C. trachomatis* the most common cause of secondary infertility. The risk of ectopic pregnancy is increased seven- to ten-fold following chlamydial PID.[1] It is noteworthy that the successful campaign in Sweden to reduce genital chlamydial infection has apparently led to a fall in ectopic pregnancies.[2]

Prevalence

Chlamydial infection of the cervix is found in 15–30% of women attending a sexually transmitted diseases clinic. Unfortunately, as is the case with gonorrhoea, 70% of cervical chlamydial infection is asymptomatic. Furthermore, 35–40% of women with gonorrhoea will have concurrent chlamydial infection.[1] A recent study of prevalence in women attending north London general practices yielded a prevalence of 2.6%.[3] Some 80% of the women who tested positive were within the age range 16–25 years. Higher prevalences have been reported from specific risk groups, such as 8–12% in women presenting for termination of pregnancy.[4,5] The reported prevalence in pregnancy ranges from 2% to 30%.[6] Risk factors for infection in pregnancy are the same as those for nonpregnant women and include age less than 25 years, recent partner change, multiple partners and unmarried status. Allaire *et al.*[7] found that, in their population, 10.4% of women were positive for *C. trachomatis* infection. They went on to note that, of women testing positive at first visit, 32% were positive at a subsequent visit and that, of women testing negative at first visit, 5.7% were positive at a subsequent visit. They concluded that, in their inner-city USA practice, most pregnant women had risk factors suggesting that rescreening later in pregnancy was prudent, a finding also emphasised in a study by Miller,[8] who correlated young maternal age with recurrent chlamydial infection in pregnancy.

Thus, the reservoir of silent chlamydial infection in women is large and therefore its potential to affect pregnancy is high. The recent report of the Chief Medical Officer's Expert Advisory Group recommended the screening of sexually active women under the age of 25 years and older women with a history of recent partner change, or any symptomatic woman.[9,10] Since most of these categories could include the pregnant woman, a case for routine antenatal screening can be made. Such a strategy was suggested in 1986.[11]

Effect on pregnancy

The effect of chlamydial infection on pregnancy is not well understood. Studies involving nontreatment of pregnant women with genital chlamydial infection are now difficult to justify ethically. Apart from causing a vaginal discharge as a consequence of mucopurulent cervicitis, the main concern is with ascending infection and its potential to cause amnionitis and perinatal endometritis. Acute non-gonococcal salpingitis is unusual in pregnancy. *C. trachomatis* infects the female urethra in 30–60% of women, either alone or concurrently with cervical infection. Urethral infection should be considered in women with dysuria and frequency who have negative bacterial cultures.

The role of chlamydial infection in preterm rupture of membranes, preterm delivery and neonatal death is not clear. While some reports have reported an association, others have not been able to confirm this. For example, Martin found that gestation was shorter in infected women and that neonatal death occurred in 33%, compared with 3.4% of non-infected women.[12] Gravett *et al.*[13] also found that antenatal colonisation with *C. trachomatis* was significantly associated with premature rupture of membranes, preterm labour and also with low-birthweight infants. In contrast, Sweet *et al.*[14] were unable to demonstrate any statistically significant difference between cases and controls for premature rupture of membranes, preterm delivery, amnionitis, intrapartum pyrexia, low birthweight, postpartum endometritis or neonatal sepsis. However, a subset of women with evidence of recent invasive chlamydial infection, characterised by specific immunoglobulin M (IgM) antibodies, were more likely to have preterm delivery or premature rupture of membranes than the IgM-negative group with chlamydial infection. Gencay *et al.*[15] found an association between raised maternal serum antichlamydial IgM and an increase in incidence of chorioamnionitis, prematurity and perinatal mortality compared with uninfected controls. Support for these findings comes from a more recent study that found that the presence of specific anti-*C. trachomatis* immunoglobulin G (IgG) was also significantly associated with a higher incidence of preterm birth, lower gestational age baby and low-birthweight baby than in seronegative women.[16]

A large intervention study compared outcomes in 2433 women who tested positive for chlamydia. Of these, 1110 were untreated. The untreated group had significantly greater incidence of premature rupture of membranes, low-birthweight infants and infant mortality than either the treated group (1323) or the chlamydia-negative control group (9111).[17] In contrast, a multicentre study involving over 6000 patients in Hungary found no direct correlation with premature rupture of membranes, low birthweight and dysmaturity with chlamydial genital infection.[18] Combined low birthweight and neonatal death was significantly greater in the group with chlamydial infection. The prevalence of chlamydial infection in antenatal patients was 17% in a recent study from India. However, there was no difference in birthweight or prematurity between infected patients and controls.[19]

The role of *C. trachomatis* in post-delivery sepsis is even less clear-cut. One widely quoted case report is that of a 17-year-old with severe post-caesarean section sepsis.[20] *C. trachomatis* was isolated from peritoneal fluid. There is no doubt that chlamydial infection is a risk factor for pelvic sepsis after therapeutic abortion. There is, however, less certainty that the organism is an important cause of puerperal sepsis.[21]

Effect on the fetus and neonate

True congenital infection has not been described. Infection, when it has occurred, has always been associated with ruptured membranes. However, as indicated above, there have been a number of studies correlating chlamydial genital infection with fetal wastage. One serological study of note looked at antibodies to 13 viruses, and to *Mycoplasma pneumoniae*, *Treponema pallidum*, *Toxoplasma gondii*, *C. trachomatis*, *C. psittaci* and *C. pneumoniae*. Antibodies to human parvovirus B19 or to *C. trachomatis* were the only ones raised in 42 women studied following delivery of a stillborn infant.[22]

Up to 70% of babies born to mothers with chlamydia infection will become colonised, with 30–40% developing conjunctivitis, and 10–20% a characteristic pneumonia.[1] The pharynx, middle ear, rectum and vagina are also targets for infection, with a delay of up to seven months before cultures become positive. The infection may persist for over two years.[23,24]

An important study by Jain[25] examined prospectively 530 children aged three months or younger with upper respiratory symptoms, of whom 13.2% (70 of 530) were chlamydia-positive in the conjunctiva or nasopharynx. Of the infants for whom full results were available (66 of 70), 73% had conjunctivitis, 20% had pneumonia and 7% had both conditions. Of particular note were the findings on examination of the maternal antenatal records. Of the 55 records available, 22% (12 of 55) had not been tested in the antenatal period. Of those tested, 44.2% (19 of 43) had tested positive but had not been treated prior to delivery, 37.2% (16 of 43) had tested negative at some point during the antenatal period, but not at term, and 18.6% (8 of 43) had tested positive and had been treated but test of cure or retest at term had not been performed.

Ophthalmia neonatorum of chlamydial aetiology is much more common than that of gonococcal aetiology. In practice, however, the conditions are usually indistinguishable and may occur together, with 50% of gonococcal ophthalmia being concurrently infected with *C. trachomatis*. The incubation period of chlamydial ophthalmia is 6–21 days, in contrast to the 48-hour incubation period for gonococcal ophthalmia. Symptoms range from a mild 'sticky eye', through mucopurulent conjunctivitis, to full-blown purulent conjunctivitis with marked periorbital oedema. Unlike in cases of trachoma, the lower conjunctival surface is more heavily infected than the upper. For this reason, samples for pathogen identification are taken by swabbing the lower everted eyelid. Although scarring has been reported, in general the condition seems to be self-limiting after a relapsing course. Treatment is with systemic erythromycin for two to three weeks, with local saline bathing. Topical antibiotics are not recommended for chlamydial ophthalmia. As indicated above, care is necessary to ensure that gonococcal ophthalmia does not mask a chlamydial infection, as treatment for the former may not be adequate for the latter.

Organisms present in the conjunctiva may pass down the nasolacrimal duct into the pharynx. Infection via the Eustachian tube may cause otitis media. In one study, 50% of babies with chlamydial pneumonia also had secretory otitis media.[26] Pneumonitis develops within three weeks to three months of birth and is characterised by a staccato cough and diffuse alveolar infiltrations on chest X-ray. A peripheral blood eosinophilia is found, as are raised specific IgM-class antibodies. There is a possible association between *C. trachomatis* pneumonitis and childhood asthma, reported at up to 30% in one series.[27]

There would seem to be little doubt that screening in pregnancy can be justified on grounds of preventing neonatal morbidity.[28]

Diagnosis

The introduction of nucleic acid amplification (NAA) tests has revolutionised the diagnosis of *C. trachomatis*. There are currently four commercially available NAA tests, which are based on polymerase chain reaction (PCR), ligase chain reaction (LCR), transcription mediated amplification (TMA) and strand displacement assay (SDA). These tests are highly sensitive and specific, and the commercially available PCR and LCR tests are of equivalent sensitivity and specificity.[29] Preliminary reports on TMA and SDA suggest that they compare favourably with PCR and LCR, but studies in pregnancy have not been reported.

The cost of NAA tests is, however, substantially greater than that of the older enzyme immunoassays (EIAs) widely used. However, the sensitivity of EIAs is around 55–65%, compared with 90–95% for NAAs. Specificity is also markedly greater with NAAs, thus obviating the routine use of a confirmatory test, which should be mandatory for EIA tests. Specificity is of particular relevance in a low-risk population, such as that which attends an antenatal clinic, where a test of lower specificity will have a proportionately much lower predictive value of a positive result.

The most convenient test for the clinician is a first-catch urine sample. However, this is far from an ideal sample for the laboratory because of the extra work required in processing the specimen. Some NAA tests require a cold chain to be maintained to the laboratory. Urine samples are very prone to inhibitors of NAA tests, which may go undetected, and thus false negative results are possible. The inhibitors are different for each technology, as is the prevalence. Thus, in a study by Mahony *et al.*[30] using spiked urine samples from pregnant and nonpregnant women, β-human chorionic gonadotrophin (β-hCG) and crystals inhibited PCR (Amplicor), nitrites inhibited LCR, and haemoglobin, nitrites and crystals inhibited TMA. In this study, PCR was the only

NAA test in which pregnancy had a greater inhibitory effect on the test than the nonpregnant state. Overall, inhibitors were found in 7.5% of TMA tests, 2.6% of LCR tests and 4.9% of PCR tests (but inhibition was 9.9% in the pregnant group and 3.1% in the nonpregnant group). Overnight storage of the sample at 4°C or –70°C will eliminate many inhibitors but reduce turnaround time. Clinicians must discuss with their local laboratory the tests available and agree a testing protocol. It is likely in the future that a vulval swab may prove to be the optimal specimen for patient, clinician and laboratory.

A recent paper commenting on the findings of the Chief Medical Officer's Expert Advisory Group[9] recommends that NAA tests are used to screen women for genital chlamydial infection.[10]

Serological tests have no place in the routine diagnosis of acute chlamydial genital infection. They are of low sensitivity and low specificity in this situation.

Treatment

For practical purposes, there are three classes of antibiotic available for treating genital chlamydial infections.[31–33] These are the tetracyclines (including doxycycline), the macrolides (erythromycin and related drugs) and the fluorinated quinolones. The specific use of amoxycillin in pregnancy, for patients intolerant of erythromycin, must also be considered. The tetracyclines and fluoroquinolones are currently contraindicated in pregnancy.

Erythromycin has long been a mainstay for treating cervical chlamydial infection as an alternative to the tetracyclines.[34] However, adverse gastrointestinal effects are common and may affect compliance, particularly in pregnancy. Furthermore, erythromycin estolate is contraindicated due to its drug-related hepatotoxicity.[32] A consequence of the pharmacokinetic difficulties surrounding oral absorption is the number of chemically different preparations available. Standard dosage in the UK is 500 mg of the base or stearate four times daily for seven days. This dosage will result in 25% of patients experiencing adverse gastrointestinal effects, which will affect compliance. Schachter et al.[11] treated 60 women with erythromycin ethylsuccinate for seven days (400 mg four times daily); 92% were cured and only 3% were intolerant of therapy. Chlamydial infection developed in 7% of the babies born to treated mothers, compared with 50% of the untreated group (P<0.001). There are limited data on the use of twice-daily regimens, with efficacy reported as 73–95%.[34] At least one study indicates that patients should be treated for 14 days.[35]

There are several newer macrolides that have pharmacological advantages over erythromycin, both with regard to adverse-effect profile and to dose frequency. A number of these have been studied for genital chlamydial infection in pregnancy, for example josamycin. Söltz-Szöts et al.[36] treated pregnant women with either 500 mg twice daily for 12 days (group A), or 500 mg three times daily for eight days (group B) of josamycin. Microbiological cure rates were 83% and 91% respectively. Failures were considered to be largely due to errors in dosage or to re-infection. They recommended the routine use of the group B regimen.

Treatment of chlamydial infection has been revolutionised by the discovery of the azalide macrolide, azithromycin. This compound has a low gastrointestinal adverse-effect profile, is concentrated within cells and has a prolonged half-life for excretion.

Furthermore, it is effective for the treatment of genital chlamydial infection in a single 1 g oral dose. Martin *et al.*[37] compared the efficacy of a single oral dose of azithromycin 1 g with standard doxycycline therapy of 100 mg twice daily for seven days, for treatment of laboratory-confirmed chlamydial urethritis or cervicitis. Cumulative results for eradication of *C. trachomatis* were 97% (95 of 98) for women treated with azithromycin, compared with 99% (185 of 187) for women in the doxycycline group. Clinical cure rates varied between centres within the range 91–98%.

There have been a number of reported studies on the use of azithromycin in pregnancy, demonstrating that the drug is highly effective and well tolerated. Bush and Rosa[38] compared the use of 500 mg of erythromycin four times daily for one week with single 1 g oral dose of azithromycin. No patient in the azithromycin group complained of gastrointestinal adverse effects, compared with all patients in the erythromycin group. Furthermore, a dose reduction was required in one-third of the erythromycin group (5 of 15). Cure rates were similar, at 100% for the azithromycin group and 98% for the erythromycin group. Miller[39] treated 146 pregnant women with a single 1 g dose of azithromycin and achieved a 95% eradication of chlamydial infection, with no reported adverse effect on the fetus. A similar study by Adair *et al.*[40] yielded cure rates of 88% for the azithromycin single-dose group, and 93% for the erythromycin course group. Gastrointestinal adverse effects were reported in 11.9% and 58.1% respectively. An interesting study by Wehbeh *et al.*[41] looked additionally at partner treatment. They stratified patients and partners into three groups:

1. Azithromycin single-dose to both

2. Erythromycin course to patient and tetracycline course to partner

3. Single-dose azithromycin to patient and tetracycline course to partner.

Cure rates were 95.5% in the azithromycin group, and 78.9% in the erythromycin group. In the erythromycin group, 38.8% complained of adverse effects sufficient to affect compliance, compared with 7.4% taking single-dose azithromycin. Thus, although azithromycin is not yet licensed for this purpose, there is a reasonable body of evidence supporting its use and confirming its efficacy.[42]

In general, the lincosamine clindamycin has not proved reliable in the treatment of genital chlamydial infection and is not recommended. However, at least one study has been conducted in pregnancy, demonstrating that clindamycin at 450 mg four times daily was as effective as an erythromycin regimen (333 mg four times daily), both given for 14 days. Cure rates were 92.7% and 83.8%, respectively. Adverse effects were related to noncompliance and to treatment failure and were significantly more common in the erythromycin group than in the clindamycin or placebo group. Placebo-controlled trials can no longer be justified in pregnancy.[43]

β-lactam antibiotics are generally regarded as unreliable for the treatment of chlamydial infection, as they may induce latency in *in vitro* cell culture experiments. However, because of the problems with licensed alternatives such as erythromycin, the use of amoxicillin may have to be considered. A recent Cochrane review[44] analysed 11 trials of amoxicillin given in pregnancy and concluded that amoxicillin as 500 mg three times daily for seven days was a suitable alternative to erythromycin. This review also noted that azithromycin or clindamycin could be considered as alternatives to erythromycin or amoxicillin.

Table 13.1 lists current recommendations for antenatal treatment. In all cases, because of the lower cure rates than those seen with nonpregnant women, a test of cure

Table 13.1.   Current national guidelines for treatment of genital chlamydial infection in pregnancy

UK[33]	USA[32]
Erythromycin 500 mg 4 times daily for 7 days	Erythromycin base 500 mg orally 4 times daily for 7 days
Erythromycin 500 mg 2 times daily for 14 days	Amoxycillin 500 mg 3 times daily for 7 days
Amoxycillin 500 mg 3 times daily for 7 days	Erythromycin base 250 mg orally 4 times daily for 14 days
	Erythromycin ethylsuccinate 800 mg orally 4 times daily for 7 days
	Erythromycin ethylsuccinate 400 mg orally 4 times daily for 14 days
	Azithromycin 1 g orally as single dose

should be carried out no earlier than three weeks after completion of treatment. As with any sexually transmitted infection, partner identification and treatment is an important component of management. The baby should be observed for signs of chlamydial infection but there is no evidence to support the use of prophylactic antibiotics.

References

1. Schachter J, Ridgway GL, Collier L. Chlamydial diseases. In: Hausler WJ, Sussman M, editors. *Topley and Wilson's Microbiology and Microbial Infections*, vol 3. London: Arnold; 1998. p. 977–94.
2. Egger M, Low N, Smith GD, Lindblom B, Herrmann B. Screening for chlamydial infections and the risk of ectopic pregnancy in a county in Sweden: ecological analysis. *BMJ* 1998;**316**:1776–80.
3. Grun L, Tassano-Smith J, Carder C, *et al.* Comparison of two methods of screening for genital chlamydial infection in women attending in general practice: cross sectional survey. *BMJ* 1997;**315**:226–30.
4. Fish AN, Fairweather DV, Oriel JD, Ridgway GL. *et al. Chlamydia trachomatis* infection in a gynaecology clinic population: identification of high-risk groups and the value of contact tracing. *Eur J Obstet Gynecol Reprod Biol* 1989;**31**:67–74.
5. Ridgway GL, Mumtaz G, Stephens RA, Oriel JD. Therapeutic abortion and chlamydial infection. *BMJ* 1983;**286**:1478–9.
6. Hammerschlag MR. *Chlamydia trachomatis* infection and pregnancy. In: Reeves P, editor. *Chlamydial Infections*. Berlin: Springer-Verlag; 1987. p. 56–71.
7. Allaire AD, Huddleston JF, Graves WL, Nathan L. Initial and repeat screening for *Chlamydia trachomatis* during pregnancy. *Infect Dis Obstet Gynecol* 1998;**6**:116–22.
8. Miller JM. Recurrent chlamydial colonization during pregnancy. *Am J Perinatol* 1998;**15**:307–9.
9. Chief Medical Officer's Expert Advisory Group. *Main Report of the CMO's Expert Advisory Group on* Chlamydia trachomatis. London: Department of Health; 1998.
10. Pimenta J, Catchpole M, Gray M, Hopwood J, Randall S. Screening for genital chlamydial infection. *BMJ* 2000;**321**:629–31.
11. Schachter J, Sweet RL, Grossman M, Landers D, Robbie M, Bishop E. Experience with the routine use of erythromycin for chlamydial infections in pregnancy. *N Engl J Med* 1986;**314**:276–9.
12. Martin DH, Koutsky L, Eschenbach DA, Daling JR, Alexander ER, Benedetti JK, *et al.* Prematurity and perinatal mortality in pregnancies complicated by maternal *Chlamydia trachomatis* infections. *JAMA* 1982;**247**:1585–8.
13. Gravett MG, Nelson HP, DeRouen T, *et al.* Independent associations of bacterial vaginosis and *Chlamydia trachomatis* infection with adverse pregnancy outcome. *JAMA* 1986;**256**:1899–903.
14. Sweet RL, Lander D, Walker C, *et al. Chlamydia trachomatis* infection and pregnancy outcome. *Am J Obstet Gynecol* 1987;**156**:824–33.

15. Gencay M, Koskiniemi M, Saikku P, *et al*. *Chlamydia trachomatis* seropositivity during pregnancy is associated with perinatal complications. *Clin Infect Dis* 1995;**21**:424–6.

16. Claman P, Toye B, Peeling RW, Jessamine P, Belcher J. Serologic evidence of *Chlamydia trachomatis* infection and risk of preterm birth. *CMAJ* 1995;**153**:259–62.

17. Ryan GM, Abdella TN, McNeeley SG, Baselski VS, Drummond DE. *Chlamydia trachomatis* infection in pregnancy and effect of treatment on outcome. *Am J Obstet Gynecol* 1990;**162**:34–9.

18. Kovacs L, Nagy E, Berbik I, Meszaros G, Deak J, Nyari T. The frequency and the role of *Chlamydia trachomatis* infection in premature labour. *Int J Gynaecol Obstet* 1998;**62**:47–54.

19. Paul VK, Singh M, Gupta U, *et al*. *Chlamydia trachomatis* infection among pregnant women: prevalence and prenatal importance. *Natl Med J India* 1999;**12**:11–14.

20. Cytryn A, Sen P, Chung HR, Raina S, Cooper R, Louria DB. Severe pelvic infection from *Chlamydia trachomatis* after caesarean section. *JAMA* 1982;**247**:1732–4.

21. McGregor JA, French JI. *Chlamydia trachomatis* infection during pregnancy. *Am J Obstet Gynecol* 1991;**164**:1782–9.

22. Koskiniemi M, Ammala P, Narvanen A, *et al*. Stillbirths and maternal antibodies to *Chlamydia trachomatis*: a new EIA test for serology. *Acta Obstet Gynecol Scand* 1996;**75**:657–61.

23. Bell TA, Stamm WE, Kuo CC, Wang SP, Holmes KK, Grayston JT. Delayed appearance of *Chlamydia trachomatis* infections acquired at birth. *Pediatr Infect Dis J* 1987;**6**:928–31.

24. Bell TA, Stamm WE, Wang SP, Kuo CC, Holmes KK, Grayston JT. Chronic *Chlamydia trachomatis* infections in infants. *JAMA* 1992;**267**:400–2.

25. Jain S. Perinatally acquired *Chlamydia trachomatis* associated morbidity in young infants. *J Matern Fetal Med* 1999;**8**:130–3.

26. Tipple MA, Beem MO, Saxon EM. Clinical characteristics of the afebrile pneumonia associated with *Chlamydia trachomatis* infection in infants less than 6 months of age. *Pediatrics* 1979;**63**:192–7.

27. Weiss SG, Newcomb RW, Beem MO. Pulmonary assessment of children after chlamydial infection of infancy. *J Pediatr* 1986;**108**:659–64.

28. Schachter J, Grossman M, Sweet RL, Holt J, Jordan C, Bishop E. Prospective study of perinatal transmission of *Chlamydia trachomatis*. *JAMA* 1986;**255**:3874–7.

29. Davies PO, Ridgway GL. The role of polymerase chain reaction and ligase chain reaction for the detection of *Chlamydia trachomatis*. *Int J STD AIDS* 1997;**8**:731–8.

30. Mahony J, Chong S, Jang D, *et al*. Urine specimens from pregnant and nonpregnant women inhibitory to amplification of *Chlamydia trachomatis* nucleic acid by PCR, ligase chain reaction, and transcription-mediated amplification: identification of urinary substances associated with inhibition and removal of inhibitory activity. *J Clin Microbiol* 1998;**36**:3122–6.

31. Robinson AJ, Ridgway GL. Concurrent gonococcal and chlamydial infection: how best to treat. *Drugs* 2000;**59**:801–13.

32. Anonymous. 1998 guidelines for treatment of sexually transmitted diseases. Centers for Disease Control and Prevention. *MMWR Morb Mortal Wkly Rep* 1998;**47**:1–111.

33. Clinical Effectiveness Group. UK national guidelines on sexually transmitted infections and closely related conditions. *Sex Transm Inf* 1999;**75** Suppl 1:S4–S8.

34. Oriel JD, Ridgway GL. Comparison of erythromycin and oxytetracycline for the treatment of cervical infection by *Chlamydia trachomatis*. *J Infect* 1980;**2**:259–62.

35. Linnemann CC Jr, Heaton CL, Ritchey M. Treatment of *Chlamydia trachomatis* infections: comparison of 1- and 2- g doses of erythromycin daily for seven days. *Sex Transm Dis* 1987;**14**:102–6.

36. Söltz-Szöts J, Schneider S, Niebauer B, Knobler RM, Lindmaier A. Significance of the dose of josamycin in the treatment of chlamydia infected pregnant patients. *Z Hautkr* 1989;**64**:129–131.

37. Martin DH, Mroczkowski TF, Dalu ZA, McCarty J, Jones RB, Hopkins SJ, *et al*. A controlled trial of a single dose of azithromycin for the treatment of chlamydial urethritis and cervicitis. *N Engl J Med* 1992;**327**:921–5.

38. Bush M, Rosa C. Azithromycin and erythromycin in the treatment of cervical chlamydial infection during pregnancy. *Obstet Gynecol* 1994;**84**:61–3.

39. Miller JM. Efficacy and tolerance of single dose azithromycin for the treatment of chlamydial cervicitis during pregnancy. *Infect Dis Obstet Gynecol* 1995;**3**:189–92.

40. Adair CD, Gunter M, Stovall TG, McElroy G, Veille JC, Ernest JM. Chlamydia in pregnancy: a randomized trial of azithromycin and erythromycin. *Obstet Gynecol* 1998;**91**:165–8.

41. Wehbeh HA, Ruggeirro RM, Shahem S, Lopez G, Ali Y. Single-dose azithromycin for chlamydia in pregnant women. *J Reprod Med* 1998;**43**:509–14.

42. Lea AP, Lamb HM. Azithromycin: a pharmacokinetic review of its use as a single-dose regimen in the treatment of uncomplicated urogenital *Chlamydia trachomatis* infections in women. *Pharmacoeconomics* 1997;**12**:596–611.

43. Alger LS, Lovchik JC. Comparative efficacy of clindamycin versus erythromycin in eradication of antenatal *Chlamydia trachomatis*. *Am J Obstet Gynecol* 1991;**165**:375–81.
44. Brocklehurst P, Rooney G. Interventions for treating genital *Chlamydia trachomatis* infection in pregnancy. *Cochrane Database Syst Rev* 2000;(2):CD000054.

Chapter 14

Bacterial vaginosis and pregnancy

Phillip Hay

Introduction

Bacterial vaginosis (BV) is a clinical syndrome of unknown aetiology characterised by an overgrowth of vaginal anaerobes and depletion of the normal lactobacillus population. This is accompanied by a rise in pH from below 4.5 to levels as high as 7.0 and a fishy smell due to increased levels of polyamines and trimethylamine. In some women it relapses and remits spontaneously. Many women are asymptomatic during transient phases of BV but some experience frequent symptomatic episodes of BV. Current antibiotic treatments restore the normal lactobacillus-dominated flora in the short term but approximately 30% of patients relapse within one month.[1,2]

BV is associated with complications of pregnancy, including miscarriage, preterm birth and postpartum endometritis. Since the association between BV and preterm birth was found, studies have not always confirmed that antibiotics are effective in improving pregnancy outcome.[3] BV is also associated with infectious morbidity following gynaecological surgery, such as hysterectomy or termination of pregnancy. In recent studies it is emerging as a co-factor for sexually transmitted infections and, importantly, acquisition of HIV in women. If ways of reducing the prevalence of BV can be found, this may be a way of reducing the incidence of sexually transmitted HIV infection.[4]

Prevalence

In the West, BV is the leading cause of abnormal vaginal discharge. In an unselected population, the prevalence rate is usually 10–20%[5] but the reported prevalence varies widely: from 5% to 51% in different populations. In the USA, Bump and Buesching[6] reported a prevalence of approximately 13% among adolescent girls. In the UK, we reported a similar prevalence in a gynaecology clinic[7] and antenatal clinic.[8] A higher incidence of 28% was found in women undergoing termination of pregnancy,[9] and 24.6% in a group of women undergoing *in vitro* fertilisation (IVF) treatment.[10] In the

USA, a high incidence was reported in some populations, for example inner-city pregnant women (32.5%).[11] The highest incidence, however, has been reported from Rakai in rural Uganda, where 50.9% of women had BV, along with a prevalence for trichomoniasis of 23.8%.[12] Eighty percent of these women were asymptomatic. Most women with trichomoniasis have intermediate flora or BV, so the role of *Trichomonas* in this high prevalence of BV needs to be determined.

These studies report point prevalences. Three studies of asymptomatic volunteers have examined self-prepared vaginal smears by Gram stain over a period of one to two months. Gram-stain changes compatible with the onset of BV occurred in 36% (9 of 25),[13] 25.5% (13 of 51)[14] and 12% (2 of 17)[15] of subjects. It may be that in most populations the majority of women will develop asymptomatic BV at some time.

Aetiology and natural history of BV

This has been reviewed in detail elsewhere.[16] The majority of studies find associations between BV and black race, receiving oral sex, smoking and the use of an intrauterine contraceptive device. Anecdotally, many women with BV report its occurrence when they changed sexual partners. There is some evidence that BV behaves as a sexually transmitted disease[17] but the original study by Bump and Buesching[6] found no difference in its prevalence between virgin and non-virgin adolescent women.

Lactobacilli are the predominant organism in the healthy vagina. They produce lactic acid, which acidifies the vaginal fluid to a pH below 4.5. It is thought that the production of H_2O_2 is an important mechanism for inhibiting the growth of the anaerobic and facultative anaerobic organisms, which usually colonise the vagina in low concentrations. When these organisms increase in concentration, by up to a thousand-fold, bacterial vaginosis develops. It is not known what initiates such a dramatic change in the vaginal flora, which is accompanied by a rise in pH. *In vitro* studies have shown that, at a pH of less than 4.5, H_2O_2-producing lactobacilli inhibit the growth of BV-associated organisms effectively, but that the effect wanes at higher pH levels.[18] It is thus likely that the vaginal flora is more vulnerable to the development of BV when the pH is elevated, such as at the time of menstruation and following unprotected intercourse. Vaginal douching has also been associated with BV in several studies but prospective studies are needed to determine whether this has a genuine aetiological role.[19,20]

Recent studies suggest that potentially transmissible lactobacillus phages may be the noxious agents of lactobacilli depletion and dysfunction.[21] Lactobacillus phages are known to affect yoghurt cultures in the food industry. They can remain in a temperate state, or become lytic, when up to 99% of the lactobacillus population may be killed. They have now been isolated from human lactobacilli from the vagina[22] and gut, and from lactobacilli in yoghurt. The latter were shown to inhibit vaginal lactobacilli.[23] Phages might be transmitted by sexual intercourse, dairy products or faeco-oral spread.

We observed that, in women with recurrent BV, the symptoms were frequently cyclical, with BV appearing soon after a vaginal candidal infection or around the time of menstruation.[24] Data from experimental animal models suggest a role for reproductive hormones.[25–27] However, other factors, such as genetic or racial predisposition and sexual behaviour, may modify susceptibility to BV.

Diagnosis

BV is diagnosed clinically on the basis of the presence of any three of Amsel's four composite criteria.[28] These are:

- a characteristic thin, homogeneous, white or yellow discharge
- detection of clue cells on microscopy of a wet mount of vaginal fluid
- pH of vaginal fluid greater than 4.5
- release of a pungent fishy odour when alkali (10% KOH) is mixed with vaginal fluid.

Microbiologically, there is an increase in concentration of many bacterial species and a decrease in the concentration of lactobacilli. The species most often identified in BV include *Gardnerella vaginalis*, *Mobiluncus* spp., *Bacteroides* spp. and *Mycoplasma hominis*. *G. vaginalis* is present in the vagina of 50–60% of healthy women without BV[29] and its isolation from cultures of vaginal swabs is not diagnostic of BV.

Gram staining of air-dried vaginal smears, if quantified according to the Nugent's criteria, provides a reliable and reproducible method of diagnosis.[30] Moreover, it detects the less florid but nevertheless abnormal intermediate flora. This flora was characterised in a study of pregnant women, and found to be genuinely intermediate in character.[31] Not all abnormal vaginal floras can be classified into a continuum from normal to BV. Inflammatory conditions such as those due to *Candida* spp., *Trichomonas vaginalis* or streptococci may occur alongside normal, intermediate or BV flora.

New rapid tests for the diagnosis of BV have been developed. Some of these are based on DNA probes for *G. vaginalis* genes while others measure metabolic products of anaerobic bacteria, such as proline aminopeptidase.[32,33]

Obstetric complications

Mechanisms

Endometritis

BV is associated with endometritis. It may be that the endometritis leads to problems in pregnancy, rather than the BV itself. BV-related organisms have been isolated from the endometrium and fallopian tubes of women with pelvic inflammatory disease, suggesting a role for BV in this disease.[34] Lund *et al.*[35] have demonstrated rhythmic contractions of the uterus in pregnant and nonpregnant women, during which contrast medium placed in the vagina travelled through the uterus and tubes into the peritoneal cavity. This suggests that ascent of microbes from the vagina into the upper genital tract is almost inevitable.

BV has been associated with subclinical endometritis. A study that used sheathed endometrial samplers to minimise contamination from vaginal material found plasma cell endometritis in 10 of 22 endometrial biopsies from symptomatic women with BV, compared with 1 of 19 of uninfected women (OR 15; 95% CI 2–686; $P<0.01$).[36] Microorganisms associated with BV were isolated from the endometria of 9 of 11 women with and 8 of 30 women without plasma cell endometritis (OR 12.4; 95% CI 2–132; $P = 0.002$), suggesting a link between BV and non-chlamydial, non-gonococcal upper genital tract infection.

Potential role of inflammatory cytokines

The release of prostaglandins leading to cervical ripening, uterine contractions and preterm birth may be mediated by pro-inflammatory cytokines such as interleukin-1, interleukin-6, and tumour necrosis factor alpha (TNF-α).[37,38] These cytokines are present in greater concentrations in the amniotic and cervicovaginal fluids of women with BV compared with controls.[39,40] The immune cells and cytokines within the amniotic cavity have recently been recognised to be of fetal origin,[41] suggesting fetal systemic inflammatory response syndrome.[42] Evidence from human and animal studies suggests that the growth and development of oligodendrocytes in the fetal brain are impaired by interleukin-6 and TNF-α.[43,44] This suggests a possible immune response or cytokine-mediated neurodevelopmental disturbance that might explain the excess incidence of cerebral palsy in babies born to women with evidence of perinatal infection[45–47] and indirectly links BV with cerebral palsy. A number of studies of preterm babies have directly related antepartum or intrapartum exposure to infection and inflammatory cytokines to periventricular leukomalacia and subsequent risk of cerebral palsy.[46,48,49] This trend was also observed in babies weighing 2.5 kg and above,[47] suggesting that preterm birth cannot independently account for all the neurodevelopmental morbidity in children born prematurely.

Other risk factors

Fibronectin is released from the choriodecidual space when there is inflammation. Its detection after 22 weeks of gestation is predictive of preterm birth and has been associated with BV.[50] As discussed below, this may be too late to achieve maximum benefit from treating BV. Another marker of inflammation has been detected as early as eight weeks of gestation and may provide a better marker. Phosphorylated insulin-like growth factor binding protein 1 is produced by the decidua. Its detection in cervical mucus was associated with peripartum infection in a study from Finland.[51] The predictive value was not reduced by the use of clindamycin cream.

Vaginal washings from a subset of women in a study from Denmark[52] were examined for additional virulence markers. Although BV was not significantly associated with preterm birth, women with high levels of prolidase, sialidase and reduced or absent anti-*Gardnerella* haemolysin antibodies were at the greatest risk of preterm birth.[53]

Preterm birth

BV is associated with an increased risk of preterm premature rupture of membranes, chorioamnionitis, amniotic fluid colonisation, low-birthweight infants and postpartum endometritis.[54,55] The most common organisms cultured from the membranes, amniotic fluid and placentas of preterm births are BV-related.[56] They include *M. hominis* and fastidious anaerobic organisms. These organisms often escape clinical and routine microbiological detection and may account for a significant proportion of previously unexplained preterm births. The aetiology of preterm birth is multifactorial and the majority of women with BV have term deliveries. Other risk factors might include the genetic predisposition of the mother to produce a strong inflammatory response to infection, cervical shortening, or the levels of sialidases and other virulence factors produced by microorganisms.

Observational studies of BV in pregnancy

Infertility and first-trimester loss

BV has not been associated with infertility, although a high prevalence (24.6%) was reported from a study of 771 women undergoing IVF in Leeds.[10] The first-trimester miscarriage rate was 31.6% for those with BV, compared with 18.5% for those with normal vaginal flora (crude OR 2.49; 95% CI 1.21–5.12). The majority of these losses were in chemical pregnancies. There was a non-significant trend associating BV with an increased incidence of loss in clinical pregnancies. A smaller study of 301 women undergoing IVF treatment in Bristol also reported a high prevalence of BV (25.6%).[57] It was more common in women with tubal (31.5%) than non-tubal (19.7%) infertility (OR 1.87; 95% CI 1.11–3.18). There was no significant difference in implantation rates when comparing BV (15.8%; OR 1.03; 95% CI 0.66–1.61) and intermediate flora (13.1%; OR 0.82; 95% CI 0.45–1.52) with normal flora (15.5%).

Second-trimester loss

In a UK study, BV detected before 16 weeks of gestation was associated with a five-fold increase in the risk of mid-trimester pregnancy loss and a three-fold increased risk of preterm birth.[8] This association was confirmed in a study from Denver, USA, that reported a more than three-fold association between BV and second-trimester loss.[11] Another study reported an association between previous second-trimester miscarriage and BV, but not between recurrent first-trimester loss and BV.[58]

Preterm birth

Many studies from different countries have confirmed the association between BV and preterm birth. These were reviewed by Hillier et al.[59] The odds ratios have varied between 1.4 in a large multicentre USA study[59] to 6.9 in a Finnish study.[60] The two studies that screened earliest in pregnancy found the greatest odds ratios,[8,60] while those screening later tended to find weaker associations. One large study from Denmark did not report a significant association, although subsequent analyses showed associations between detection of particular organisms such as M. hominis and adverse outcome.[52]

Postpartum endometritis

One study examined risk factors for endometritis following caesarean section.[61] The strongest predictor of endometritis was an interval of greater than 24 hours between rupture of membranes and delivery, but BV was associated with endometritis with an odds ratio of 5.8 in the multivariate analysis. No studies have been performed to evaluate the role of screening and prophylactic treatment.

Treatment of BV in pregnancy

Published studies are summarised in Table 14.1.

High-risk pregnancies

A history of preterm birth is the strongest predictor of subsequent preterm birth. Intervention studies of systemic antibiotic treatment of BV in high-risk pregnancies suggest that treatment reduces the risk of preterm birth and infectious morbidity.[11,62,63] However, these studies have been criticised either for their small sample sizes or design flaws.

In the first published study, 80 pregnant women with BV and at high risk of preterm birth because of a previous preterm birth or preterm premature rupture of membranes were randomised at 13–20 weeks of gestation to take oral metronidazole 250 mg three times daily for seven days or placebo.[62] Compared with the placebo group, women in the treatment arm had significantly fewer admissions for preterm labour: 12 of 44 (27%) versus 28 of 36 (78%); preterm birth: 8 of 44 (18%) versus 16 of 36 (39%); and preterm premature rupture of membranes: 6 of 44 (14%) versus 12 of 36 (33%).

In another intervention trial, 624 pregnant women at high risk of preterm birth because of a previous preterm birth and/or maternal weight of less than 50 kg were randomised at a mean gestational age of 23 weeks to take metronidazole and erythromycin or placebo.[63] In the 258 women with BV, the antibiotic treatment reduced the preterm birth rate compared with placebo (31% versus 49%; $P = 0.006$), while there was no significant benefit from treatment in women who did not have BV. It is unclear which component of the combination therapy was effective, and the benefit from treating BV was drawn from a subgroup analysis.

Pregnancy outcome was observed in a non-randomised study of 1138 women from 20 weeks of gestation.[11] In the observational (control) phase of the trial, BV was treated with oral clindamycin 300 mg twice daily for seven days only in symptomatic women. All women were screened for chlamydia, gonorrhoea and syphilis and appropriate treatment prescribed. In the treatment phase, women were screened for BV and treated with the same clindamycin regimen, while trichomoniasis was treated with oral metronidazole. The rate of preterm birth was reduced by 50% in the treatment phase compared with the observational phase (9.8% of 194 versus 18.8% of 171). The population studied, however, had a high prevalence of BV and sexually transmitted diseases, and the methodology was not considered to be as valid as a randomised double-blind placebo-controlled trial.

The current recommendation by the Centers for Disease Control and Prevention[64] and the *Drug and Therapeutics Bulletin*[65] is that it is reasonable to screen and treat BV in high-risk pregnancies, based on the findings of the above studies.

Table 14.1.   Published trials of antibiotic treatment for bacterial vaginosis (BV) in pregnancy

Study	Design	Population	Diagnosis	Intervention	Active drug	Control	P
Systemic treatment							
Morales[62]	RDBPCT 13–20 weeks	Prior PTB and BV	Amsel	Metronidazole 250 mg tds 7 days	n = 44 PTL: 27% PTB: 18%	n = 36 PTL: 78% PTB: 39%	<0.05 <0.05
Hauth[63]	RDBPCT 22–24 weeks	Prior PTB or weight <50 kg	Amsel	Metronidazole 250 mg tds and erythromycin 333 mg tds 7 days Repeated[a]	n = 426 PTB: 26%	n = 190 PTB: 36%	= 0.01
McDonald[66]	RPCT 16–26 weeks	Asymptomatic BV	Gram stain or GV >10⁷/ml	Metronidazole 400 mg bd 2 days Repeated[a]	n = 429 PTB: 7.2% SPTB: 4.7% PPROM: 2.8%	n = 428 PTB: 7.5% SPTB: 5.6% PPROM: 3.3%	= 0.9 = 0.5 = 0.7
Carey[3]	RDBPCT 23 weeks	Asymptomatic BV	Gram stain	Metronidazole 2 g day 1 and 3 Repeated[a]	n = 946 PTB: 12.2% <32 wk: 2.3%	n = 955 PTB: 12.4% <32 wk: 2.6%	>0.05 >0.05
McGregor[11]	Prospective cohort 22–29 weeks	All women	Modified Amsel and Gram stain	Clindamycin 300 mg bd 7 days for women with BV	n = 559 <30 wk: 0.9% PPROM: 3.4%	n = 579 <30 wk: 1.8% PPROM: 3.4%	= 0.1 = 0.9
Topical treatment							
McGregor[74]	RDBPCT 16–27 weeks	All BV	Modified Amsel and Gram stain	Clindamycin cream od 7 days	n = 60 PTB: 15% PPROM: 15%	n = 69 PTB: 7.2% PPROM: 16.2%	= 0.16 = 0.85
Joesoef[73]	RDPCT 14–26 weeks	All BV	Gram stain and pH >4.5	Clindamycin cream od 7 days	n = 340 PTB: 15%	n = 341 PTB: 13.5%	= 0.6

[a] treatment repeated after 2–4 weeks in women with persistent BV; bd = twice daily; GV = concentration of *Gardnerella vaginalis* in vaginal fluid; od = once daily; PPROM = preterm prelabour rupture of the membranes; PTB = preterm birth; PTL = preterm labour; RDBPCT = randomised double-blind placebo-controlled trial; RPCT = randomised placebo-controlled trial; SPTB = spontaneous preterm birth; tds = three times daily

Unselected pregnancies

In a large randomised controlled trial from Australia, oral metronidazole therapy did not significantly reduce the risk of preterm birth in low-risk pregnant women.[66] This study, however, introduced therapy at 24 weeks of gestation using a two-day course of oral metronidazole 400 mg twice daily. Repeat therapy was required in more than 60% of the women in the treatment arm because of treatment failure. Women considered to be at high risk for preterm birth were usually treated by their obstetrician and not randomised. A subgroup analysis showed a benefit for treatment particularly in women with a prior preterm birth who reported adherence to the medication.

The largest randomised controlled trial of treatment of asymptomatic BV in pregnancy is a multicentre study from the USA.[3] No reduction in preterm birth, or even a trend, was found from treating BV in pregnancy (Table 14.2). There was a non-significant trend for treatment to be associated with a reduction in very low birthweight (less than 1.5 kg). Does this mean that antibiotic therapy is not the answer?

The study has limitations. Only a small proportion of potential subjects were randomised. A total of 29 625 women were considered for screening at a gestational age between eight and 23 weeks. Reasons for exclusion included vaginal symptoms (1437), antibiotics (1037), medical conditions (1303) and refused consent (1294), leaving 21 965 to be screened. The investigators identified 7393 women with BV: a further 853 were excluded because of co-infection with *Trichomonas*. Further exclusions were due to the following: ineligible (3339), refused consent (651), missed appointment (421) and results only available after recruitment ended (193). Thus only 1953 women from the original 29 625 were randomised. The exclusion of symptomatic women may also be important.

The intervention was 2 g metronidazole or placebo, taken under supervision in the clinic and repeated at home two days later. The course was repeated four weeks later. This is an unconventional treatment and may not be optimal for treating upper genital tract infection. If the mechanism for preterm birth is due to chorioamnionitis caused by a spectrum of BV-associated organisms, using metronidazole late in gestation may not be sufficient to improve outcome. For instance, it has limited activity against *M. hominis*, *G. vaginalis* and *Mobiluncus* spp. The treatment was administered relatively late, often after 20 weeks of gestation. In summary, the intervention may be 'too little, too late'. Despite that, it is disappointing that there was not even a trend for a reduction in preterm birth. This study should not, however, be used as justification for therapeutic nihilism, as there are other studies that have shown a benefit from antibiotic treatment.

BV is also associated with late miscarriages[8,11] and tends to resolve spontaneously as pregnancy progresses.[67,68] If screening and treatment are performed around the 24th

Table 14.2. Results of a multicentre study of metronidazole 2 g stat, repeated after 48 hours; both treatments were repeated four weeks later[3]

Outcome	Metronidazole % (n = 953)	Placebo % (n = 966)	RR (95% CI)
PTB < 37 weeks	12.2	12.5	1.0 (0.8–1.2)
PTB < 35 weeks	5.0	5.1	1.0 (0.7–1.5)
PTB < 32 weeks	2.3	2.7	0.9 (0.5–1.5)
Birthweight < 2.5 kg	10.9	11.4	1.0 (0.7–1.2)
Birthweight < 1.5 kg	2.0	2.7	0.7 (0.4–1.3)

PTB = preterm birth

week of gestation, the opportunity to prevent late miscarriage and to treat cases in which BV has resolved spontaneously has been missed. Such spontaneous resolution, however, does not modify the risk of preterm birth. In a follow-up study of 92 pregnant women with BV, it resolved spontaneously in approximately 50% but the risk of preterm birth was unaltered.[69] An unpublished study looked at the risk of preterm delivery in women not randomised because their BV spontaneously resolved after screening.[70] Their incidence of preterm birth was similar to that of women randomised to the placebo arm. The question still remains whether screening for and treating BV very early in the second trimester may yet be beneficial, even in the so-called low-risk pregnancy. The optimal time to introduce therapy is, however, unknown. Moreover, the efficacy of short-course treatments such as single-dose or two-day course has not been established for pregnant women. Longer courses of treatment may be better.

Treatment agent and route of administration

Antibiotic treatment of BV in nonpregnant women

The treatment of BV was reviewed in 1998.[2] Overall, the cure rates immediately after treatment with oral metronidazole may reach 95%, dropping off to 80% after four weeks in open studies and to less than 70% in blinded studies.[1] Following successful treatment, 14–41% of women experience a recurrence. The high rate of recurrence of BV makes comparisons between trials using different lengths of follow-up impossible. There is no uniformly agreed method of defining clinical cure or 'improvement'.

Lactobacillus replacement therapy

The therapeutic replacement of *Lactobacillus acidophilus* and the application of yoghurt into the vagina have both failed to provide relief beyond the next menstrual period.[1] *L. acidophilus* may not be the optimum organism for H_2O_2 production and colonisation of the vagina. A preparation of *L. crispatus and L. jensenii* is being evaluated as adjunctive therapy, with promising results.[71]

Rationale for choice in pregnancy

Topical metronidazole 0.75% gel and clindamycin 2% cream, dosed for five and seven nights respectively, have shown similar short-term efficacy to oral metronidazole. Unlike clindamycin, metronidazole is not active against lactobacilli and may allow a quicker restoration of normal vaginal flora. However, while anaerobic bacteria are highly sensitive to metronidazole, *G. vaginalis*, *M. hominis* and *Mobiluncus* spp. are not. Failure to eradicate *G. vaginalis* has been suggested as the cause of recurrence of BV.[72]

Women with BV may also have endometrial colonisation by BV organisms and subclinical endometritis.[36] Although topical clindamycin cream eradicates BV in pregnancy and reduces the activity of mucinase and sialidase in the vagina, it has not been shown to reduce the risk of preterm birth, presumably because intravaginal medication may not eradicate BV organisms in the endometrial cavity.[73,74] Macrolide antibiotics such as erythromycin, clindamycin and azithromycin have anti-inflammatory properties. They have been shown to downregulate TNF production in response to infection. This could be useful in minimising release of cytokines in the uterus when treatment for BV is prescribed in pregnancy.

However, an unpublished randomised controlled trial of clindamycin intravaginal cream in 404 pregnant women with BV showed a trend towards reduction of preterm birth in the 199 women treated with topical clindamycin compared with 205 women treated with placebo (8 of 199 [4.1%] versus 18 of 205 [9%]; $P = 0.06$).[70] Initially a three-day course was administered, followed by a seven-day course one month later if BV persisted. The success of this treatment, compared with the previously reported studies of clindamycin cream that showed no reduction in preterm birth,[73,74] might be due to early administration with the majority of subjects treated at less than 16 weeks of gestation, and the re-treatment. Despite this as-yet unpublished study, if treatment is indicated in pregnancy the oral route is recommended.

BV and HIV acquisition

Acquisition of HIV in pregnancy or the puerperium is a potential risk for the fetus and infant. It would seem unlikely that BV could increase the efficiency of HIV transmission as it is not an ulcerative or inflammatory genital condition.[75] However, there are *in vitro* data demonstrating the ability of H_2O_2-producing lactobacilli to kill HIV.[76] A study of 144 female sex workers in Thailand found an association between BV and HIV seropositivity (OR 2.7; 95% CI 1.3–5.0).[77] In a cross-sectional study of 4718 Ugandan women, Sewankambo *et al.*[78] demonstrated a two-fold increase in the prevalence of HIV-1 in women with severe BV ($P < 0.0001$) and interpreted their results to imply that BV was a risk factor for HIV acquisition.

Taha *et al.*[79] addressed the temporal relationship between BV and HIV seroconversion in a longitudinal follow-up study of 1196 pregnant and postnatal women in Malawi. In women followed antenatally for a median of 3.4 months, 27 seroconverted by the time of delivery. Postnatally, there were 97 seroconversions among 1169 seronegative women followed for a median of 2.5 years. BV was significantly associated with antenatal and postnatal HIV seroconversion (OR 3.7 and 2.3 respectively). Such acquisition during pregnancy or the puerperium represents a high risk of transmission to the fetus, particularly in a population in which prolonged breastfeeding is the norm.

These studies suggest that women with disturbances of vaginal flora have an increased risk of HIV acquisition or seroconversion and that the severity of the BV (the degree of lactobacilli depletion) is directly correlated with an increased risk of seropositivity. Intervention studies are required to examine the potential benefit of the treatment of BV in reducing susceptibility to HIV.

Conclusions

BV is associated with adverse pregnancy outcome and infectious morbidity following gynaecological surgery. Intervention studies in women who are BV-positive and at high risk of preterm birth show benefit. In low-risk pregnant women, the role of antibiotic treatment of BV is yet to be established. Future treatment studies should use markers of additional risk to identify women who might benefit most from treatment. Good cure rates are achieved with either metronidazole or clindamycin, although recurrence is also common. If treatment is indicated in pregnancy, it should be systemic rather than topical. Increasingly, good laboratory and clinical evidence suggest that BV may be a risk factor for heterosexual HIV transmission. Further studies are required to clarify these areas.

References

1. Larsson PG. Treatment of bacterial vaginosis. *Int J STD AIDS* 1992;**3**:239–47.
2. Hay PE. Therapy of bacterial vaginosis. *J Antimicrob Chemother* 1998;**41**:6–9.
3. Carey JC, Klebanoff MA, Hauth JC, Hillier SL, Thom EA, Ernest JM, *et al.* Metronidazole to prevent preterm delivery in pregnant women with asymptomatic bacterial vaginosis. *N Engl J Med* 2000;**342**:534–40.
4. Mayaud P. Tackling bacterial vaginosis and HIV in developing countries. *Lancet* 1997;**350**:530–1.
5. Mead PB. Epidemiology of bacterial vaginosis. *Am J Obstet Gynecol* 1993;**169**:446–9.
6. Bump RC, Buesching WJ. Bacterial vaginosis in virginal and sexually active adolescent females: evidence against exclusive sexual transmission. *Am J Obstet Gynecol* 1988;**158**:935–9.
7. Hay PE, Taylor-Robinson D, Lamont RF. Diagnosis of bacterial vaginosis in a gynaecology clinic. *Br J Obstet Gynaecol* 1992;**99**:63–6.
8. Hay PE, Lamont RF, Taylor-Robinson D, Morgan DJ, Ison C, Pearson J. Abnormal bacterial colonisation of the genital tract and subsequent preterm delivery and late miscarriage. *BMJ* 1994;**308**:295–8.
9. Blackwell AL, Thomas PD, Wareham K, Emery SJ. Health gains from screening for infection of the lower genital tract in women attending for termination of pregnancy. *Lancet* 1993;**342**:206–10.
10. Ralph SG, Rutherford AJ, Wilson JD. Influence of bacterial vaginosis on conception and miscarriage in the first trimester: cohort study. *BMJ* 1999;**319**:220–3.
11. McGregor JA, French JI, Parker R, Draper D, Patterson E, Jones W, *et al.* Prevention of premature birth by screening and treatment for common genital tract infections: results of a prospective controlled evaluation. *Am J Obstet Gynecol* 1995;**173**:157–67.
12. Paxton LA, Sewankambo N, Gray R, Serwadda D, McNairn D, Li C, *et al.* Asymptomatic non-ulcerative genital tract infections in a rural Ugandan population. *Sex Transm Infect* 1998;**74**:421–5.
13. Priestley CJ, Jones BM, Dhar J, Goodwin L. What is normal vaginal flora? *Genitourin Med* 1997;**73**:23–8.
14. Schwebke JR, Richey CM, Weiss HL. Correlation of behaviors with microbiological changes in vaginal flora. *J Infect Dis* 1999;**180**:1632–6.
15. Keane FE, Ison CA, Taylor-Robinson D. A longitudinal study of the vaginal flora over a menstrual cycle. *Int J STD AIDS* 1997;**8**:489–94.
16. Hay PE. Recurrent bacterial vaginosis. *Dermatol Clin* 1998;**16**:769–74.
17. Nilsson U, Hellberg D, Shoubnikova M, Nilsson S, Mardh PA. Sexual behavior risk factors associated with bacterial vaginosis and *Chlamydia trachomatis* infection. *Sex Transm Dis* 1997;**24**:241–6.
18. Klebanoff SJ, Hillier SL, Eschenbach DA, Waltersdorph AM. Control of the microbial flora of the vagina by H_2O_2-generating lactobacilli. *J Infect Dis* 1991;**164**:94–100.
19. Hawes SE, Hillier SL, Benedetti J, Stevens CE, Koutsky LA, Wolner-Hanssen P, *et al.* Hydrogen peroxide-producing lactobacilli and acquisition of vaginal infections. *J Infect Dis* 1996;**174**:1058–63.
20. Rajamanoharan S, Low N, Jones SB, Pozniak AL. Bacterial vaginosis, ethnicity, and the use of genital cleaning agents: a case control study. *Sex Transm Dis* 1999;**26**:404–9.
21. Blackwell AL. Vaginal bacterial phaginosis? *Sex Transm Infect* 1999;**75**:352–3.
22. Pavlova SI, Kilic AO, Mou SM, Tao L. Phage infection in vaginal lactobacilli: an *in vitro* study. *Infect Dis Obstet Gynecol* 1997;**5**:36–44.
23. Tao L, Pavlova SI, Mou SM, Ma W, Kilic AO. Analysis of *Lactobacillus* products for phages and bacteriocins that inhibit vaginal lactobacilli. *Infect Dis Obstet Gynecol* 1997;**5**:244–51.
24. Hay PE, Ugwumadu A, Chowns J. Sex, thrush and bacterial vaginosis. *Int J STD AIDS* 1997;**8**:603–8.
25. Furr PM, Taylor-Robinson D. Oestradiol-induced infection of the genital tract of female mice by *Mycoplasma hominis*. *J Gen Microbiol* 1989;**135**:2743–9.
26. Levison ME, Corman LC, Carrington ER, Kaye D. Quantitative microflora of the vagina. *Am J Obstet*

Gynecol 1977;**127**:80–5.

27. Kornman KS, Loesche WJ. Effects of estradiol and progesterone on *Bacteroides melaninogenicus* and *Bacteroides gingivalis*. *Infect Immun* 1982;**35**:256–63.

28. Amsel R, Totten PA, Spiegel CA, Chen KC, Eschenbach D, Holmes KK. Nonspecific vaginitis. Diagnostic criteria and microbial and epidemiologic associations. *Am J Med* 1983;**74**:14–22.

29. Sobel JD. Vaginitis. *N Engl J Med* 1997;**337**:1896–903.

30. Nugent RP, Krohn MA, Hillier SL. Reliability of diagnosing bacterial vaginosis is improved by a standardized method of Gram stain interpretation. *J Clin Microbiol* 1991;**29**:297–301.

31. Rosenstein IJ, Morgan DJ, Sheehan M, Lamont RF, Taylor-Robinson D. Bacterial vaginosis in pregnancy: distribution of bacterial species in different Gram-stain categories of the vaginal flora. *J Med Microbiol* 1996;**45**:120–6.

32. Thomason JL, Gelbart SM, Wilcoski LM, Peterson AK, Jilly BJ, Hamilton PR. Proline aminopeptidase activity as a rapid diagnostic test to confirm bacterial vaginosis. *Obstet Gynecol* 1988;**71**:607–11.

33. O'Dowd TC, West RR, Winterburn PJ, Hewlins MJ. Evaluation of a rapid diagnostic test for bacterial vaginosis. *Br J Obstet Gynaecol* 1996;**103**:366–70.

34. Sweet RL. Sexually transmitted diseases. Pelvic inflammatory disease and infertility in women. *Infect Dis Clin North Am* 1987;**1**:199–215.

35. Lund KS, McGregor JA Parsons A Williamson L. Uterine transport of ultrasound contrast medium in nonpregnant women: A key to understanding bacterial vaginosis (BV) associated endometritis and salpingitis. Second International Conference on Bacterial Vaginosis, 17–20 September 1998, Aspen, Colorado, USA.

36. Korn AP, Bolan G, Padian N, Ohm-Smith M, Schachter J, Landers DV. Plasma cell endometritis in women with symptomatic bacterial vaginosis. *Obstet Gynecol* 1995;**85**:387–90.

37. Baumann P, Romero R. Intra-amniotic infection, cytokines and premature labor. *Wien Klin Wochenschr* 1995;**107**:598–607.

38. Gibbs RS, Romero R, Hillier SL, Eschenbach DA, Sweet RL. A review of premature birth and subclinical infection. *Am J Obstet Gynecol* 1992;**166**:1515–28.

39. Platz-Christensen JJ, Mattsby-Baltzer I, Thomsen P, Wiqvist N. Endotoxin and interleukin-1 alpha in the cervical mucus and vaginal fluid of pregnant women with bacterial vaginosis. *Am J Obstet Gynecol* 1993;**169**:1161–6.

40. Yoon BH, Jun JK, Romero R, Park KH, Gomez R, Choi JH, *et al*. Amniotic fluid inflammatory cytokines (interleukin-6, interleukin-1beta, and tumor necrosis factor-alpha), neonatal brain white matter lesions, and cerebral palsy. *Am J Obstet Gynecol* 1997;**177**:19–26.

41. Sampson JE, Theve RP, Blatman RN, Shipp TD, Bianchi DW, Ward BE, *et al*. Fetal origin of amniotic fluid polymorphonuclear leukocytes. *Am J Obstet Gynecol* 1997;**176**:77–81.

42. Gomez R, Ghezzi F, Romero R, Yoon BH, Mazor M, Berry SM. Two thirds of human fetuses with microbial invasion of the amniotic cavity have a detectable systemic cytokine response before birth. *Am J Obstet Gynecol* 1998;**176** Suppl:S14.

43. Kahn MA, De Vellis J. Regulation of an oligodendrocyte progenitor cell line by the interleukin-6 family of cytokines. *Glia* 1994;**12**:87–98.

44. Robbins DS, Shirazi Y, Drysdale BE, Lieberman A, Shin AS, Shin ML. Production of cytotoxic factor for oligodendrocytes by stimulated astrocytes. *J Immunol* 1987;**139**:2593–7.

45. Murphy DJ, Hope DL, Johnson A. Neonatal risk factors for cerebral palsy in very preterm babies: case–control study. *BMJ* 1997;**314**:404–8.

46. Murphy DJ, Sellers S, Mackenzie IZ, Yudkin PL, Johnson AM. Case–control study of antenatal and intrapartum risk factors for cerebral palsy in very preterm singleton babies. *Lancet* 1995;**346**:1449–54.

47. Grether JK, Nelson KB. Maternal infection and cerebral palsy in infants of normal birth weight. *JAMA* 1997;**278**:207–11.

48. Perlman JM, Risser R, Broyles RS. Bilateral cystic periventricular leukomalacia in the premature infant: associated risk factors. *Pediatrics* 1996;**97**:822–7.

49. Zupan V, Gonzalez P, Lacaze-Masmonteil T, Boithias C, d'Allest AM, Dehan M, *et al*. Periventricular leukomalacia: risk factors revisited. *Dev Med Child Neurol* 1996;**38**:1061–7.

50. Goldenberg RL, Thom E, Moawad AH, Johnson F, Roberts J, Caritis SN. The preterm prediction study: fetal fibronectin, bacterial vaginosis, and peripartum infection. NICHD Maternal Fetal Medicine Units Network. *Obstet Gynecol* 1996;**87**:656–60.

51. Kekki M, Kurki T, Paavonen J, Rutanen EM. Insulin-like growth factor binding protein-1 in cervix as a marker of infectious complications in pregnant women with bacterial vaginosis [letter]. *Lancet* 1999;**353**:1494.

52. Thorsen P, Jensen IP, Jeune B, Ebbesen N, Arpi M, Bremmelgaard A, *et al*. Few microorganisms associated with bacterial vaginosis may constitute the pathologic core: a population-based microbiologic

study among 3596 pregnant women. *Am J Obstet Gynecol* 1998;**178**:580–7.

53. Cauci S, Thorsen P, Schendel D, Bremmelgaard A, Quadrifoglio F, Guaschino S. IgA mucosal response, sialidase and prolidase activities as markers for low birth weight in women with BV. Third International Meeting on Bacterial Vaginosis, 14–17 September 1998, Ystad, Sweden.

54. Silver HM, Sperling RS, St Clair PJ, Gibbs RS. Evidence relating bacterial vaginosis to intraamniotic infection. *Am J Obstet Gynecol* 1989;**161**:808–12.

55. Martius J, Eschenbach DA. The role of bacterial vaginosis as a cause of amniotic fluid infection, chorioamnionitis and prematurity – a review. *Arch Gynecol Obstet* 1990;**247**:1–13.

56. Hillier SL, Martius J, Krohn M, Kiviat N, Holmes KK, Eschenbach DA. A case–control study of chorioamnionic infection and histologic chorioamnionitis in prematurity. *N Engl J Med* 1988;**319**:972–8.

57. Liversedge NH, Turner A, Horner PJ, Keay SD, Jenkins JM, Hull MG. The influence of bacterial vaginosis on *in vitro* fertilization and embryo implantation during assisted reproduction treatment. *Hum Reprod* 1999;**14**:2411–15.

58. Llahi-Camp JM, Rai R, Ison C, Regan L, Taylor-Robinson D. Association of bacterial vaginosis with a history of second trimester miscarriage. *Hum Reprod* 1996;**11**:1575–8.

59. Hillier SL, Nugent RP, Eschenbach DA, Krohn MA, Gibbs RS, Martin DH, *et al.* Association between bacterial vaginosis and preterm delivery of a low-birth-weight infant. The Vaginal Infections and Prematurity Study Group. *N Engl J Med* 1995;**333**:1737–42.

60. Kurki T, Sivonen A, Renkonen OV, Savia E , Ylikorkala O. Bacterial vaginosis in early pregnancy and pregnancy outcome. *Obstet Gynecol* 1992;**80**:173–7.

61. Watts DH, Krohn MA, Hillier SL, Eschenbach DA. Bacterial vaginosis as a risk factor for post-cesarean endometritis. *Obstet Gynecol* 1990;**75**:52–8.

62. Morales WJ, Schorr S, Albritton J. Effect of metronidazole in patients with preterm birth in preceding pregnancy and bacterial vaginosis: a placebo-controlled, double-blind study. *Am J Obstet Gynecol* 1994;**171**:345–7.

63. Hauth JC, Goldenberg RL, Andrews WW, DuBard MB, Copper RL. Reduced incidence of preterm delivery with metronidazole and erythromycin in women with bacterial vaginosis. *N Engl J Med* 1995;**333**:1732–6.

64. Centers for Disease Control and Prevention. 1998 guidelines for treatment of sexually transmitted diseases. *MMWR Morb Mortal Wkly Rep* 1998;**47**:1–111.

65. Anonymous. Management of bacterial vaginosis. *Drug Ther Bull* 1998;**36**:33–5.

66. McDonald HM, O'Loughlin JA, Vigneswaran R, Jolley PT, Harvey JA, Bof A, *et al.* Impact of metronidazole therapy on preterm birth in women with bacterial vaginosis flora (*Gardnerella vaginalis*): a randomised, placebo controlled trial. *Br J Obstet Gynaecol* 1997;**104**:1391–7.

67. Hay PE, Morgan DJ, Ison CA, Bhide SA, Romney M, McKenzie P, *et al.* A longitudinal study of bacterial vaginosis during pregnancy. *Br J Obstet Gynaecol* 1994;**101**:1048–53.

68. Platz-Christensen JJ, Pernevi P, Hagmar B, Andersson E, Brandberg A, Wiqvist N. A longitudinal follow-up of bacterial vaginosis during pregnancy. *Acta Obstet Gynecol Scand* 1993;**72**:99–102.

69. Gratacos E, Figueras F, Barranco M, Vila J, Cararach V, Alonso PL, *et al.* Spontaneous recovery of bacterial vaginosis during pregnancy is not associated with an improved perinatal outcome. *Acta Obstet Gynecol Scand* 1998;**77**:37–40.

70. Lamont RF, Duncan SLB, Mandal D, Morgan DJ, Sheehan M. Pregnancy outcome following use of clindamycin intravaginal cream (CVC) for the treatment of BV. A prospective, randomised, double-blind placebo controlled study. *Perinatal and Neonatal Medicine* 1998;**3** Suppl 2. Abstract 4.2 (a).

71. Hillier S. Recolonization of the vagina with an exogenous strain of *Lactobacillus crispatus*. Second International Conference on Bacterial Vaginosis, 17–20 September 1998, Aspen, Colorado, USA.

72. Ferris DG, Litaker MS, Woodward L, Mathis D, Hendrich J. Treatment of bacterial vaginosis: a comparison of oral metronidazole, metronidazole vaginal gel, and clindamycin vaginal cream. *J Fam Pract* 1995;**41**:443–9.

73. Joesoef MR, Hillier SL, Wiknjosastro G, Sumampouw H, Linnan M, Norojono W, *et al.* Intravaginal clindamycin treatment for bacterial vaginosis: effects on preterm delivery and low birth weight. *Am J Obstet Gynecol* 1995;**173**:1527–31.

74. McGregor JA, French JI, Jones W, Milligan K, McKinney PJ, Patterson E, *et al.* Bacterial vaginosis is associated with prematurity and vaginal fluid mucinase and sialidase: results of a controlled trial of topical clindamycin cream. *Am J Obstet Gynecol* 1994;**170**:1048–59.

75. Ugwumadu A, Hay P, Taylor-Robinson D. HIV-1 infection associated with abnormal vaginal flora morphology and bacterial vaginosis. *Lancet* 1997;**350**:1251.

76. Klebanoff SJ, Coombs RW. Viricidal effect of Lactobacillus acidophilus on human immunodeficiency virus type 1: Possible role in heterosexual transmission. *J Exp Med* 1991;**174**:289–92.

77. Cohen CR, Duerr A, Pruithithada N, Rugpao S, Hillier S, Garcia P, *et al*. Bacterial vaginosis and HIV seroprevalence among female commercial sex workers in Chiang Mai, Thailand. *AIDS* 1995;**9**:1093–7.
78. Sewankambo N, Gray RH, Wawer MJ, Paxton L, McNaim D, Wabwire-Mangen F, *et al*. HIV-1 infection associated with abnormal vaginal flora morphology and bacterial vaginosis. *Lancet* 1997;**350**:546–50.
79. Taha TE, Hoover DR, Dallabetta GA, Kumwenda NI, Mtimavalye LA, Yang LP, *et al*. Bacterial vaginosis and disturbances of vaginal flora: association with increased acquisition of HIV. *AIDS* 1998;**12**:1699–706.

Chapter 15

Toxoplasmosis and pregnancy

Richard E Holliman

Introduction

The protozoan parasite *Toxoplasma gondii* is an established cause of fetal loss and severe neonatal disease. Sequelae of congenital infection include mental retardation and ocular disease.[1] A number of European countries have introduced national, regional or local screening programmes intended to reduce the incidence of congenital toxoplasmosis,[2] although the effectiveness of such an approach is controversial.[3] Routine screening for toxoplasmosis during pregnancy is not recommended in most countries worldwide, including the UK. This chapter considers the evidence base influencing these decisions.

Toxoplasmosis in pregnancy

Pregnant women acquire toxoplasmosis by ingestion of one of the life forms of the parasite. Sporocysts are excreted in the faeces of the primary host of the parasite, members of the cat family, and may contaminate inadequately washed vegetables and salad plants. Similarly, contaminated soil may allow the transfer of sporocysts to the mouth via the hands while gardening. In addition, food animals, notably sheep and pigs, can become infected by ingestion of infected pasture leading to human infection through eating inadequately cooked meat containing viable parasitic tissue cysts (Figure 15.1). The relative importance of these routes of transmission may vary between geographical regions. One French study[4] found poor hand hygiene to be the major risk factor for acquiring toxoplasmosis in pregnancy whereas consumption of undercooked meats was the most important route of transmission among women of reproductive age in Yugoslavia.[5] Risk-factor data are not available for the UK, although viable *Toxoplasma gondii* has been isolated from ready-to-eat cured meat in London.[6] Following penetration of the gut epithelium, the parasite spreads around the body in the blood and lymphatic system. In most instances, the duration of parasitaemia is less than three weeks. Consequently, it is proposed that placental infection is only a

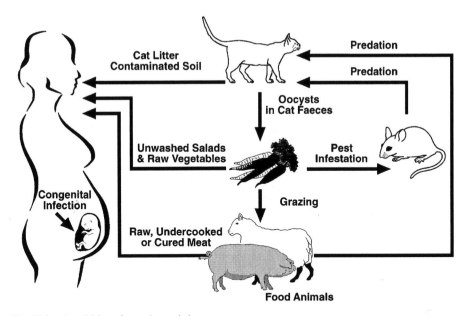

Fig. 15.1.   Acquisition of toxoplasmosis in pregnancy

significant risk if the mother acquires her infection during or immediately before the onset of pregnancy. Only a minority of maternal infections break the placental barrier to establish an infection of the fetus.[1] The risk of congenital transmission is greatest when maternal infection is acquired in late pregnancy. Overall, approximately 30–40% of maternal infections acquired during pregnancy result in congenital toxoplasmosis.[7] Acute maternal toxoplasmosis is usually asymptomatic. The incidence of toxoplasmosis acquired in pregnancy in the UK is not fully established. Localised studies suggest a rate of 1–2 infections per 1000 pregnancies.[8] Extrapolation from data acquired from the nonpregnant population indicates that the incidence of infection is falling in many developed countries including the UK, reflecting changes in farming techniques, food preparation and the use of deep freezing to store meats, a process that destroys the cysts of the parasite.[9] However, mathematical modelling shows that such changes may lead to an initial increase in the number of cases of congenital toxoplasmosis as the proportion of women of childbearing age susceptible to infection rises.[10] Approximately 85% of pregnant women in the UK are susceptible to toxoplasmosis at booking. Higher rates of toxoplasmosis have been found in women born outside the UK, notably Africa, the Caribbean, Ireland and Pakistan,[11] which may reflect differences in dietary habit, cat population and soil contact.

The relative importance of long-standing maternal preconceptual infection leading to congenital toxoplasmosis remains poorly defined. Consensus opinion is that maternal infection acquired before the onset of the pregnancy is rarely transmitted to the fetus unless the mother is significantly immunosuppressed.[1,3] However, case reports of this phenomenon continue to appear[12] and prospective studies have not been performed.[13]

Congenital toxoplasmosis

Whereas the risk of transmission is greatest in the third trimester and smallest in the first trimester, the converse is true of the risk of severe congenital disease as a result of toxoplasmosis infection. Only 10% of congenitally infected babies are significantly affected at birth.[1] The most recent study of the incidence of congenital toxoplasmosis in the UK, performed by the British Paediatric Surveillance Unit in 1989–90, found 14 cases, not all of which were severely affected.[14] Calculations based on an incidence of acute toxoplasmosis in pregnancy of 2 per 1000, 40% transmission to the fetus and 10% of congenitally infected babies showing severe disease at birth predict approximately 50 cases of severe congenital toxoplasmosis in the UK each year.[15]

The classical triad of congenital toxoplasmosis comprises hydrocephalus, intracranial calcification and choroidoretinitis. Non-specific signs include rash, growth restriction, jaundice, hepatosplenomegaly and thrombocytopenia.[13] Intrauterine death can occur, particularly in association with infection established during the first trimester. Late-onset sequelae of congenital toxoplasmosis include mental restriction and ocular defects. The frequency of these sequelae is uncertain. One small study found that four out of five children with significant toxoplasmosis at birth who subsequently received antiparasitic therapy went on to develop eye lesions as did four out of six children who were asymptomatic at birth and remained untreated.[16,17] A similarly poor prognosis was found in a USA study where three of 13 children, asymptomatic at birth, developed unilateral blindness, five had bilateral choroidoretinitis and three had unilateral retinitis. In addition, five of the 13 children developed neurological defects.[18] Partly based on findings such as these, it was generally accepted that the great majority of cases of toxoplasmosis-associated eye disease seen in children and adults represented late sequelae of congenital infection rather then a consequence of acute, postnatal toxoplasmosis.[1,19] This dogma has, however, been challenged. Calculations based on prevalence data proposed that the proportion of cases of ocular toxoplasmosis resulting from postnatal infection to those resulting from congenital infection is in the range 2:1 to 5:1.[20] Studies in the southern region of Brazil have detected a large number of cases of ocular toxoplasmosis clinically and serologically linked to acute postnatal infection.[21]

Uncertainty over the incidence of congenital toxoplasmosis in the UK and over the frequency of clinical sequelae makes it difficult to determine the level of morbidity associated with this condition. Furthermore, advances in the general management of diseases such as hydrocephalus, deafness and visual impairment are likely to have reduced the degree of handicap resulting from congenital toxoplasmosis.

Diagnosis

The diagnosis of acute toxoplasmosis in pregnant women usually relies on laboratory testing as the great majority of cases are asymptomatic or associated with only a mild non-specific illness. Most reliable is the documentation of immunoglobulin G (IgG) seroconversion in closely paired sera but this information is routinely available only in regions where antenatal screening is performed. The detection of maternal *Toxoplasma*-specific immunoglobulin M (IgM) can present interpretation difficulties.

Depending on the sensitivity of the assay used, IgM may be detected for a minimum of three months to more than 18 months after the onset of infection.[22] Consequently, it is necessary to understand the performance of the IgM assay used locally in order to define the clinical significance of positive findings. Most reference laboratories use a sequence of tests in order to establish the likely duration of maternal toxoplasmosis and, by comparison with the gestational age, calculate the risk of congenital infection and neonatal damage. Various combinations of immunoglobulin M, A, E and/or G avidity tests may be employed but the optimum approach is not defined.[23] Where the risk of toxoplasmosis acquired during pregnancy cannot be excluded it becomes necessary to attempt to establish the status of the fetus. Ultrasound investigation will detect most cases of symptomatic infection[24] but is not helpful in the 90% of cases of congenital toxoplasmosis that are subclinical up to the time of delivery.[1]

Serological testing of fetal blood obtained by cordocentesis used to be widely promoted.[25] However, the advent of gene amplification has led to a shift to testing amniotic fluid using the polymerase chain reaction (PCR), thus reducing fetal mortality and morbidity associated with sampling.[26] While some groups have claimed good results,[27] the incidence of assay contamination remains of concern, with up to one-third of all reactions proving to be false positive results.[28]

Extended postnatal investigation of the child is usually required to confirm or refute the diagnosis of congenital toxoplasmosis and persistence of specific IgG at the age of 12 months remains the 'gold standard'.[1,3] Comparison of mother-to-baby immune profiles by Western blot or enzyme-linked immunofiltration assay has shown encouraging results and may allow reliable diagnosis of infected children soon after birth (see Table 15.1).[29]

Table 15.1.   Investigation of toxoplasmosis associated with pregnancy

Population	Purpose of investigation	Specific test
Female population	Preconceptual serotesting	IgG
Pregnant woman	Prenatal testing: routine screening, anxiety but no specific symptoms, compatible clinical illness	IgG/IgM
Pregnant woman with clinical/laboratory evidence of recent infection	Assessment of the duration of infection	IgM with defined sensitivity IgG avidity IgA Differential agglutination
Fetus with enhanced risk of congenital toxoplasmosis	Detection of acute infection	Detailed ultrasound examination Parasitological culture of amniotic fluid Molecular studies on amniotic fluid
Baby with suspected congenital toxoplasmosis	Detection of acute immune response	Serial IgG measurement Mother–baby serological comparison (Western blot, ELIFA[a])
	Detection of acute infection	Parasitological culture of placental tissue and neonatal blood

[a] enzyme-linked immunofiltration assay

Management

Antiparasitic therapy can be given to acutely infected mothers to attempt to prevent congenital transmission, or to limit fetal damage after congenital infection has been established. None of the current drugs available has reliable activity against the cyst form of *T. gondii* so it is not possible to eradicate infection. Treatment is aimed at destroying the actively dividing trophozoite life-form of the parasite, thus limiting tissue damage.

When acute maternal infection is diagnosed, termination of pregnancy is often requested. Women who elect to continue the pregnancy are given spiramycin therapy each day until delivery in an attempt to prevent congenital transmission. Unfortunately, the efficacy of such treatment is unclear, with studies reporting conflicting results.[30] Other groups have found that, although fetal transmission is not affected, therapeutic intervention may reduce the severity of congenital disease.[31] In cases of confirmed congenital infection, the more active but toxic combination of sulphadiazine plus pyrimethamine is used for both prenatal and postnatal therapy, continuing until the child is 12 months of age, in an attempt to minimise tissue damage in early life until the child's immune system matures sufficiently to control the infection. Short courses of combination therapy are alternated with courses of spiramycin in a repeating cycle. Systemic steroids may be given to the neonate if neurological damage is marked.[32]

There are no randomised, controlled trials assessing the efficacy of treatment for congenital toxoplasmosis.[33] A number of studies have monitored the outcome after antiparasitic therapy with or without comparison to historical controls.[34,35] Major defects of this approach include bias in case inclusion and the failure to consider the effect of therapeutic abortion when calculating disease rates. Acute exacerbation of ocular toxoplasmosis in later life following congenital infection may be treated with short-course antiparasitic and anti-inflammatory therapy, particularly if the lesion is sited centrally on the retina.[30]

Prevention

As discussed, congenital toxoplasmosis may be managed by termination of pregnancy or antiparasitic therapy given to mothers with acute infection. Such intervention constitutes secondary prevention.[3] Alternatively, primary prevention is aimed at reducing the number of women who acquire toxoplasmosis during their pregnancy. This may be achieved by providing health education, reducing the infective load in the environment or vaccinating susceptible individuals (Figure 15.2).

Health education

As human toxoplasmosis is acquired by ingestion of one of the life forms of the parasite, specific health education emphasising good hygiene and appropriate diet might reduce the incidence of infection in pregnancy. Recommendations to pregnant women should include:

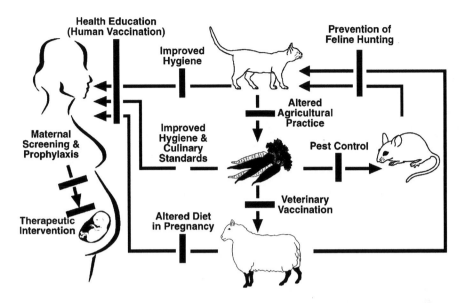

Fig. 15.2. Prevention of congenital toxoplasmosis

- avoiding raw or undercooked meat and unpasteurised dairy products
- washing or peeling fruit and vegetables before eating
- wearing gloves when gardening
- maintaining good kitchen hygiene and hand washing
- avoiding the handling of cat litter if possible. If avoidance is not possible, the litter should be changed daily, wearing gloves and washing hands thoroughly afterwards.

It has been demonstrated that health education can reduce 'risk' behaviour[36] but there are no published studies showing the effect on infection rates. Poorly designed health education material can be counterproductive, raising anxiety levels or promoting dangerous practices such as cleaning cat-litter trays with boiling water. A survey of health education material concluded that most leaflets and booklets had not received the necessary scientific appraisal and commitment required to make them effective.[37]

Environmental infective load

The level of environmental contamination with viable *T. gondii* may be reduced by measures such as vaccination of food animals,[38] protecting animal feeds from cat faeces and elimination of infectious cysts in raw meats by freezing to −20° C. The benefits of this approach have not been subject to prospective study.

Human vaccination

In the past, some regions in the UK undertook deliberate exposure of prepubescent girls to *Toxoplasma*-infected meat, thus rendering these individuals immune to acute infection during pregnancy in later life.[1] Such an approach is now considered unethical due to establishment of chronic quiescent infection that can reactivate in states of immune suppression such as malignancy, steroid therapy, organ graft/transplant or HIV infection. Research is aimed at producing a subunit vaccine that provides solid, long-lasting protection without the formation of toxoplasmosis tissue cysts in the recipient. Animal studies have shown promising results using modern genetic methods[39] but problems of toxicity and breakthrough 'wild-strain' infection remain. Nonetheless, a human vaccine is likely to be made available before 2010.

Screening

In the context of congenital toxoplasmosis, screening can be considered at the different stages of transmission of the parasite, from the environment to pregnant women, to the placenta and to the fetus (primary, secondary and tertiary prevention). The national antenatal screening programmes adopted in Austria and France incorporate elements of both primary (health education) and secondary prevention (identification of acutely infected mothers and therapeutic intervention). In these two countries, routine, preconceptual testing of women is performed, often at the time of marriage, followed by serial testing of seronegative individuals during pregnancy in an attempt to detect seroconversion.[2]

An alternative screening approach through tertiary prevention (identification of infected babies with therapeutic intervention) has been adopted in New England.[40] This system uses the routine collection of neonatal blood samples, which are stored on Guthrie cards. Serum is extracted from the cards and tested for *Toxoplasma*-specific IgM. This method will not detect IgM-negative, asymptomatic individuals, who may comprise up to one-third of all cases of congenital toxoplasmosis.[41] In an attempt to improve case capture, the Danish screening programme incorporates comparison of *Toxoplasma*-specific IgG tests on maternal first-trimester (booking) samples to that of the neonatal (Guthrie card) samples. All apparent instances of seroconversion are followed up by clinical and laboratory testing of the baby.[42] A parallel study found that IgM testing of neonatal sera alone would have detected 70–80% of cases of congenital toxoplasmosis. The major disadvantage of postnatal screening is the questionable efficacy of treatment of the infected baby in reducing the late sequelae of congenital infection.

Most models of screening have assumed full compliance with the programme when calculating the likely benefit of intervention. However, prospective studies suggest suboptimal compliance is a major problem. One UK study found only half of a group of self-selected, motivated women, previously shown to be a high risk of congenital transmission, actually completed the series of investigations required to establish the status of the child.[43] One-third of Dutch women advised to have repeat blood tests for suspected toxoplasmosis in pregnancy dropped out of the study[44] while in France over 40% of infants under investigation for congenital toxoplasmosis were followed up for no more than six weeks.[45] Consequently, improved standards of pre- and postnatal healthcare services are required to obtain the potential benefits of routine screening for toxoplasmosis in pregnancy.

Harm versus benefit

Any proposed screening programme should be assessed using the World Health Organization's 'principles of screening'. In order to establish the harm:benefit ratio of the proposed programme, information regarding the disease, diagnostic tests, treatment and administrative structure must be determined.[46] Only when there is a clear balance of benefit over harm can screening be promoted on an ethical basis. Unfortunately, there are many unanswered questions regarding screening for toxoplasmosis in pregnancy that hamper this harm:benefit assessment. The incidence of acute toxoplasmosis acquired during pregnancy is not well established and there are doubts over the rate of transmission between mother and fetus. Similarly, the proportion of children with congenital toxoplasmosis who develop disease is unclear and there is even less knowledge regarding the degree of handicap suffered.[1,7,8] Diagnostic tests for detecting acute infection have improved in recent years but most exhibit acceptable sensitivity with suboptimal specificity. As a result, many women who are not at significant risk would be subject to unnecessary tests and therapeutic intervention.[10] Detection of fetal infection has been improved by the implementation of PCR testing of amniotic fluid[27,28] but postnatal confirmation of congenital toxoplasmosis still largely relies on serial testing until 12 months of age. Patient acceptance of this prolonged diagnostic procedure is relatively poor.[43] Efficacy of therapeutic intervention remains uncertain due to the lack of properly controlled, randomised prospective studies.

Potential benefits from the initiation of routine screening for toxoplasmosis in pregnancy include a reduction in the number of babies born with congenital infection and a decrease in the severity of disease in those infected. Most women can be reassured that there is no evidence of enhanced risk of congenital infection. Many health workers find it more difficult to appreciate harm associated with a screening programme. However, every screening programme carries with it harmful sequelae. In the instance of toxoplasmosis in pregnancy, such harm includes misdiagnosis of acute maternal infection, anxiety induced by the screening procedure, diversion of finite medical resources from better established initiatives, drug toxicity and ethical concerns such as amelioration when, for example, a baby with otherwise fatal disease obtains sufficient benefit from therapy to survive with gross physical and mental handicap.[3]

In view of the complexity of the assessment and the areas of uncertainty identified, it is not surprising that health economic calculations have reached conflicting conclusions regarding the validity of screening for toxoplasmosis in pregnancy. Some have proposed that the benefits of routine screening exceed the harm.[47–50] Other authorities have considered similar data and yet concluded that routine screening would do more harm than good.[33,51,52] Little progress has been made in resolving this debate.[3]

Conclusions

At the beginning of the 21st century, the approach to toxoplasmosis in the UK remains unchanged from that defined by a multidisciplinary working group a decade before.[53] Pregnant women with cervical lymphadenopathy or 'glandular fever' syndrome should have tests for acute toxoplasmosis included in the investigations. Women expressing anxiety regarding toxoplasmosis should be given specific counselling so that only selected individuals progress to serological testing. Health education promoting good hygiene and a sensible diet should be given to all pregnant women. There is no place for routine prenatal screening for toxoplasmosis outside of ethically approved, properly constructed studies incorporating informed consent from all participants.

While further research might help to resolve at least some of the controversy in this subject, it would seem increasingly likely that the future introduction of an effective human vaccine will consign the debate over toxoplasmosis screening to the pages of history.

References

1. Remington JS, McLeod R, Desmonts G. Toxoplasmosis. In: Remington JS, Klein J, editors. *Infectious Diseases of the Fetus and Newborn Infant*, 4th ed. Philadelphia: WB Saunders; 1995. p. 140–267.
2. Thulliez P. Screening programme for congenital toxoplasmosis in France. *Scand J Infect Dis Suppl* 1992;**84**:43–5.
3. Holliman RE. Congenital toxoplasmosis: prevention, screening and treatment. *J Hosp Infect* 1995;**30**:179–90.
4. Baril L, Ancelle T, Goulet U, Thulliez P, Tirard-Fleury V, Carme B. Risk factors for *Toxoplasma* infection in pregnancy: A case–control study in France. *Scand J Infect Dis* 1999;**31**:305–9.
5. Bobic B, Jevremovic I, Marinkovic J, Sibalik D, Djurkovic-Djakovic O. Risk factors for *Toxoplasma* infection in a reproductive age female population in the area of Belgrade, Yugoslavia. *Eur J Epidemiol* 1998;**14**:605–10.
6. Warnekulasuriya MR, Johnson JD, Holliman RE Detection of *Toxoplasma gondii* in cured meats. *Int J Food Microbiol* 1998;**45**:211–15.
7. Dunn D, Wallon M, Peyron R, Petersen E, Peckham C, Gilbert R. Mother-to-child transmission of toxoplasmosis: risk estimates for clinical counselling. *Lancet* 1999;**353**:1829–33.
8. Allain JP, Palmer CR, Pearson G. Epidemiological study of latent and recent infection by *Toxoplasma gondii* in pregnant women from a regional population in the UK. *J Infect* 1998;**36**:189–96.
9. Walker J, Nokes DJ, Jennings R. Longitudinal study of *Toxoplasma* seroprevalence in South Yorkshire. *Epidemiol Infect* 1992;**108**:99–106.
10. Ades AE. Methods for estimating the incidence of primary infection in pregnancy: a reappraisal of toxoplasmosis and cytomegalovirus data. *Epidemiol Infect* 1992;**108**:367–75.
11. Gilbert RE, Tookey PA, Cubitt WD, Ades AE, Masters J, Peckham CS. Prevalence of *Toxoplasma* IgG among pregnant women in west London according to country of birth and ethnic group. *BMJ* 1993;**306**:185.
12. Villena I, Chemla C, Quereux C, Dupouy D, Leroux B, Foudrinier F, *et al*. Prenatal diagnosis of congenital toxoplasmosis transmitted by an immunocompetent woman infected before conception. *Prenat Diagn* 1998;**18**:1079–81.
13. Holliman RE. Clinical sequelae of chronic maternal toxoplasmosis. *Rev Med Microbiol* 1994;**5**:47–55.
14. Hall SM. Congenital toxoplasmosis. *BMJ* 1992;**305**:291–7.
15. Peckham CS, Logan S. Screening for toxoplasmosis during pregnancy. *Arch Dis Child* 1993;**68**:3–5.
16. Koppe JG, Loewer-Sieger DH, de Roever-Bonnet H. Results of 20-year follow-up of congenital toxoplasmosis. *Lancet* 1986;**i**:254–6.
17. Koppe JG, Rothova A. Congenital toxoplasmosis. A long-term follow-up of 20 years. *Int Ophthalmol* 1989;**13**:387–90.
18. Wilson CB, Remington JS, Stagno S, Reynolds DW. Development of adverse sequelae in children born with subclinical congenital toxoplasma infection. *Pediatrics* 1980;**66**:767–74.
19. Perkins ES. Ocular toxoplasmosis. *Br J Ophthalmol* 1973;**57**:1–17.
20. Gilbert RE, Stanford M. Is ocular toxoplasmosis caused by prenatal or postnatal infection? *Br J Ophthalmol* 2000;**84**:224–6.
21. Glasner PD, Silveira C, Kruszon-Moran D, Martins MC, Burnier Junior M, Silveira S, *et al*. An unusually high prevalence of ocular toxoplasmosis in southern Brazil. *Am J Ophthalmol* 1992;**114**:136–44.
22. Duffy KT, Wharton PJ, Johnson JD, New L, Holliman RE. Assessment of immunoglobulin-M

immunosorbent agglutination assay (ISAGA) for detecting *Toxoplasma* specific IgM. *J Clin Pathol* 1989;**42**:1291–5.

23. Holliman RE, Johnson JD. Duration of *Toxoplasma* infection. *J Clin Pathol* 1991;**44**:525.

24. Desai MB, Kurtz AB, Martin ME, Wapner RJ. Characteristic findings of toxoplasmosis *in utero*. *J Ultrasound Med* 1994;**13**:60–2.

25. Desmonts G, Forestier F, Thulliez P, Daffos F, Capella-Pavlovsky M, Chartier M. Prenatal diagnosis of congenital toxoplasmosis. *Lancet* 1985;**ii**:500–4.

26. Hezard N, Marx-Chemla C, Foudrinier F, Villena I, Quereux C, Leroux B, *et al*. Prenatal diagnosis of congenital toxoplasmosis in 261 pregnancies. *Prenat Diagn* 1997;**17**:1047–54.

27. Forestier F, Hohfeld P, Sole Y, Daffos F. Prenatal diagnosis of congenital toxoplasmosis by PCR: extended experience. *Prenat Diagn* 1998;**18**:405–15.

28. Jenum PA, Holberg-Petersen M, Melby KK, Stray-Pedersen B. Diagnosis of Toxopl*asma gondii* by polymerase chain reaction (PCR) on amniotic fluid samples. The Norwegian experience. *APMIS* 1998;**106**:680–6.

29. Pinon JM, Chemla C, Villena I, Foudrinier F, Aubert D, Puygauthier-Toubas D, *et al*. Early neonatal diagnosis of congenital toxoplasmosis: value of comparative enzyme-linked immunofiltration assay immunological profiles and anti-*Toxoplasma gondii* immunoglobulin M (IgM) or IgA immunocapture and implications for postnatal therapeutic strategies. *J Clin Microbiol* 1996;**34**:579–83.

30. Wallon M, Liou C, Garner P, Peyron F. Congenital toxoplasmosis: systematic review of evidence of efficacy of treatment in pregnancy. *BMJ* 1999;**318**:1511–14.

31. Foulon W, Villena I, Stray-Pedersen B, Decoster A, Lappalainen M, Pinon JM, *et al*. Treatment of toxoplasmosis during pregnancy: a multicentre study of impact on fetal transmission and children's sequelae at age 1 year. *Am J Obstet Gynecol* 1999;**180**:410–15.

32. Holliman RE. Uncommon infections: 4. Toxoplasmosis, toxocariasis and cryptosporidiosis. *Prescribers J* 1992;**32**:127–32.

33. Eskild A, Oxman A, Magnus P, Bjorndal A, Bakketeig LS. Screening for toxoplasmosis in pregnancy: what is the evidence for reducing a health problem? *J Med Screen* 1996;**3**:188–94.

34. Hohfeld P, Daffos F, Thulles P. Fetal toxoplasmosis: outcome of pregnancy and infant follow-up after *in utero* treatment. *J Pediatr* 1989;**115**:765–9.

35. Villena I, Aubert D, Leroux B, Dupouy D, Talmud M, Chemla C, *et al*. Pyrimethamine-sulfadoxine treatment of congenital toxoplasmosis: follow-up of 78 cases between 1980 and 1997. *Scand J Infect Dis* 1998;**30**:295–300.

36. Carter AO, Gelmon SB, Wells GA, Toepell AP. The effectiveness of a prenatal education programme for the prevention of congenital toxoplasmosis. *Epidemiol Infect* 1989;**103**:539–45.

37. Newton LH, Hall SM. A survey of health education material for the primary prevention of congenital toxoplasmosis. *Commun Dis Rep CDR Rev* 1995;**5**:21–7.

38. Buxton D, Innes EA. A commercial vaccine for ovine toxoplasmosis. *Parasitology* 1995;**110** Suppl:S11–16.

39. Aosai F, Mun HS, Narose K, Chen M, Hata H, Kobayashi M, *et al*. Protective immunity induced by vaccination with SAG1 gene transfected cells against *Toxoplasma gondii* infection in mice. *Microbiol Immunol* 1999;**43**:87–91.

40. Guerina NG, Hsu HW, Meissner HC. Neonatal serologic screening and early treatment for congenital *Toxoplasma gondii* infection. *N Engl J Med* 1994;**33**:1858–63.

41. Holliman RE, Johnson JD. The post-natal diagnosis of congenital toxoplasmosis. *Serodiagn Immunother Infect Dis* 1989;**3**:323–7.

42. Lebech M, Andersen O, Christensen NC, Hertel J, Nielsen HE, Peitersen B, *et al*. Feasibility of neonatal screening for *Toxoplasma* infection in the absence of prenatal treatment. *Lancet* 1999;**353**:1834–7.

43. Hartup C, Johnson JD, Holliman RE. Medical audit of the investigation of toxoplasmosis associated with pregnancy. *Lancet* 1992;**340**:118.

44. Conyn-van Spaendonck MA. *Prevention of Congenital Toxoplasmosis in the Netherlands*. Bilthoven: National Institute of Public Health and Environmental Protection; 1991.

45. Pujol M, Malbruny B, Morel C, Exmelin L. [Recall of the importance of serological monitoring of children with suspected congenital toxoplasmosis.] *Pathol Biol (Paris)* 1992;**40**:238–41. French.

46. Wilson JM, Junger G. *Principles and Practice of Screening for Disease*. Geneva: WHO; 1968. Public Health Papers No. 34.

47. Joss AW, Chatterton JM, Ho-Yen DO. Congenital toxoplasmosis: to screen or not to screen? *Public Health* 1990;**104**:9–20.

48. McCabe R, Remington JS. Toxoplasmosis: the time has come. *N Engl J Med* 1988;**318**:313–15.

49. Joynson DH, Payne R. Screening for toxoplasmosis in pregnancy. *Lancet* 1988;**ii**:795–6.

50. Lappalainen M, Sintonen H, Koskiniemi M, Hedman K, Hiilesmaa V, Ammala P, *et al*. Cost–benefit

analysis of screening for toxoplasmosis during pregnancy. *Scand J Infect Dis* 1995;**27**:265–72.

51. Henderson JB, Beattie CP, Hale EG, Wright T. The evaluation of new services: Possibilities for preventing congenital toxoplasmosis. *Int J Epidemiol* 1984;**13**:65–72.

52. Bader TJ, Macones GA, Asch DA. Prenatal screening for toxoplasmosis. *Obstet Gynecol* 1997;**90**:457–64.

53. Royal College of Obstetricians and Gynaecologists. *Prenatal Screening for Toxoplasmosis in the UK. Report of a Multidisciplinary Working Group.* London; 1992.

Chapter 16

Bacterial and other infections during pregnancy II

Discussion

Discussion following Dr Ridgway's presentation

Smith: I understand why you are suggesting the third trimester for screening for genital chlamydial infection but, in practical terms, you are likely to achieve a much higher strike rate by targeting the booking visit.

Ridgway: Yes, I wondered about that. I was influenced by the two papers showing that there were women returning after treatment who were positive, and women who were negative in the first trimester who were positive in the third trimester. That was my only reason for that and it is certainly something I am not totally clear about.

Smith: With reference to your third recommendation concerning contact tracing, would I be right in thinking that it is the fact that very few gynaecologists actually get involved in treatment of the partner which means that the problem keeps coming back?

Ridgway: Yes. I would be happy to modify my first recommendation to say that we should screen all antenatal women for genital chlamydia infection with a nucleic acid amplification test, provided that we do carry out the third recommendation.

Regan: Is there a hospital that is screening all pregnant women for chlamydia? This is an excellent suggestion and it follows on logically from your presentation but, if we are to recommend it as a group, we have to realise that it will have a massive impact on both workload and expense in every hospital in the country.

Ridgway: The groups I highlighted are in fact the groups that the Chief Medical Officer is currently recommending should be included in the screening programme, subject to the trials that are currently in progress. These encompass pregnant women.

MacLean: One of the paradoxes is that we all screen women who choose to terminate their pregnancy, but those who choose to continue their pregnancy are not being screened.

Carrington: Dr Ridgway, in your first recommendation you have not mentioned the specimen type. We know that urine samples in women are not particularly useful. We know that obstetricians are reluctant to perform cervical visualisation. As you have suggested, the best data come from nucleic acid amplification of vulvovaginal swabs taken by the patient. What is your recommendation as to the appropriate specimen?

Ridgway: Unfortunately, as you are well aware, the vulval swab is not formally approved by the manufacturers.

By attrition, I think we will move to vulval swabs but if the College is issuing mandatory recommendations from this Study Group I do not think that we can recommend something for which the manufacturer does not have a licence. All we have officially are urine tests, which is why I have suggested that you should discuss protocols with your laboratory.

Carrington: I agree, but what is your relative sensitivity of nucleic acid amplification on urine samples in pregnant women, as opposed to patients who have been diagnosed by other methods as having chlamydia?

Ridgway: I have not specifically looked at patients who are pregnant but, in a study[1] we did comparing different specimen types, urine came out bottom. I would much prefer never to test another urine sample for chlamydia.

Hay: We are just finishing a study that is evaluating early-pregnancy screening (less than 10 weeks of gestation). We have had about 25 women who have tested positive for chlamydia and there has been one discrepancy so far between the self-administered swab and the urine sample, so the tests seem to be reasonably equivalent when taken in the first trimester.

Brocklehurst: I am concerned that amoxycillin may encourage latency. None of the randomised trials that have used amoxycillin have even bothered following up any of the children to see whether they ever developed chlamydia. One of the recommendations could be that we should further investigate the use of amoxycillin in the treatment of chlamydia, to see whether it is as effective as erythromycin, or azithromycin.

Ridgway: It is comforting to see that consideration of the use of azithromycin is entering into the Cochrane database.

Hughes: Women attending an antenatal clinic are quite different from women requesting termination of pregnancy. The Chief Medical Officer's recommendations are that women under 25 years, or with a new partner or with multiple partners, should be screened. The average age at an antenatal clinic is the late-20s now, so you cannot justify screening all pregnant women on that basis. Perhaps we should select women at the booking clinic according to age or sexual history.

Ridgway: It depends where you take your cut-off. You will find about 80% of chlamydia-positive patients if you look for those between the ages of 16 and 25 years. If you want to pick up nearer 100%, you need to extend the age to 35 years, which would cover your antenatal patients.

Hay: One possible risk factor, which you did not mention, is ethnic origin. In the study[2] Pippa Oakeshott did in Wandsworth, and in other studies as well, black race at any age was a strong risk factor for chlamydia.

Smith: On the practical consideration of contact tracing, at Chelsea and Westminster Hospital we have gone down the route of being very firmly allied with the genitourinary medicine department. Thus, all the contact tracing is directly performed by that department, and we have a health adviser who is split between the two departments.

Ridgway: I support that wholeheartedly.

Soothill: It is not that easy, and I would rather support what Dr Hughes said. If you are going to apply such a policy of contact tracing to all patients, it will discourage some women from seeking antenatal care. You have to be careful about that. We would have great difficulty in getting the midwives to accept that first proposal.

Discussion following Dr Hay's paper

Ridgway: I am surprised that you are recommending a macrolide–metronidazole combination. The one organism that will not be touched by a macrolide, unless you use midecamycin acetate, which is not available in the UK, is *Mycoplasma hominis* – this organism is resistant. The differential sensitivity is remarkable: ureaplasmas are erythromycin-macrolide-sensitive, and clindamycin-resistant, while *Mycoplasma hominis* is the other way around, being clindamycin-sensitive and macrolide-resistant.

Brocklehurst: I obviously have a different slant on the evidence that is available at the moment. I would dispute quite strongly your comment that bacterial vaginosis (BV) is causally related to preterm birth. While there is certainly a strong association, there is not yet sufficient evidence that one is causally related to the other. The trials evidence is conflicting.

The strongest evidence comes from the Carey study[3], which showed absolutely no difference in preterm birth, with a very effective treatment for bacterial vaginosis, in that 80% of women having the active treatment had normal bacterial flora afterwards. In the substantial subgroup of women who had a previous preterm delivery, the incidence of subsequent preterm delivery was identical.

We do not yet have sufficient evidence to say that BV causes preterm delivery, although it is certainly strongly associated with it. However, there may be maternal factors that lead women to be predisposed to BV and preterm birth, or there must be something happening in some women, in association with BV, which may not be caused by it, which leads to the increase in preterm birth. I am not sure yet whether we are ready to do another large multicentre treatment study, at least not until we can elucidate some of these mechanisms. I am concerned that we could do another large study that would come out with exactly the same results as Carey. I am not convinced by the argument that intervening at an earlier gestation will make a big difference.

Hay: If you look at the studies that have shown benefits, I know that the Morales study[4] has been criticised methodologically in many ways and is clearly much smaller than the Carey study.[3] The Hauth study,[5] certainly the one that I was involved in, ran out of both time and money and had to stop at 500 women instead of the 800 we had initially wanted to study. However, as a proof of concept, these studies do show that perhaps there are some interventions (the right one, at the right time) that may be able to produce a benefit. So, despite the Carey study, I do not think we should be totally nihilistic about it. We should not delay for too long because this is a very important area. I believe it is causing a great deal of devastation in pregnancies, and we should try to sort out a treatment that will work.

Regan: I would just make a comment similar to Dr Brocklehurst's about preterm birth. I also do not think you can say that BV is causally related to early loss. The only data that suggested that are the studies from Leeds,[6] where they were looking at *in vitro* fertilisation patients, who have a totally different vaginal pH after the stimulation techniques.

Hay: I was not referring to those – I was referring to second-trimester loss.

Regan: There are no prospective data, are there? Our group published data[7] demonstrating that there was a higher prevalence in women who were nonpregnant and then, when we followed them through, the course of BV remits and relapses spontaneously in pregnancy. We could not make head nor tail of their results if we followed them through sequentially on monthly swabs.

Hay: There have been two studies. There was our Northwick Park Hospital screening study[8] where, if you looked at the women recruited prior to 16 weeks, they had a 5.5-fold increased risk of second-trimester loss between 16 and 24 weeks of gestation. McGregor[9] in Denver reported a 3.3-fold increased risk in his observational cohort.

Soothill: There is a good deal more evidence that may be coming out soon. One example would be the Premet study, which is related to fetal fibronectin, but there is a correlation between that and BV, at least in our data. The other aspect that has been hard to study has been the confounding factors, of which I am sure one is cervical length. If you have a large amount of infection in the vagina and a short cervix, that may be more of a risk than if you have a long cervix. Separating that out may give the studies a good deal more power, and we are working on that.

Perhaps I could also mention that a paper[10] has just been published, using the sialidase assay, which is potentially a simple colour change assay. This is a very high predictor of BV and could be quite useful if we could follow some of your ideas and your work on women self-testing. That may make it slightly easier to get power into the studies.

Ridgway: I would like to see more gynaecologists using narrow-range pH papers prior to initiating more sophisticated tests. How you can have a gynaecology outpatient clinic without using pH papers is beyond me, but perhaps I am being naive.

Hay: That is one of the points I did not address. Reference has been made to having a simple, robust diagnostic test. We have had an international workshop recently on reading Gram stains for BV. People who have been doing a good deal of work on it were getting reasonably good kappa values, the lowest being about 0.7 and the highest up at 0.8 or 0.9. However, when you try to get a group of so-called 'experts' to agree on whether a slide is BV or not, you do not always find good agreement. You could not have highly trained technicians going out to every antenatal clinic to read Gram stains all day – we need good, simple, bedside tests. There is the PAP test, where you look at a pH change and measure proline aminopeptidase, which is produced by anaerobes, so perhaps we should be evaluating those kinds of tests in screening.

I have seen a presentation from Germany, where they manufacture a glove with some pH paper on the end of it. They are getting women to examine themselves, wearing these gloves, twice a week to see whether their pH is changing. If it changes, they go to their obstetrician. This, again, is empowering the women to do the testing.

Discussion following Dr Holliman's paper

Jauniaux: This is a practical comment. I fully agree with your first point. The problem is that patients find a way of getting screened – especially non-UK-born patients such as the French, Germans, Italians, Spanish, Greeks and Belgians that I see, and also the Americans. It is a real nightmare, because they end up with obstetricians who have no idea how to interpret the results and no idea how to prevent the consequences of the test and of the disease if it is really acquired during the pregnancy. Perhaps as a group we should make some recommendation about what to do with those patients who have been screened and who have been found to have a positive result.

Holliman: I would agree with you. I used to spend a great deal of my working life trying to deal with cases like that, where a woman had read an article, seen a television programme or spoken to a friend who had told her that all she needed was this simple test that doctors were withholding in order to save money. The nightmare then arises when the test – whatever that test might be – comes back as positive.

This illustrates the fact that, if you are going to do a test, you should have the facilities and the approach in place to react to a positive test, rather than assuming that it will be negative. It also draws attention to the difficulties of our current advice, which is that a woman who asks for a test should be counselled. That is all very well, and it sounds wonderful in a textbook, but the reality of the situation is that it is far simpler and quicker to do the test and hope that it will be negative, than it is to counsel a woman. You would need to go through what are quite complicated arguments, hoping to convince her that you would probably be doing her more harm than good by giving her the test that she thought she wanted.

There is a great deal of room for improvement there. I am not sure what the answer is, but we need to broaden the debate beyond just medical circles, and try to encourage our colleagues in the media that their intervention in debates, such as screening for toxoplasmosis, can be extremely harmful. It may sell newspapers, but it may also cause a considerable amount of anxiety and, indeed, terminations as a result. In the last five years I have dealt with at least three cases where a woman was tested for toxoplasmosis in pregnancy because she asked for the test. The result indicated that she was immunoglobulin G (IgG) positive: no further tests were done and the pregnancy was terminated.

Jauniaux: That raises the medico-legal impact of this. Can we refuse to test a patient? If a patient asks for screening for toxoplasmosis, and if we agree, how often do we do it? In some countries, such as France, it is done every month, while in other countries, such as the USA, it is done every three months.

Holliman: Exactly. In France and Austria there is variation in the frequency of testing, but, because of the difficulties of trying to decide when a woman acquired the infection, their objective is to try to test every month. Thus, the initial negative test, while it is good news, means that you are then committed to testing repeatedly during the pregnancy to try to pick up a seroconversion.

In the UK situation, where 85% or more of women are susceptible, huge numbers of women would have to be tested repeatedly. Again, if you do a one-off test on a pregnant woman, in my view you should be committed to doing that test repeatedly – so it is not just the one test.

Jauniaux: Can we refuse to do it?

Holliman: As some of you will be aware, UK law – or certainly English and Welsh law – is based on case law and not on theory. I am not aware of any of these cases going to court yet, but sooner or later one will. We will then find out.

At the moment, the professional advice is that if you properly counsel the woman, but at the end of that she still refuses and insists on the test, you then have to make a professional judgement about whether you are doing more harm than good. If you feel that you are doing more harm, you should refer the patient on. That sounds wonderful from a lawyer's point of view, but I have severe reservations about how practical it might be.

Jauniaux: The situation is similar in Down syndrome. There was a recent UK legal case where a woman was denied amniocentesis after a positive biochemical test for Down syndrome, and the obstetrician was found negligent. It is exactly the same situation with toxoplasmosis.

MacLean: One of the questions along that line is if a laboratory received a specimen, would they do the test, or would they choose not to do the test? Presumably, these tests are done within the local hospital, and only the positive results are referred to you.

Holliman: Most laboratories in the UK have the capability of doing initial testing and deciding whether the woman has ever had toxoplasmosis or not. Then it moves on to trying to decide whether she has toxoplasmosis, when did she have it? Again, most laboratories can say, using a very sensitive immunoglobulin M (IgM) test, that she has had it for a considerable period of time. The problem arises, however, when the woman tests positive for both IgG and IgM. Then, if we are honest about it, even in the most advanced reference laboratories it is not really possible to give an accurate answer to that question, which is, of course, absolutely crucial.

Carrington: Do you see the benefits of affinity testing, and a place for that in the determination of acute toxoplasmosis, as being relevant to the question of following these patients through?

Holliman: It is certainly an advance – affinity/avidity testing is a way of looking at IgG to try to get a handle on how actively it binds to its target. The fact is that, the longer a patient has been infected with the disease, the better adapted the antibody is to that disease and therefore the better it binds on. Thus, antibody that has been around for a relatively short period of time has low affinity or avidity, whereas a longstanding infection would be associated with high avidity and affinity.

It is generally agreed that in toxoplasmosis, and indeed in other diseases, it is an advance over straight IgM testing, in that some women will produce IgM for a very long period of time, idiosyncratically, both in toxoplasmosis and indeed in other conditions. Avidity can often help to sort those out. Even with the most accurate avidity test, however, you can probably only get down to saying that she acquired this infection in the last three months, but often that is not as precise an answer as the obstetrician, and indeed the woman, would require.

Peckham: Screening was introduced in the belief that there was an intervention that would reduce mother-to-child transmission. The knowledge that is now emerging, that, in fact, the treatment is no good, is quite awkward. As has already been said, it is very difficult to discontinue a screening programme once it is in place.

We are thinking about introducing something. If you have an infection where there is no intervention and nothing is done, because nothing is useful, then that changes the whole situation. We are looking at it now as if there is a screening programme that works, but things are changing. Perhaps other countries may reconsider their programmes too – I do not know.

Holliman: I would like to agree with you – and certainly personally I would agree with you. However, the experience of colleagues working on the Continent is quite the reverse. They look at the same data and say that perhaps the evidence for interrupting transmission is not that good, but that there are problems with the studies and so on. However, there is evidence coming through that it reduces the severity of disease and this is therefore the justification for continuing the screening programme.

This illustrates the point you referred to. Once you have started to do something, the politics of it becomes possibly more important than the science.

Peckham: I would just like to add that some countries are beginning to perform newborn screening for congenital toxoplasmosis rather than antenatal screening.[11] They feel that if you can identify an infected child at birth, you can then treat with the advantage of knowing that the child is infected. Then there is the issue as to whether you can do a trial to see whether treatment of the newborn, or the child, is effective and, if so, for how long treatment is beneficial.

Holliman: Absolutely. That approach has been carried out for some time in Massachusetts and New England.[12] It was also adopted in Denmark in the late 1990s. The problem is that there is no good evidence that treating an infected child has any effect on the child's ultimate handicap. I would like to reiterate that point: handicap is the important issue, not infection. It is not even disease, but whether that disease process has actually caused a significant reduction in the quality of life. There is no published evidence, to my knowledge, that treating a child in the postnatal period reduces handicap.

Jauniaux: Toxoplasmosis is probably the best example of a condition where we have to get the recommendation absolutely right. If you draw a parallel with Down syndrome screening, you probably know that most health authorities have not endorsed nuchal translucency evaluation, which is one of the new tests to screen for Down syndrome. Can we say that, at a national level, we are not providing any screening at all for toxoplasmosis in pregnancy? I go back to my initial question: can we therefore refuse to test for it in the NHS? There would then be the danger that, after some time, patients would obtain the tests privately, as they do for nuchal translucency. You would be creating a huge business there, but with poor counselling because most of the people who perform the nuchal translucency test – or the people who would be performing the screening for toxoplasmosis in the private sector – would have no facilities for counselling and would not provide any for the patient.

Holliman: Just to clarify, the Chief Medical Officer's advice is not that toxoplasmosis testing should never be done in pregnancy. Clearly, for the woman who presents with an illness – a syndrome – that is compatible with acute toxoplasmosis, which is normally a glandular fever-type syndrome, such testing is perfectly appropriate. Indeed, it would probably be poor practice not to try to discover what the cause of the glandular fever syndrome is – it could be toxoplasma, or it could be cytomegalovirus. Glandular fever syndrome is an accepted criterion for investigating for toxoplasmosis in pregnancy.

As you infer, the really difficult area is the woman who comes and asks for the test. I am not clear what backing you would receive if you followed the scientific evidence and tried to persuade the woman not to have the test – and if you could not persuade her but then refused to do the test on the medical grounds that the evidence showed that you were actually doing her more harm than good. I do not know what the legal outcome would be but I would not personally want to be the test case.

References

1. Carder C, Robinson AJ, Broughton C, Stephenson JM, Ridgway GL. Evaluation of self-taken samples for the presence of genital *Chlamydia trachomatis* infection in women using the ligase chain reaction assay. *Int J STD AIDS* 1999;**10**:776–9.
2. Oakeshott P, Kerry S, Hay S, Hay P. Opportunistic screening for chlamydial infection at time of cervical smear testing in general practice: prevalence study. *BMJ* 1998;**316**:351–2.
3. Carey JC, Klebanoff MA, Hauth JC, Hillier SL, Thom EA, Ernest JM, *et al*. Metronidazole to prevent preterm delivery in pregnant women with asymptomatic bacterial vaginosis. *N Engl J Med* 2000;**342**:534–40.
4. Morales WJ, Schorr S, Albritton J. Effect of metronidazole in patients with preterm birth in preceding pregnancy and bacterial vaginosis: a placebo-controlled, double-blind study. *Am J Obstet Gynecol* 1994;**171**:345–7.
5. Hauth JC, Goldenberg RL, Andrews WW, DuBard MB, Copper RL. Reduced incidence of preterm delivery with metronidazole and erythromycin in women with bacterial vaginosis. *N Engl J Med* 1995;**333**:1732–6.
6. Ralph SG, Rutherford AJ, Wilson JD. Influence of bacterial vaginosis on conception and miscarriage in the first trimester: cohort study. *BMJ* 1999;**319**:220–3.
7. Llahi-Camp JM, Rai R, Ison C, Regan L, Taylor-Robinson D. Association of bacterial vaginosis with a history of second trimester miscarriage. *Hum Reprod* 1996;**11**:1575–8.
8. Hay PE, Lamont RF, Taylor-Robinson D, Morgan DJ, Ison C, Pearson J. Abnormal bacterial colonisation of the genital tract and subsequent preterm delivery and late miscarriage. *BMJ* 1994;**308**:295–8.

9. McGregor JA, French JI, Parker R, Draper D, Patterson E, Jones W, *et al*. Prevention of premature birth by screening and treatment for common genital tract infections: results of a prospective controlled evaluation. *Am J Obstet Gynecol* 1995;**173**:157–67.

10. Wiggins R, Crowley T, Horner PJ, Soothill PW, Millar MR, Corfield AP. Use of 5-bromo-4-chloro-3-indolyl-alpha-D-N-acetylneuraminic acid in a novel spot test To identify sialidase activity in vaginal swabs from women with bacterial vaginosis. *J Clin Microbiol* 2000;**38**:3096–7.

11. Lebech M, Andersen O, Christensen CN, Hertel J, Neilsen HE, Peitersen B, *et al*. Feasibility of neonatal screening for toxoplasma infection in the absence of prenatal treatment. Danish Congenital Toxoplasmosis Study Group. *Lancet* 1999;**353**:1834–7.

12. Guerina NG, Hsu HW, Meissner HC, Maguire JH, Lynfield R, Stechenberg B, *et al*. Neonatal serologic screening and early treatment for congenital *Toxoplasma gondii* infection. The New England Regional Toxoplasma Working Group. *N Engl J Med* 1994;**330**:1858–63.

SECTION 5

VIRUSES AND PREGNANCY I

Chapter 17

Effects of viruses on the placenta

Harold Fox

Introduction

Viruses almost invariably infect the placenta from the maternal blood. Infection of the placenta from a lesion in the endometrium is uncommon, if only because endometritis tends to militate against successful implantation. This is not, however, an invariable rule and there is certainly the possibility of a chronic viral infection of the endometrial glands, which may serve as a potential reservoir for placental infection without seriously diminishing fertility (this is known to occur in some animals). Viral infection is therefore always secondary to an overt or subclinical maternal infection by a pathogenic organism. This is in sharp contrast to bacterial infections, which are commonly due to normal inhabitants of the birth canal.

Morphology of viral infections of the placenta

Viral infections involve the placental parenchyma rather than the membranes and often evoke no detectable inflammatory response. When an inflammatory reaction does occur, it is seen within the villous substance and is known as a villitis. The villitis may be focal, with lesions present in random isolated villi, or diffuse, with extensive involvement of contiguous villi. The focal form is the more common and very few villi may be involved, to the extent that the lesions may be missed unless the placenta is extensively sampled.

A villitis is usually characterised by a mixed villous infiltrate of lymphocytes, plasma cells and histiocytic cells and granulomas of either histiocytic or tuberculoid type are occasionally seen. Necrosis may also be present. Eventually, the inflammatory lesion within the villi undergoes organisation and repair, with granulation tissue formation and fibroblastic proliferation, leading to villous fibrosis and scarring. The placental findings in any particular viral infection will thus vary with, and depend upon, the stage reached in the evolution and repair of the inflammatory lesion at the time of delivery.

Specific patterns of placental inflammation

The patterns of placental pathological changes have been defined for a number of viral infections.

Rubella[1–8]

In the acute stage of the infection there is a focal necrotising villitis and a necrotising endarteritis of the fetal villous vessels. The villitis is highly variable: some affected villi exhibit only focal necrosis of the trophoblast. In others, the trophoblast is completely necrotic, with perivillous deposition of fibrin and polymorphs. Small groups of villi are sometimes agglutinated by fibrin. The villous stroma can be hypercellular or oedematous and often contains prominent Hofbauer cells, which may have eosinophilic granules in their cytoplasm. The villous fetal vessels characteristically show endothelial necrosis, while fragmented erythrocytes may be present in their lumina. There is sometimes also a well-marked perivasculitis. Eosinophilic inclusion bodies may be seen in the endothelial cells or, less frequently, in the villous trophoblast.

In placentas obtained after the acute stage of the disease has passed there may be only scattered, avascular, shrunken fibrotic villi, but in some both active and healed lesions are present simultaneously, which suggests continuing and progressive villous damage.

Vaccinia

Vaccinial infection of the placenta is characterised by the presence of minute, pinhead-sized greyish-white scattered nodules, which, on histological examination, are seen to consist of foci of necrotic villi surrounded by fibrin and polymorphs.[9–11] Eosinophilic inclusion bodies may also be seen.

Variola

In variola minor infection, tiny yellowish nodules having a creamy consistency are present both on the surface and within the parenchyma. Histological examination reveals multiple necrotising tuberculoid granulomas, patchy necrosis of villi and an intervillous accumulation of fibrin, polymorphs and inflammatory debris.[12]

Varicella zoster

In placentas infected with varicella there is an acute necrotising villitis in early and severe cases, with a progression via a lymphocytic/granulomatous villitis, in which histiocytic giant cells are present, to stromal fibrosis with obliteration of fetal vessels.[5,7,12–15] Groups of agglutinated inflamed villi may be macroscopically visible and have been described as resembling rice seed. Eosinophilic intranuclear inclusions may be present in decidual cells and within the histiocytic giant cells.

Herpes simplex

Herpes simplex virus causes necrosis of the trophoblast of scattered villi and agglutination of groups of involved villi but, interestingly enough, often without provoking any significant inflammatory reaction,[16] although there may be a mild lymphocytic villitis.[7]

Enteroviruses

The enteroviruses cause an extensive vasculitis of the fetal vessels of the placenta and a focal or extensive lymphocytic and histiocytic infiltration of the villous stroma, with trophoblastic necrosis.[17]

Mumps virus

In placentas infected with mumps virus there is widespread necrotising villitis with an accumulation of necrotic material and mononuclear cells in the intervillous space. Necrotising granulomas containing giant cells and epithelioid cells are present in some villi. There is a necrotising endarteritis of the fetal villous vessels and inclusion bodies can be observed in the cytoplasm of villous stromal cells and in decidual cells.[18]

Measles

Measles results in an intervillous mononuclear cell, fibrinous exudate, villous adhesions and villous syncytial necrosis. Measles virus antigen can be demonstrated immunohistologically in villous syncytiotrophoblast.[19]

Parvovirus

Placentas infected by parvovirus B19 tend to be large and may be oedematous. Histological examination reveals a markedly increased number of nucleated red blood cells within the fetal vessels. Often, but not invariably, some of the erythrocytes contain intranuclear inclusions consisting of a central clear or eosinophilic area with peripheral chromatin condensation.[7,20] Patchy villous immaturity and oedema is common and a vasculitis, affecting villous capillaries and occasionally stem arteries, is a common finding, often associated with a perivascular round-cell inflammatory infiltrate.[21]

Cytomegalovirus

In cases of cytomegalovirus (CMV) infection, the placenta is often unremarkable but can sometimes appear bulky and oedematous. Histological examination will characteristically show a low-grade focal or diffuse lymphoplasmacytic villitis.[22–29] The villi undergo a wide range of histological changes, from a focal necrotising and proliferative villitis, sometimes with granulomatous features[7] in the early stages, to atrophy and fibrosis in the later stages. The brunt of the inflammatory damage is borne by the villous stroma rather than by the trophoblast. While there is usually an infiltration of lymphocytes into the stroma, it is not uncommon also to find plasma cells, which are often most numerous in the immediately perivascular areas. The lymphocytes appear to be all T cells while the plasma cells may be immunoglobulin M- or immunoglobulin G-secreting.[30] An increased number of Hofbauer cells may be present. Focal or generalised villous oedema is sometimes seen and thrombosis of fetal vessels may occur. Deposition of haemosiderin pigment in the villi is often a striking feature. CMV inclusion bodies can often be found in the infected placenta, although they are usually few in number and are sometimes only detected after a prolonged search. These inclusion bodies are usually seen in the endothelial cells of the fetal vessels but may occasionally be located in the stromal cells or in the trophoblast.

In many cases of documented intrauterine fetal CMV infection, the placenta appears normal on histological examination[31] and it is known that CMV can be isolated from such placentas.[32,33] Furthermore, a villitis evoked by CMV infection may show no specific features and can masquerade as a villitis of unknown aetiology.

Hepatitis B virus

In placentas of women with infective hepatitis there is deposition of bilirubin in the villous macrophages and there may be focal syncytial necrosis without any inflammatory reaction.[34,35] The presence of hepatitis B surface antigen (HBsAg) can be demonstrated by immunocytochemistry in the villous Hofbauer cells and fetal villous vessel endothelial cells of asymptomatic HBsAg carriers. Hepatitis B core antigen is demonstrable in the Hofbauer and endothelial cells.[36,37]

Influenza virus

In influenza infection, the placenta is characterised by villous trophoblastic necrosis, a villous lymphocytic infiltrate, necrosis of the endothelium of fetal stem vessels and intracellular cytoplasmic inclusions.[38]

Human immunodeficiency virus

This virus can be identified within placental tissue by a variety of techniques. It is detected most frequently in the Hofbauer cells but also occasionally in the trophoblast and fetal endothelial cells.[39–49]

Placentas of women who are seropositive for HIV usually appear macroscopically normal although in a few studies the placentas have been unusually heavy.[39,50] Chorioamnionitis is common[39,51–53] but this is almost certainly because of a secondary opportunistic infection. There is a widespread consensus that a villitis is not seen histologically and that no specific abnormalities are present.[39,45,47,50–52,54] In one study,[44] villous immaturity, villous oedema, focal trophoblastic necrosis, an excess of villous Hofbauer cells, necrosis of Hofbauer cells, excessive intravillous fibrin deposition and chorangiosis were noted as features, albeit non-specific ones, of placentas exposed to possible infection by HIV. There were, however, numerous confounding factors to dilute the significance of these findings.

Non-specific patterns of placental inflammation

Although it is clearly established that many infections reaching the placenta from either the maternal bloodstream or the endometrium result in villitis, it remains true that in the vast majority of cases of villitis no specific infective organism can be identified. The noted incidence of villitis of unknown aetiology is variable: it is influenced by ethnic, environmental and socio-economic factors.[55] The inflammatory process often involves only 2–4% of the villus population and is detected only in extensively sampled and thoroughly examined placentas. Even among experienced pathologists there is a significant degree of inter-observer variation in the recognition of villitis.[56]

Nevertheless, it is clear that villitis of unknown aetiology is a relatively common finding: it is present in 6–14% of unselected series of third-trimester placentas in Western countries.[57–60] It has been suggested that villitis of this type is not, in fact, infective in nature but is the morphological expression of an immunological reaction within villous tissue – a marker of either a maternal graft rejection or a graft-versus-host reaction.[61–65] However, this concept remains unproven and, although not discounted, a majority view would still be that many, probably most, cases of villitis of unknown aetiology are due to an infection, usually viral in nature.[35,66,67] Certainly, the application of immunocytochemical, molecular and genetic techniques has identified a viral infection in many cases of villitis which would otherwise have been considered of unknown aetiology.[29,31,68–74]

The placenta as a barrier to viral infection of the fetus

The placenta is often considered to be a barrier to the free passage of organisms from the maternal circulation to the fetus. It must be conceded, however, that any barrier-like function of the placenta is not manifested with any great degree of consistency or success. A large variety of organisms is known to be able to pass through the placenta and infect the fetus. Indeed, it is doubtful whether there is any infective agent that invariably fails to penetrate the defences of the placenta.

The available evidence suggests, therefore, that the placenta can act only as a partial barrier to fetal infection. This partial resistance could be based on one or more of the following mechanisms:

1. The placenta may mount an immunological attack against infecting organisms.

2. The placenta could possess specific antiviral properties that enable it to resist infection.

3. Placental phagocytosis of infecting organisms.

4. The placenta may simply function as a non-specific physical barrier.

The first of these possibilities has little to recommend it, as the placenta is a fetal organ and there is no convincing evidence that it possesses any immunological defence mechanism against infection that is either specific or differs significantly from that of other fetal tissues.

There is evidence, however, that the placenta does possess specific non-immunologically mediated defence mechanisms against infection that are independent of those of the fetus. The placenta, in particular the trophoblast and the Hofbauer cells, produces a wide range of cytokines when stimulated by viruses, including interferons, interleukins and tumour necrosis factor.[75-83] Placental interferon synthesis is autonomous for, while cell cultures of other fetal tissues produce higher levels of interferon when challenged by Sendai virus than when attacked by rubella virus, the reverse is true for cultured placental tissue.[84] Whether placental interferon synthesis is an important factor in limiting transplacental viral spread is far from being fully clear. Various strains of rubella virus have differing abilities to stimulate placental, but not fetal, interferon synthesis and their capacity in this respect is inversely proportional to their ability to cross the placenta.[85] High placental interferon-α levels appear to inhibit transmission of herpes simplex virus to the fetus[86] but, conversely, placental interferons do not inhibit HIV transmission.[87] Under *in vitro* conditions, it has not proved possible to correlate placental interferon synthesis with constitutively expressed placental viral resistance.[88] The role played by other placental cytokines in resisting viral infections is also obscure. Indeed, locally produced cytokines may increase the permissiveness of trophoblast for viral replication.[89]

A novel placental mechanism for limiting the ability of viruses to cross the placenta may be increased apoptosis: infection of trophoblast with human T-lymphotropic virus leads to a significant increase in apoptosis of trophoblastic cells.[90] The Hofbauer cells of the placental villi have all the characteristics of macrophages and are present in sufficient numbers for the placenta almost to be considered a reticulo-endothelial organ – this may be an overstatement but it is nevertheless likely that the phagocytic capacity of the placenta is of considerable importance in limiting transplacental spread of infection.[91] This role has been emphasised by *in vitro* studies, which have shown that when Hofbauer cells are infected with herpes simplex virus or echovirus the viruses are rapidly destroyed.[92]

The placenta also acts as a simple physical barrier to prevent the spread of infection to the fetus. In most infections, however, the placenta appears only to delay the passage of organisms to the fetus, this delay being accounted for by the time taken for the organism to establish a focus of infection in the placental tissue, from which the fetus is subsequently infected. Viruses must replicate in placental cells and, in theory, any virus unable to multiply in such cells would not pass through the placenta. In practice, however, most viruses appear to replicate readily in placental tissue[93-96] and are thus able to establish a focus from which the fetus is later involved. This is readily seen in rubella, in which the virus reaches, and proliferates in, the endothelium of fetal placental vessels, a site from which they can pass with ease into the fetal circulation.

Two further points should be mentioned. Firstly, not all investigators have found that specific viruses can infect the trophoblast and it has been suggested that transmission of viruses from mother to fetus can only occur if there are breaks in the placental barrier.[97] Secondly, in experimental studies, maternal factors such as maternal age and uteroplacental bloodflow appear to affect virus spread to the fetus.[98]

Mechanisms of placental damage in viral infections

Viral infections could, in theory, cause placental damage by a variety of mechanisms. The infecting organisms could:

- directly cause cell death and tissue damage
- produce lesions in the uteroplacental vessels
- provoke an immune response that is directed against placental tissue.

In infections of animal placentas, there is often extensive necrosis of the placental parenchyma but, in the human placenta, a necrotising inflammation rarely involves more than scattered individual villi or small groups of villi. In rare instances the necrosis may be widespread, with extensive villous destruction,[99] but in the vast majority of cases the proportion of villi damaged is insufficient to compromise the functional ability of the placenta, due to the considerable reserve capacity of the placenta. Necrosis of villous tissue may, of course, be secondary to infective damage to the uteroplacental vasculature with widespread thrombosis. This occurs in a variety of animal infections but is not, as far as is known, a feature of infection in humans.

Some studies have found activated macrophages and T lymphocytes in a villitis[100–102] and it has been suggested that finding such cells in this lesion is indicative of allogeneic recognition and a rejection reaction in the placenta.[103] The possibility that infection triggers off a cell-mediated immune attack on placental tissues cannot be firmly excluded but would, if true, still only damage a small proportion of the placental villi.

Effects and clinical significance of viral infection

The most obvious consequence of a haematogenous viral placental infection is that the establishment of an inflammatory lesion in the placental tissue serves as a focus from which the fetus is later infected.

That many cases of placental infection are associated with intrauterine fetal death or abortion is an established fact but in most instances the demise of the fetus appears to be linked more to the direct effects of the infection on either the mother or the fetus than to placental damage. It has been shown experimentally that, in mice, placental CMV infection *per se*, without fetal infection or severe maternal illness, can be associated with a high incidence of fetal loss.[104] There are, however, no well-defined examples of this phenomenon in humans. Furthermore, the degree of tissue damage seen in most viral placental infections in humans is such that its effects could be easily neutralised by the organ's considerable functional reserve.

The above remarks apply to those cases of villitis that are clearly due to a specific infection, such as rubella. What, however, is the clinical significance of a villitis of unknown aetiology that is presumed but not proven to be indicative of a viral infection? There is certainly an association between villitis of unknown aetiology and an increased incidence of intrauterine fetal growth restriction,[57–63,105–111] although it must be stressed that in prospective studies the vast majority of neonates whose placentas show a villitis are of normal weight. Thus, in a personally studied series only 6.8% of neonates from cases of villitis had a birthweight for gestational age that was below the fifth centile.[60] A villitis of unknown aetiology can recur in successive pregnancies and it has been maintained that this recurrent form of villitis tends to be unusually extensive and shows a particularly strong association with fetal growth restriction.[99,112,113] Such cases are, however, rare and, of course, a pathologist examining a placenta usually does not know whether any villitis present is recurrent or not.

The nature of the link between villitis of unknown aetiology and diminished fetal growth is far from being clear. Benirschke and Kaufmann,[35] while pointing out that there is no absolute relationship between the severity of the villitis and the severity of growth restriction, consider nevertheless that the restriction of fetal growth is related to the elimination of a considerable amount of placental parenchyma from nutrient transfer. This may be true in occasional rare cases but is clearly not true in the vast majority of cases of villitis, in which the inflammatory damage wreaked upon the placenta is far too limited in extent to diminish the functional reserve of the organ. Hence, some other cause must be sought. If chronic villitis is due to an unrecognised viral infection then it is perfectly possible that the virus passes through the inadequate barrier of the placenta to infect the fetus and restrict its growth (the inhibitory effect of viruses on fetal DNA synthesis is well established). It is true that neonates whose placentas show evidence of villitis usually have no clinical evidence of infection but the infection may have been relatively transitory and the growth restriction temporary. If, on the other hand, some cases of villitis are due to an immunological interaction between maternal and fetal tissues then this may be associated with abnormal placentation with consequent restriction of fetal growth.

References

1.   Tondury GT, Smith DW. Fetal rubella pathology. *J Pediatr* 1996;**68**:867–79.
2.   Driscoll SG. Histopathology of gestational rubella. *Am J Dis Child* 1969;**118**:49–53.
3.   Ornoy A, Segal S, Nishmi M, Simcha A, Polishuk WZ. Fetal and placental pathology in gestational rubella. *Am J Obstet Gynecol* 1973;**116**:949–56.
4.   Garcia AGP, Marques RLS, Lobato YY, Fonseca MEF, Wigg MD. Placental pathology in congenital rubella. *Placenta* 1985;**6**:281–95.
5.   Kaplan C. The placenta and viral infections. *Clin Obstet Gynecol* 1990;**33**:232–41.
6.   Horn LC, Becker V. [Morphologic placenta findings in clinico-serologically verified and suspected rubella infection in the 2nd half of pregnancy]. *Z Geburtshilfe Perinatol* 1992;**196**:199–204. German.
7.   Kaplan C. The placenta and viral infections. *Semin Diagn Pathol* 1993;**10**:232–50.
8.   Horn LC, Buttner W, Horn E. Rotelnbedingte Plazentaveranderungen. *Perinat Med* 1993;**5**:5–10.
9.   Wielenga G, van Tongeren HAE, Ferguson AH, van Rijssel TG. Prenatal infection with vaccinia virus. *Lancet* 1961;**i**:258–60.
10. Entwistle DM, Bray PT, Laurence KM. Prenatal infection with vaccinia virus: report of a case. *BMJ* 1962;**ii**:238–9.
11. Hood CK, McKinnon GE. Prenatal vaccinia. *Am J Obstet Gynecol* 1963;**85**:238–40.
12. Garcia AGP. Fetal infection in chickenpox and alastrim, with histopathologic study of the placenta. *Pediatrics* 1963;**32**:895–901.
13. Blanc WA. Pathology of the placenta and cord in some viral infections. In: Hanshaw JB, Dudgeon JA, editors. *Viral Diseases of the Fetus and Newborn*. Philadelphia: Saunders; (1978). p. 237–58.
14. Robertson NJ, McKeever PA. Fetal and placental pathology in two cases of maternal varicella infection. *Pediatr Pathol* 1992;**12**:545–50.
15. Qureshi F, Jacques SM. Maternal varicella during pregnancy: correlation of maternal history and fetal outcome with placental histopathology. *Hum Pathol* 1996;**27**:191–5.
16. Witzleben CL, Driscoll SG. Possible transplacental transmission of herpes simplex infection. *Pediatrics* 1965;**36**:192–9.
17. Garcia APG, Basso NGD, Fonseca MEF, Zuardi JAT, Otanni HN. Enterovirus associated placental morphology: a light, virological, electron microscopic and immunohistologic study. *Placenta* 1991;**12**:533–47.
18. Garcia AGP, Pereira JMS, Vidigal N, Lobato YY, Pegado CS, Branco JPC. Intrauterine infection with mumps virus. *Obstet Gynecol* 1980;**56**:756–9.
19. Moroi K, Saito S, Kurata T, Sata T, Yanagida M. Fetal death associated with measles virus infection of the placenta. *Am J Obstet Gynecol* 1991;**164**:1107–8.

20. Rogers BB, Mark Y, Oyer CE. Diagnosis and incidence of fetal parvovirus infection in an autopsy series. I. Histology. *Pediatr Pathol* 1993;**13**:371–9.

21. Morey AL, Keeling JW, Porter HJ, Fleming KA. Clinical and histopathological features of parvovirus B19 infection in the human fetus. *Br J Obstet Gynaecol* 1992;**99**:566–74.

22. Lepage F, Schramm B. Aspects histologiques du placenta et des membranes dans la maladie des inclusions cytomégaliques. *Gynécol Obstét* 1958;**57**:273–9.

23. Quan A, Strauss L. Congenital cytomegalic inclusion disease: observations in a macerated fetus with a congenital defect, including a study of the placenta. *Am J Obstet Gynecol* 1962;**83**:1240–8.

24. Cochard AM, Tan-Vinh L, Lelong M. Le placenta dans la cytomegalie; étude anatomoclinque de 3 observations personelles. *Arch Franc Pédiat* 1963;**20**:35–46.

25. Rosenstein DL, Navarrete-Reyna A. Cytomegalic inclusion disease: observation of the characteristic inclusion bodies in the placenta. *Am J Obstet Gynecol* 1964;**89**:220–4.

26. Altshuler G, McAdams AJ. Cytomegalic inclusion disease of a nineteen-week fetus: case report including a study of the placenta. *Am J Obstet Gynecol* 1971;**111**:295–8.

27. Benirschke K, Mendoza GR, Bazeley PL. Placental and fetal manifestations of cytomegalovirus infection. *Virchows Arch B Cell Pathol* 1974;**16**:121–39.

28. Mostoufi-Zadeh M, Driscoll SG, Biano SA, Kundsi RB. Placental evidence of cytomegalovirus infection of the fetus and neonate. *Arch Pathol Lab Med* 1984;**108**:403–6.

29. Garcia, AGP, Fonseca MEF, Marques RLS, Lobato YY. Placental morphology in cytomegalovirus infection. *Placenta* 1989;**10**:1–19.

30. Schwartz DA, Khan R, Stoll B. Characterizaton of the fetal inflammatory response to cytomegalovirus placentitis. *Arch Pathol Lab Med* 1992;**116**:221–7.

31. Muhlemann K, Miller RK, Metlay L, Menegus MA. Cytomegalovirus infection of the human placenta: an immunocytochemical study. *Hum Pathol* 1992;**23**:1234–7.

32. Davis LE, Tweed GV, Steward JA, Bernstein MT, Miller GL, Gravelle CR, *et al*. Cytomegalovirus mononucleosis in a first trimester pregnant female with transmission to the fetus. *Pediatrics* 1971;**48**:200–6.

33. Strulovici D, Copelovici Y, Bedivan M, Maior E, Teodoru GC. Isolation of cytomegalic virus from the placenta in a case of inapparent human infection. *Rev Roum Virol* 1974;**25**:265–70.

34. Khudr G, Benirschke K. Placental lesion in viral hepatitis. *Obstet Gynecol* 1972;**40**:381–4.

35. Benirschke K, Kaufmann P. *The Pathology of the Human Placenta*, 4th ed. New York: Springer Verlag; 2000.

36. Lucifore G, Calabro S, Carroccio G, Brigandi A. Immunocytochemical HBsAg evidence in placentas of asymptomatic carrier mothers. *Am J Obstet Gynecol* 1988;**159**:839–42.

37. Lucifore G, Martines F, Calabro S, Carroccio G, Brigandi A, de Pasquale A. HBcAg identificaton in the placental cytotypes of symptom-free HBsAg-carrier mothers: a study with the immunoperoxidase method. *Am J Obstet Gynecol* 1990;**163**:235–9.

38. Mel'nikova VF, Tsinzerling AV, Aksenov OA, Vydumkina SP, Kalinina NA. [Involvement of the afterbirth in influenza]. *Arkh Patol* 1987;**49**:19–25. Russian.

39. Jauniaux E, Nessmann C, Imbert MC, Meuris S, Puissant F, Hustin J. Morphological aspects of the placenta in HIV pregnancies. *Placenta* 1988;**8**:633–42.

40. Lewis SH, Reynolds-Kohler C, Fox HE, Nelson J. HIV-1 in trophoblastic and villous Hofbauer cells, and haematological precursors in eight-week fetuses. *Lancet* 1990;**335**:565–8.

41. Backe E, Jiminez E, Unger M, Schafer A, Jauniaux E, Vogel M. Demonstration of HIV-1 infected cells in human placenta by *in situ* hybridization and immunostaining. *J Clin Pathol* 1992;**45**:871–4.

42. Martin AW, Brady K, Smith SI, DeCoste D, Page DV, Malpica A, *et al*. Immunohistochemical localization of human immunodeficiency virus p24 antigen in placental tissue. *Hum Pathol* 1992;**23**:411–14.

43. Mattern CFT, Murray K, Jensen A. Localization of human immunodeficiency virus core antigen in term human placentas. *Pediatrics* 1992;**89**:207–9.

44. Anderson VM, Zevallos E, Gu J. The HIV-exposed placenta: morphologic observations and interpretation. *Troph Res* 1994;**8**:47–65.

45. Backe E, Jimenez E, Unger M, Schafer A, Vocks-Hauck M, Grosch-Worner I, *et al*. Vertical human immunodeficiency virus transmission: a study of placental pathology in relation to maternal risk factors. *Am J Perinatol* 1994;**11**:326–30.

46. Zevallos EA, Anderson VM, Bard E, Gu J. Detection of HIV-1 sequences in placentas of HIV infected mothers by *in situ* polymerase chain reaction. *Cell Vis* 1994;**1**:116–21.

47. Villegas-Castrejon H, Carrillo-Farga J, Paredes Y, Barron A, Karchmer S. [Ultrastructural study of placentas from HIV seropositive women]. *Ginecol Obstet Mex* 1994;**62**:136–42. Spanish.

48. Katz JM, Fox CH, Eglington GS, Meyers WA, Queenan JT. Relationship between human

immunodeficiency virus-1 RNA identification in placenta and perinatal transmission. *J Perinatol* 1997;**17**:119–24.

49. Sheikh AU, Polliotti BM, Miller RK. Human immunodeficiency virus infection: *in situ* polymerase chain reaction localization in human placentas after *in utero* and *in vitro* infection. *Am J Obstet Gynecol* 2000;**182**:207–13.

50. Caretti N, Bertolin A, Dalla Pria S. Placental alterations and fetal conditions in relation to the presence of anti-human immunodeficiency virus (HIV) in pregnant mothers. *Panminerva Med* 1988;**30**:77–80.

51. Chandwani S, Greco MA, Mittal K, Antoine C, Krasinski K. Borkowsky W. Pathology and human immunodeficiency virus expression in placentas of seropositive women. *J Infect Dis* 1991;**163**:1134–8.

52. Chandwani S, Greco MA, Krasinski K, Borkowsky W. Pathology of the placenta in HIV-1 infection. *Prog AIDS Pathol* 1992;**3**:65–81.

53. Gichangi PB, Nyongo AO, Temmerman M. Pregnancy outcome and placental weights: their relationship to HIV-1 infection. *East Afr Med J* 1993;**70**:85–9.

54. Schwartz DA, Nahmias AJ. Human immunodeficiency virus and the placenta: current concepts of vertical transmission in relation to other viral agents. *Ann Clin Lab Sci* 1991;**21**:264–74.

55. Loga EM, Driscoll SG, Munro HN. Comparison of placentae from two socio-economic groups. I. Morphometry. *Pediatrics* 1972;**50**:24–31.

56. Khong TY, Staples A, Moore L, Byard RW. Observer reliability in assessing villitis of unknown aetiology. *J Clin Pathol* 1993;**46**:208–10.

57. Altshuler G, Russell P. The human placental villitides: a review of chronic intrauterine infection. *Curr Top Pathol* 1975;**60**:64–112.

58. Russell P. Inflammatory lesions of the human placenta. II. Villitis of unknown etiology in perspective. *Am J Diagn Gynecol Obstet* 1979;**1**,:339–46.

59. Russell P. Inflammatory lesions of the human placenta. III. The histopathology of villitis of unknown aetiology. *Placenta* 1980;**1**:227–44.

60. Knox WF, Fox H. Villitis of unknown aetiology: its incidence and significance in placentae from a British population. *Placenta* 1984;**5**:395–402.

61. Labarrere C, Althabe O, Telenta M. Chronic villitis of unknown aetiology in placentae of idiopathic small for gestational age infants. *Placenta* 1982;**3**:309–18.

62. Labarerre C, Althabe O, Calenti E, Musculo D. Deficiency of blocking factors in intrauterine growth retardation and its relationship with chronic villitis. *Am J Reprod Immunol Microbiol* 1986;**10**:14–19.

63. Althabe O, Labarrere CA. Chronic villitis of unknown aetiology and intrauterine growth retarded infants of normal and low ponderal index. *Placenta* 1985;**6**:369–73.

64. Michaud P, Michenet P, Lemaire B, Maitre F, Tescher M. [Placental villitis]. *Rev Fr Gynecol Obstet* 1991;**86**:225–8. French.

65. Redline RW. Placental pathology: a neglected link between basic disease mechanisms and untoward pregnancy outcome. *Curr Opin Obstet Gynecol* 1995;**7**:10–15.

66. Fox H. *Pathology of the Placenta*, 2nd ed. London; Saunders; 1997.

67. Hyde SR, Altshuler G. Infectious disorders of the placenta. In: Lewis SH, Perrin E, editors. *Pathology of the Placenta*, 2nd ed. New York: Churchill Livingstone; 1999. p. 317–42.

68. Borisch B, Jahn G, Scholl BC, Filger-Brillinger J, Heymer B, Fleckenstein B, et al. Detection of human cytomegalovirus DNA and viral antigens in tissues of different manifestations of CMV infection. *Virchows Arch B Cell Pathol Incl Mol Pathol* 1988;**55**:93–9.

69. Chehab FF, Xiao X, Kan YW, Yen TSB. Detection of cytomegalovirus infection in paraffin-embedded tissue specimens with the polymerase chain reaction. *Mod Pathol* 1989;**2**:75–8.

70. Sachdev R, Nuovo GR, Kaplan C, Greco MA. *In situ* hybridization analysis for cytomegalovirus in chronic villitis. *Pediatr Pathol* 1990;**10**:909–17.

71. Sinzger C, Muntefering H, Loning T, Stoss H, Plachter B, Jahn G. Cell types infected in human cytomegalovirus placentitis identified by immunohistochemical double staining. *Virchows Arch A Pathol Anat Histopathol* 1993;**423**:249–56.

72. Muhlemann K, Miller RA, Metlay L, Menegus MA. Characterization of cytomegalovirus infection by immunocytochemistry. *Troph Res* 1994;**8**:,215–22.

73. Nakamura Y, Sakuma S, Ohta Y, Kawano K, Hashimoto T. Detection of the human cytomegalovirus gene in placental chronic villitis by polymerase chain reaction. *Hum Pathol* 1994;**25**:815–18.

74. Benirschke K, Coen R, Patterson B, Key T. Villitis of known origin: varicella and toxoplasmosis. *Placenta* 1999;**20**:395–9.

75. Main EK, Strizki J, Schochet P. Placental production of immunoregulatory factors: trophoblast is a source of interleukin-1. *Troph Res* 1987;**2**:149–60.

76. Toth FD, Juhl BC, Norskov-Lauritsen N, Aboagye-Mathiesen G, Ebbesen P. Interferon production by cultured human trophoblasts and choriocarcinoma cell lines by Sendai virus. *J Gen Virol* 1990;**71**:3067–9.

77. Reuben JM, Gonik B, Li S, Loo L, Turpin J. Induction of cytokines in normal placental cells by the human immunodeficiency virus. *Lymphokine Cytokine Res* 1991;**10**:195–9.

78. Chen HL, Yang Y, Hu XL, Yelavartchi KK, Fishback JL, Hunt JS. Tumor necrosis factor-alpha and protein are present in human placental and uterine cells at early and late stages of gestation. *Am J Pathol* 1991;**139**:327–35.

79. Vince G, Shorter S, Starkey P, Humphreys J, Clover L, Wilkins T, *et al*. Localization of tumor necrosis factor production in cells at the materno/fetal interface in human pregnancy. *Clin Exp Immunol* 1992;**88**:174–80.

80. Aboagye-Mathiesen G, Toth FD, Hager H, Human trophoblast interferons. *Antiviral Res* 1993;**22**:91–105.

81. Guilbert L, Robertson SA, Wegmann TG. The trophoblast as an integral component of macrophage-cytokine network. *Immunol Cell Biol* 1993;**71**:49–57.

82. Whaley AE, Reddy Meka CS, Harbison LA, Hunt JS, Imakawa K. Identification and cellular localization of unique interferon mRNA from human placenta. *J Biol Chem* 1994;**269**:10864–8.

83. Steinborn A, von Gall C, Hildebrand R, Stutte H-J, Kaufmann M. Identification of placental cytokine-producing cells in term and premature labour. *Obstet Gynecol* 1998;**91**:329–35.

84. Banatvala JE, Potter JE, Best JM. Interferon response to Sendai and rubella viruses in human foetal cultures. *J Gen Virol* 1971;**13**:193–201.

85. Banatvala JE, Potter JE, Webster MJ. Foetal interferon responses induced by rubella virus. In: *Intrauterine Infections CIBA Foundation Symposium 10*. Amsterdam: Associated Scientific Publishers; 1973. p. 77–99.

86. Zdravkovic M, Knudsen HJ, Liu X, Hager H, Zachar V, Aboagye-Mathiesen G, *et al*. High interferon alpha levels in placenta, maternal, and cord blood suggest a protective effect against intrauterine herpes simplex infection. *J Med Virol* 1997;**51**:210–13.

87. Zachar V, Fazio-Tirrozzo G, Fink T, Roberts DJ, Broadhead RL, Brabin B, *et al*. Lack of protection against vertical transmission of HIV-1 by interferons produced during pregnancy in a cohort from East African republic of Malawi. *J Med Virol* 2000;**61**:195–200.

88. Paradowska E, Blach-Olszewska Z, Sender J, Jarosz W. Antiviral nonspecific immunity of human placenta at term: possible role of endogenous tumor necrosis factors and interferons. *J Interferon Cytokine Res* 1996;**16**:941–8.

89. Bacsi A, Aranyosi J, Beck Z, Ebbesen P, Andirko I, Szabo J, *et al*. Placental macrophage contact potentiates the complete replicative cycle of human cytomegalovirus in syncytiotrophoblast cells: role of interleukin-B and transforming growth factor-beta 1. *J Interferon Cytokine Res* 1999;**19**:1153–60.

90. Fujino T, Iwamoto I, Otsuka H, Ikeda T, Takesako S, Nagata Y. Apoptosis in placentas from human t-lymphotropic virus type 1 seropositive pregnant women: a possible defence mechanism against transmission from mother to fetus. *Obstet Gynecol* 1999;**94**:279–83.

91. Vince GS, Johnson PM. Immunobiology of human uteroplacental macrophages – friend or foe? *Placenta* 1996;**17**:191–9.

92. Oliveira LHS, Fonseca MEF, de Bonis M. Placental phagocytic cells infected with Herpes simplex type 2 and echovirus type 19: virological and ultrastructural aspects. *Placenta* 1992;**13**:405–16.

93. Ebbesen P, Toth F, Aboagye-Mathiesen G, Zachar V, Hager H, Norskov-Lauritsen N, *et al*. Vertical transmission of HIV: possible mechanisms and placental response. *Troph Res* 1994;**8**:1–17.

94. Norskov-Lauritsen N, Aboagye-Mathiesen G, Dalsgaard AM, Gildberg A, Petersen PM, Toth F, *et al*. Vaccinia virus infection of cultured human first trimester trophoblast. *Troph Res* 1994;**8**:151–60.

95. Hemmings DG, Kilani R, Nykiforuk C, Preiksaitis J, Gilbert LJ. Permissive cytomegalovirus infection of primary villous term and first trimester trophoblasts. *J Virol* 1998;**72**:4970–9.

96. Zachar V, Zacharova V, Fink T, Thomas RA, King BR, Ebbesen P, *et al*. Genetic analysis reveals ongoing HIV type 1 evolution in infected human placental trophoblast. *AIDS Res Hum Retroviruses* 1999;**15**:1673–83.

97. Tscherning-Casper C, Papadogiannakis N, Anvret M, Stolpe L, Lindgren S, Bohlin AB, *et al*. The trophoblastic epithelial barrier is not infected in full-term placentae of human immunodeficiency virus-seropositive mothers undergoing antiretroviral therapy. *J Virol* 1999;**73**:9673–8.

98. Abzug MJ. Maternal factors affecting the integrity of the late gestation placental barrier to murine enterovirus infection. *J Infect Dis* 1997;**176**:41–9.

99. Russell P, Atkinson K, Krishnan L. Recurrent reproductive failure due to severe placental villitis of unknown etiology. *J Reprod Med* 1980;**24**:93–8.

100.   Labarerre CA, Faulk WP, McIntyre JA. Villitis in normal human term placentae: frequency of the lesion determined by monoclonal antibody to HLA-DR antigen. *J Reprod Immunol* 1989;**16**:127–35.
101.   Labarerre CA, McIntyre JA, Faulk WP. Immunohistologic evidence that villitis in human normal term placentas is an immunologic lesion. *Am J Obstet Gynecol* 1990;**162**:515–22.
102.   Altemani AM. Immunohistochemical study of the inflammatory infiltrate in villitis of unknown etiology: a qualitative and quantitative analysis. *Pathol Res Pract* 1992;**188**:303–9.
103.   Labarerre CA, Faulk WP. Immunopathology of human extraembryonic tissues. In: Coulam CB, Faulk WP, McIntyre JA, editors. *Immunological Obstetrics*. New York: Norton; 1992. p. 439–63.
104.   Johnson KP. Mouse cytomegalovirus: placental infection. *J Infect Dis* 1969;**120**:445–50.
105.   Altshuler G, Russell P, Ermocilla R. The placental pathology of small-for-gestational age infants. *Am J Obstet Gynecol* 1975;**121**:351–9.
106.   Bjoro KJ, Myhre E. The role of chronic non-specific inflammatory lesions of the placenta in intrauterine growth retardation. *Acta Pathol Microbiol Immunol Scand [A]* 1984;**92**:133–7.
107.   Mortimer G, MacDonald DJ, Smeeth A. A pilot study of the frequency and significance of placental villitis. *Br J Obstet Gynaecol* 1985;**92**:629–33.
108.   Altemani AM, Fassoni A, Marba S. Cord IgM levels in placentas with villitis of unknown etiology. *J Perinat Med* 1989;**17**:465–8.
109.   Nordenvall M, Sandstedt B. Placental villitis and intrauterine growth retardation in a Swedish population. *APMIS* 1990;**98**:19–24.
110.   Salafia CM, Vintzileos AM, Silberman L, Bantham KF, Vogel CA. Placental pathology of idiopathic intrauterine growth retardation at term. *Am J Perinatol* 1992;**9**:179–84.
111.   Redline RW, Patterson P. Patterns of placental injury: correlations with gestational age, placental weight, and clinical diagnoses. *Arch Pathol Lab Med* 1994;**118**:698–701.
112.   Redline RW, Abramowsky CR. Clinical and pathologic aspects of recurrent placental villitis. *Hum Pathol* 1985;**16**:727–31.
113.   Labarrere CA, Althabe O. Chronic villitis of unknown aetiology in recurrent intrauterine fetal growth retardation. *Placenta* 1987;**8**:167–73.

Chapter 18

Cytomegalovirus infection in pregnancy

Paul D Griffiths

Introduction

The focus of this chapter is on intrauterine transmission of cytomegalovirus (CMV). However, it should also be recognised that perinatal transmission is common when neonates acquire virus from their mother through contact with infected maternal genital secretions or through breast milk. The clinical course of such perinatal infections is nearly always benign and thus their medical importance is in the diagnostic confusion caused when children with suspected congenital infection are investigated and found to be infected with CMV. At present, there is no way of differentiating between congenital and perinatal CMV infection, once the child has passed three weeks of age.

The virus

The Ad169 strain of CMV has been sequenced in its entirety. It has the largest genome of any virus known to infect humans and only a small minority of its genes are used to produce the physical virion. The majority of the remaining genes probably are important for interaction with the host, and thus are potential pathogenicity genes, but the function of approximately only one-third has been delineated so far. In addition, wild strains of CMV contain an additional 22 genes,[1] which are lost when the virus is passaged in the laboratory. Some genes are known to help the virus to evade immune responses (Table 18.1). In particular, CMV contains a series of genes that co-ordinate the downregulation of class I human leukocyte antigen (HLA) molecules so that the target cell cannot be recognised efficiently by the cytotoxic T lymphocyte. To avoid lysis by natural killer cells, which recognise major histocompatibility complex molecules in a non-antigen-specific way, the virus encodes at least two other genes that provide a negative signal to the natural killer cell. CMV can infect the cytotrophoblast cells of the placenta, which lack the normal array of class I molecules. It is interesting to note that the classical HLA-C – and the non-classic HLA-G – molecules found in

Table 18.1.   Human cytomegalovirus immune evasion strategies

Defence	Response
Antibody	Fc receptor
Complement	CD55/CD46/CD59
T-cytotoxic	*UL83/US3/US6/US2/US11*
Natural killer cells	*UL18*
Chemokines	*US28*

the cytotrophoblast are not downregulated by two of the genes (*US2* and *US11*) that together potently downregulate class I in other cells.[2] It is possible that other genes within CMV are responsible for dealing with HLA-C and HLA-G molecules in the placenta, or that these molecules confer some protective function to the placenta. This might help to explain why the majority of women with primary infection do not transmit virus to the fetus *in utero*.

It should also be noted that classical studies of CMV in the laboratory have produced a series of misleading impressions of CMV, which are nevertheless enduring.

1.   Key genes have been lost from the virus in strain Ad169, as mentioned earlier.

2.   Strain Ad169 grows only slowly in fibroblast cell cultures in the laboratory, typically taking two to three weeks to produce cytopathic effect. This led to the assumption that its replication *in vivo* was slow, whereas more recent studies using modern molecular methods demonstrate rapid dynamics of CMV in the blood of patients,[3] with a doubling time (virus load on the increase) or a half-life (virus load on the decrease) of approximately one day, parameters which are rather similar to those of HIV.

3.   Studies in fibroblast cell cultures indicated that ganciclovir was the most potent compound and that aciclovir had no activity. Nevertheless, controlled clinical trials have demonstrated that aciclovir is able to inhibit CMV replication, although high doses of the compound must be given, either intravenously or through the use of the prodrug valaciclovir.[4,5]

4.   In patients treated with ganciclovir, resistant strains have been reported to be rare, although this is partly because mixed populations of mutant and wild-type virus compete in the laboratory during the two- to three-week incubation period. Modern molecular methods show that resistance is more common than previously thought[6] and this is thus an emerging clinical problem that must be taken into account when designing treatment algorithms.

Epidemiology

Sero-epidemiological studies show that CMV infection is common, with approximately 60% of women of childbearing age in developed countries[7] showing evidence of past infection and virtually 100% of those brought up in developing countries. In almost all cases, the virus is acquired asymptomatically, so that only testing for immunoglobulin G-specific antibodies can indicate which women have been infected in the past. CMV can thus be thought of as a virus that is very well adapted to its natural human host. However, if that host has impaired cell-mediated immunity, either due to HIV infection or the immunosuppressive drugs required for transplantation, or because the T-cell system is immature in the case of the fetus, then CMV can cause severe multi-system disease. It has been shown in all of these patient populations that the individuals who develop disease are those with the highest quantity of virus. Indeed, multivariate statistical models demonstrate that the quantity of virus explains all the risk factors for CMV disease previously described in classical clinical studies.[8,9,10] Furthermore, the regression line of peak quantity of virus against risk of disease is nonlinear and shows a marked threshold transition once the viral load exceeds approximately 10^5 genomes/ml of body fluid, be that blood or urine.[8,9] It is clear from this observation that, in medical practice, antiviral and vaccine strategies should be deployed to prevent patients in each of these individual groups having viral loads that rise above this threshold value. This observation is a source of optimism for the future control of CMV, since it will be easier to control high viral loads of CMV than to completely eradicate it from patients.

Congenital CMV

Neonates born with symptoms of intrauterine CMV infection may have any or all of the following problems:

- intrauterine growth restriction
- hepatosplenomegaly
- thrombocytopenic purpura
- jaundice
- microcephaly
- chorioretinitis.

The prognosis for such children is appalling, with the vast majority suffering severe mental impairment and/or hearing loss. Those born without symptoms at birth do not necessarily escape the ravages of CMV. Approximately 15% of children develop symptoms later, with the brain and inner ear being the major target organs.[11] It is thought that the progressive loss of hearing is caused by continuing CMV replication in the organ of Corti. If this is so, it could explain why CMV causes disease when maternal infection occurs in all three trimesters of pregnancy, and could suggest that neonates given effective antiviral therapy might have some of their hearing function preserved. Unfortunately, the only drug available to date has been ganciclovir. Although this is potent, it has the distinct disadvantage of requiring intravenous infusion, and causes neutropenia and thrombocytopenia. In addition, its preclinical profile shows carcinogenicity in rodents and thus caution is required when considering whether treatment would be in the patient's best interests. As part of a randomised, controlled clinical trial, Whitley et al.[12] conducted a phase II study that compared two doses of ganciclovir. The drug was administered intravenously for six weeks and the higher dose was found to be no worse in terms of tolerable neutropenia and thrombocytopenia than the lower dose. It was noted that hearing improved or stabilised in five of the 30 children who were evaluable and, since this observation was different from historical cases of untreated congenital CMV, improvement of hearing was taken forward as the primary endpoint in a controlled phase III trial of the higher dose of ganciclovir. This second study, conducted by the Collaborative Antiviral Study Group, has recently reported its results.[13] The primary endpoint of improved hearing (as measured by brainstem-evoked responses) or normal hearing that was still normal at six months showed that neonates randomised to ganciclovir did better than those randomised to no treatment, with a *P* value of approximately 0.05. In addition, the proportion of neonates whose hearing was found to be worse at follow-up was significantly lower in those randomised to ganciclovir. While a full report of the study is still awaited, I believe that these results should be acted upon now that a clinical endpoint has shown benefit from intervention and this treatment should be offered to all neonates born with the criteria used in the trial, i.e. those with central nervous system (CNS) signs present at birth. Due to the toxicity of ganciclovir mentioned above, these results should not be assumed to apply to children with no CNS symptoms, and further work should be taken forward to find an orally bioavailable compound with a better safety profile than ganciclovir. It should be noted that the availability of this treatment will have only a minor effect on the total disease caused by CMV,[14] since treatment can only be given to the minority of neonates born with symptoms (Table 18.2). Since the economic cost of congenital CMV in the USA has been reported by the Institute of Medicine to be nearly one billion dollars annually, the results of this study provide an important first step towards controlling this problem.

Primary CMV infection during pregnancy

A series of prospective studies in the 1970s and 1980s used immunoglobulin G seroconversion to detect primary CMV infection during pregnancy (Table 18.3). Overall, they show that primary infection occurs in approximately 1.3% of initially seronegative women during pregnancy, almost always without producing any symptoms. Thus, obstetricians should consider primary CMV infection to be of the same frequency as placenta praevia and placental abruption, although, as with those conditions, it does not necessarily produce disease in every case.

Intrauterine infection occurs after primary infection in all trimesters with, overall, approximately 37% of neonates being born with congenital infection (Table 18.4). It is not clear why primary infection does not cross the placenta in approximately two-thirds of infected women, but it is reasonable to suggest that those mothers able to mount immune responses may be able to moderate this infection. There is some evidence in support of this possibility.[15] Damage can result from primary infection in

Table 18.2. Annual public health impact of congenital cytomegalovirus (after Stagno, 1990[14])

	USA	UK
Number of live births	4 000 000	700 000
Number congenitally infected	40 000	2100
Proportion congenitally infected	1%	0.3%
Number with cytomegalic inclusion disease	2800	147
Number fatal	336	18
Number with sequelae	2218	116
Number asymptomatic	37 200	1953
Number with sequelae	5580	293
Total number damaged	8134	427

Table 18.3. Primary cytomegalovirus infection during pregnancy

| | | Antenatal testing | | | | | | |
| | | Total women | Seronegative women | | Seronegative women followed to delivery | | Seroconversions | |
Study	Year	(n)	(n)	(%)	(n)	(%)	(n)	(%)
Stern and Tucker[26]	1973	1040	347	33	270	78	11	4.07
Grant et al.[27]	1981	4446	2026	46	1841	91	13	0.71
Ahlfors et al.[28]	1982	4382	1218	28	1175	96	14	1.19
Griffiths and Baboonian[7]	1984	10847	4550	42	3716	82	32	0.86
Kumar et al.[29]	1984	3253	1404	43	1089	78	14	1.29
Stagno et al. (high)[30]	1986	12140	5645	47	4692	83	77	1.64
Stagno et al. (low)[30]	1986	4078	954	23	507	53	19	3.75
Yow et al.[31]	1988	4578	2181	48	1940	89	21	1.08
Totals		44754	18325	41	15220	83	201	1.32

Table 18.4. Cytomegalovirus transmission at different gestational stages

| | | Number of neonates positive/number tested | |
Study	Year	First or second trimester	Third trimester
Stern and Tucker[26]	1973	4/6	1/3
Grant et al.[27]	1981	3/4	2/7
Ahlfors et al.[28]	1982	1/1	3/8
Griffiths and Baboonian[7]	1984	2/30	6/15
Kumar et al.[29]	1984	2/6	5/8
Stagno et al.[30]	1986	23/43	12/26
Yow et al.[31]	1988	7/21	3/20
Bodeus et al.[32]	1999	31/74	38/49
Liesnard et al.[17]	2000	38/151	17/59
Totals		111/336 (33%)	87/197 (44%)

all trimesters and thus CMV is not like rubella, which acts as a teratogen; instead, CMV allows fetal organs to develop normally but then secondarily lyses them to produce disease by loss of function. Thus, unlike rubella, there is no strong gradient of neonatal disease linked to the trimester in which primary infection occurs. This is partially explained by an excess of spontaneous fetal loss when infections occur early in pregnancy, with the result that some of the cases of most severe disease do not present to paediatricians.

Since two-thirds of women do not transmit virus *in utero* and since the majority of infected neonates do not develop disease, the risk to a woman with primary infection of having a baby damaged by congenital CMV is only about 7%. This calculation led us to propose in 1984 that documented maternal primary infection on its own was not a sufficient criterion to recommend termination of pregnancy[7] and that further studies were required to provide better discrimination between those fetuses destined to develop disease. It is now clear that intrauterine infection can be diagnosed by amniocentesis.[16,17] Unfortunately, this procedure cannot be performed for this purpose before 21 weeks of pregnancy because the pathogenesis involves fetal infection of the kidneys, with excretion of virus into the amniotic fluid, and fetal renal function is not sufficiently well established before this time. Nevertheless, it is now clear that polymerase chain reaction (PCR) methods can reliably detect intrauterine infection provided that multiple replicates of amniotic fluid are tested.[18] In addition, there is emerging information that the quantity of CMV DNA found by PCR in the amniotic fluid can provide prognostic information,[16] just as it does in the transplant and AIDS populations. Further studies of this nature are required to provide evidence-based recommendations as to when termination of pregnancy is indicated.

Recurrent maternal infection during pregnancy

It has been clear for many years that women who have been infected with CMV before they become pregnant can nevertheless deliver a baby with congenital CMV infection. Indeed, a woman can deliver two babies from consecutive pregnancies congenitally infected with CMV.[19] Where such strains have been examined, they have always been indistinguishable, suggesting that it may be maternal reactivation of latent CMV that is important, although reinfection from a common source, such as the father, remains a possibility. There are no tests that can be performed on the mother to indicate whether she is experiencing recurrent infection that could transmit virus *in utero*. Nevertheless, clinical studies have recruited women who were 'immune' before they conceived and followed them in subsequent pregnancies. The incidence of such recurrent infections with transmission may be as high as 1.5% of seropositive women in highly prevalent areas, decreasing to one-tenth of that value in seropositive women from populations with a prevalence of 60%.[19] This suggests that circulation of CMV in a community is a risk factor, not just for primary infection during pregnancy but also for recurrent maternal infection. Although these percentages are low, it must be remembered that the majority of women are seropositive, so that, in some populations, approximately half of neonates born with congenital CMV infection may have acquired it following recurrent maternal infection.

Relative impact of primary and recurrent maternal infection on congenital CMV disease

If all the neonates infected *in utero* following recurrent maternal infection were born without symptoms then this route of transmission would be simply a medical curiosity. However, in 1981, Ahlfors[20] in Sweden reported a case with disease, and a few years later a second case was reported from London.[21] Since then, a series of studies has reported that substantial numbers of neonates may be damaged by recurrent and by primary maternal infections (Table 18.5). This observation is sometimes used to weaken the case for development of a CMV vaccine or for studies designed to focus on primary infection during pregnancy. However, it must be remembered that there are no laboratory tests to detect recurrent infection during pregnancy, so primary infection is the only one amenable to study and/or intervention.

No specific therapy for CMV has been studied in pregnancy. In perinatal HIV infection, the PACTG076 study demonstrated that anti-retroviral drugs given during pregnancy can greatly reduce vertical transmission of virus. Several anti-CMV drugs

Table 18.5. Cytomegalovirus disease in neonates born to mothers with known type of infection during pregnancy

Study	Year	Neonates screened (n)	Congenital infection (n)	Congenital infection %	Cases with symptoms at birth (n)	Symptomatic cases where maternal infection was defined (n)	Cases of disease/cases of maternal infection (n) primary	Cases of disease/cases of maternal infection (n) recurrent
Peckham et al.[33]	1983	14200	42	0.3	1	1	1/1	
Griffiths et al.[34]	1991	2737	9	0.33	2	2	0/4	2/5
Fowler et al.[11]	1992	N/A	197		24	24	24/132	0/65
Boppana et al.[35]	1999	20885	246	1.18	47	20	8/8	12/12
Casteels et al.[36]	1999		15		5	5	3/9	2/5
Ahlfors et al.[37]	1999		76		22	18	9/30	9/32

are now licensed, with more compounds that are orally bioavailable entering phase I clinical trials. By deploying antiviral agents to prevent the viral load increasing above the threshold value, the viral load pathogenesis model[9] predicted that a beneficial effect on CMV disease would be expected, disproportionate to the actual ability of the drug to control virus replication, i.e. a drug with moderate anti-CMV activity could transform CMV disease into asymptomatic CMV infection in most cases. This prediction is supported by the results of a trial in AIDS patients where significant reduction of CMV disease was seen when valaciclovir reduced the median viral load by only 1.3 logs.[4] If a similar threshold effect holds for transplacental transmission of CMV, this would facilitate the future recruitment of women with primary CMV infection during pregnancy into a placebo-controlled trial to determine if vertical transmission can be reduced by moderate doses of antiviral drugs. Although considerable time (and a compound with a suitable safety profile) will be required to develop the concept, the conducting of a double-blind, placebo-controlled trial should be encouraged.

Prospects for a vaccine

The details of the natural history during pregnancy have in the past been considered to provide formidable barriers to the development of a CMV vaccine. Taken together with the slow growth of virus *in vitro* and low yields of virus from cell culture, it was considered impracticable to try to develop a live attenuated vaccine in the way that was done for rubella, measles, mumps and poliomyelitis. Indeed, the pioneering results in renal allograft recipients of Plotkin et al.[22] showed no reduction in the incidence of infection. This suggested to some that a CMV vaccine would never be developed, although a reduction in the severity of disease was seen, implying some control of viral replication. However, it is now known that passage of this virus produces a strain that is not representative of the virus found *in vivo*, and molecular techniques for producing recombinant DNA vaccines now allow this slow growth *in vitro* to be bypassed. The development of a CMV vaccine should now be reconsidered, especially since the costs of CMV congenital disease have been shown to be so high that a successful vaccine would be rapidly cost-effective.

Although CMV contains approximately 225 genes, the humoral immune response is conveniently focused largely upon one protein, glycoprotein B (gB), while the cell-mediated immune response is largely focused upon a second protein, ppUL83 (pp65). It would therefore be relatively straightforward to use standard molecular techniques to produce immunogens from these two proteins and question whether they could produce protection against CMV infection. A phase I trial of recombinant, soluble gB in normal individuals was reported in 1999.[23] The results showed that this protein produced antibodies not just measurable by enzyme immunoassay but also by neutralisation. Furthermore, this soluble protein boosted the neutralising antibody titres found in individuals with natural immunity. This suggests the possibility that the gB presented in the natural environment of the virus may be poorly immunogenic, so that molecular techniques may indeed be able to produce an immune response that is superior to that found in nature. Unfortunately, the company developing this preparation abandoned all of its vaccine development work, for reasons unrelated to the CMV programme. Glycoprotein B has also been incorporated into a canarypox vector. These avian poxviruses undergo abortive infection in humans, so they stimulate cell-mediated immunity without being able to go through a full round of viral replication. At the time of writing, a combination approach using priming with the canarypox gB construct and boosting with the soluble recombinant gB is being considered. Other prototype immunogens have also been considered.

The conducting of vaccine trials with the clinical endpoint of CMV disease would require impracticably large numbers of volunteers. However, modern molecular biology can help by providing viral load as a surrogate marker of control of CMV replication.[3,6,8] It would therefore be straightforward to immunise patients on a waiting list for organ transplantation with either vaccine or placebo and then measure their viral load once they receive a transplant and become immunocompromised. In this way, evidence of emerging efficacy could be obtained, allowing optimisation of the immunisation schedule in subsequent cohorts of patients. Thus, although protection of pregnant women represents a major target for a CMV vaccine, the vaccine does not have to be evaluated in the early stages in such women.

If a vaccine preparation that is safe and is able to prevent infection effectively in immunocompromised patients is developed, then it should be deployed to interrupt transmission in the community. The standard way of doing this would be to immunise children in the first year of life, as with other viral vaccines. It is true that perinatal infection would mean that some children would become infected before the vaccine was administered and thus CMV could only be eradicated from the community after two or three generations of children had been immunised. However, this is not a fatal blow to an immunisation campaign since it also applies to the varicella-zoster virus (VZV) vaccine, which can likewise establish latency and give recurrent infection, and which represents a source of primary chickenpox. VZV vaccine is now licensed in the USA and is being used to immunise all children.

If an effective CMV vaccine were given to all children, is it possible that it might do more harm than good by altering herd immunity? This was an important consideration in the case of rubella because instituting a vaccine programme always raises the average age at which unimmunised children encounter infectious individuals and so become infected. Where the risk of disease is age-related, as is obviously the case with infections acquired during pregnancy, increasing the mean age of infection might precipitate a future epidemic of intrauterine disease.[24] The scientific knowledge that this effect of herd immunity would only damage those individuals who did not volunteer for immunisation would not necessarily provide much comfort for government and health officials who would have to manage the resulting public disquiet. However, CMV is not like rubella: the average age at which people acquire CMV is 26 years compared with seven years for rubella. It can therefore be shown using population modelling techniques that any effect of a CMV vaccine on herd immunity would be beneficial rather than deleterious.[25]

Overall, in my view, the perceived problems of developing a CMV vaccine are due more to reluctance to commit to tackle what is a difficult problem than to genuine overwhelming impediments to success.

References

1. Cha TA, Tom E, Kemble GW, Duke GM, Mocarski ES, Spaete RR. Human cytomegalovirus clinical isolates carry at least 19 genes not found in laboratory strains. *J Virol* 1996;**70**:78–83.
2. Schust DJ, Tortorella D, Seebach J, Phan C, Ploegh HL. Trophoblast class I major histocompatibility complex (MHC) products are resistant to rapid degradation imposed by the human cytomegalovirus (HCMV) gene products US2 and US11. *J Exp Med* 1998;**188**:497–503.
3. Emery VC, Cope AV, Bowen EF, Gor D, Griffiths PD. The dynamics of human cytomegalovirus replication *in vivo*. *J Exp Med* 1999;**190**:177–82.
4. Emery VC, Sabin C, Feinberg JE, Gryzwacz M, Knight S, Griffiths PD, *et al*. Quantitative effects of valaciclovir on the replication of cytomegalovirus in patients with advanced human immunodeficiency virus disease: baseline cytomegalovirus load dictates time to disease and survival. *J Infect Dis* 1999;**180**:695–701.
5. Lowance D, Neumayer HH, Legendre CM, Squifflet JP, Kovarik J, Brennan PJ, *et al*. Valacyclovir for the prevention of cytomegalovirus disease after renal transplantation. International Valacyclovir Cytomegalovirus Prophylaxis Transplantation Study Group. *N Engl J Med* 1999;**340**:1462–70.
6. Emery VC, Griffiths PD. Prediction of cytomegalovirus load and resistance patterns after antiviral chemotherapy. *Proc Natl Acad Sci U S A* 2000;**97**:8039–44.
7. Griffiths PD, Baboonian C. A prospective study of primary cytomegalovirus infection during pregnancy: final report. *Br J Obstet Gynaecol* 1984;**91**:307–15.
8. Cope AV, Sabin C, Burroughs A, Rolles K, Griffiths PD, Emery VC. Interrelationships among quantity of human cytomegalovirus (HCMV) DNA in blood, donor-recipient serostatus, and administration of methylprednisolone as risk factors for HCMV disease following liver transplantation. *J Infect Dis* 1997;**176**:1484–90.
9. Cope AV, Sweny P, Sabin C, Rees L, Griffiths PD, Emery VC. Quantity of cytomegalovirus viruria is a major risk factor for cytomegalovirus disease after renal transplantation. *J Med Virol* 1997;**52**:200–5.
10. Gor D, Sabin C, Prentice HG, Vyas N, Man S, Griffiths PD, *et al*. Longitudinal fluctuations in cytomegalovirus load in bone marrow transplant patients: relationship between peak virus load, donor/recipient serostatus, acute GVHD and CMV disease. *Bone Marrow Transplant* 1998;**21**:597–605.
11. Fowler KB, Stagno S, Pass RF, Britt WJ, Boll TJ, Alford CA. The outcome of congenital cytomegalovirus infection in relation to maternal antibody status. *N Engl J Med* 1992;**326**:663–7.
12. Whitley RJ, Cloud G, Gruber W, Storch GA, Demmler GJ, Jacobs RF, *et al*. Ganciclovir treatment of symptomatic congenital cytomegalovirus infection: results of a phase II study. National Institute of Allergy and Infectious Diseases Collaborative Antiviral Study Group. *J Infect Dis* 1997;**175**:1080–6.
13. Kimberlin DW, *et al*. 40th Interscience Conference on Antimicrobial Agents and Chemotherapy, 17–20 September 2000, Toronto, Canada. Abstract 1942.
14. Stagno S. Cytomegalovirus. In: Remington JS, Klein JO, editors. *Infectious Diseases of the Fetus and Newborn Infant*. Philadelphia (PA): WB Saunders; 1990. p. 240–81.
15. Stern H, Hannington G, Booth J, Moncrieff D. An early marker of fetal infection after primary cytomegalovirus infection in pregnancy. *BMJ* 1986;**292**:718–20.
16. Lazzarotto T, Varani S, Guerra B, Nicolosi A, Lanari M, Landini MP. Prenatal indicators of congenital cytomegalovirus infection. *J Pediatr* 2000;**137**:90–5.
17. Liesnard C, Donner C, Brancart F, Gosselin F, Delforge ML, Rodesch F. Prenatal diagnosis of congenital cytomegalovirus infection: prospective study of 237 pregnancies at risk. *Obstet Gynecol* 2000;**95**:881–8.
18. Revello MG, Sarasini A, Zavattoni M, Baldanti F, Gerna G. Improved prenatal diagnosis of congenital

human cytomegalovirus infection by a modified nested polymerase chain reaction. *J Med Virol* 1998;**56**:99–103.

19. Stagno S, Reynolds DW, Huang ES, Thames SD, Smith RJ, Alford CA. Congenital cytomegalovirus infection. *N Engl J Med* 1977;**296**:1254–8.

20. Ahlfors K, Harris S, Ivarsson S, Svanberg L. Secondary maternal cytomegalovirus infection causing symptomatic congenital infection. *N Engl J Med* 1981;**305**:284.

21. Rutter D, Griffiths P, Trompeter RS. Cytomegalic inclusion disease after recurrent maternal infection. *Lancet* 1985;**i**:1182.

22. Plotkin SA, Smiley ML, Friedman HM, Starr SE, Fleisher GR, Wlodaver C, *et al.* Towne-vaccine-induced prevention of cytomegalovirus disease after renal transplants. *Lancet* 1984;**i**:528–30.

23. Pass RF, Duliege AM, Boppana S, Sekulovich R, Percell S, Britt W, *et al.* A subunit cytomegalovirus vaccine based on recombinant envelope glycoprotein B and a new adjuvant. *J Infect Dis* 1999;**180**:970–5.

24. Knox EG. Strategy for rubella vaccination. *Int J Epidemiol* 1980;**9**:13–23.

25. Griffiths PD, McLean AR, Emery VC. Encouraging prospects for immunisation against primary cytomegalovirus infection. *Vaccine* 2001;**19**:1356–62.

26. Stern H, Tucker SM. Prospective study of cytomegalovirus infection in pregnancy. *BMJ* 1973;**2**:268–70.

27. Grant S, Edmond E, Syme J. A prospective study of cytomegalovirus infection in pregnancy. I. Laboratory evidence of congenital infection following maternal primary and reactivated infection. *J Infect* 1981;**3**:24–31.

28. Ahlfors K, Ivarsson SA, Johnsson T, Svanberg L. Primary and secondary maternal cytomegalovirus infections and their relation to congenital infection. Analysis of maternal sera. *Acta Paediatr Scand* 1982;**71**:109–13.

29. Kumar ML, Gold E, Jacobs IB, Ernhart CB, Nankervis GA. Primary cytomegalovirus infection in adolescent pregnancy. *Pediatrics* 1984;**74**:493–500.

30. Stagno S, Pass RF, Cloud G, Britt WJ, Henderson RE, Walton PD, *et al.* Primary cytomegalovirus infection in pregnancy. Incidence, transmission to fetus, and clinical outcome. *JAMA* 1986;**256**:1904–8.

31. Yow MD, Williamson DW, Leeds LJ, Thompson P, Woodward RM, Walmus BF, *et al.* Epidemiologic characteristics of cytomegalovirus infection in mothers and their infants. *Am J Obstet Gynecol* 1988;**158**:1189–95.

32. Bodeus M, Hubinont C, Goubau P. Increased risk of cytomegalovirus transmission *in utero* during late gestation. *Obstet Gynecol* 1999;**93**:658–60.

33. Peckham CS, Chin KS, Coleman JC, Henderson K, Hurley R, Preece PM. Cytomegalovirus infection in pregnancy: preliminary findings from a prospective study. *Lancet* 1983;**i**:1352–5.

34. Griffiths PD, Baboonian C, Rutter D, Peckham C. Congenital and maternal cytomegalovirus infections in a London population. *Br J Obstet Gynaecol* 1991;**98**:135–40.

35. Boppana SB, Fowler KB, Britt WJ, Stagno S, Pass RF. Symptomatic congenital cytomegalovirus infection in infants born to mothers with pre-existing immunity to cytomegalovirus. *Pediatrics* 1999;**104**:55–60.

36. Casteels A, Naessens A, Gordts F, De Catte L, Bougatef A, Foulon W. Neonatal screening for congenital cytomegalovirus infections. *J Perinat Med* 1999;**27**:116–21.

37. Ahlfors K, Ivarsson SA, Harris S. Report on a long-term study of maternal and congenital cytomegalovirus infection in Sweden. Review of prospective studies available in the literature. *Scand J Infect Dis* 1999;**31**:443–57.

Chapter 19

Chickenpox (varicella) and herpes zoster (shingles) in pregnancy

David Carrington

Introduction

Varicella-zoster virus (VZV) is a DNA virus within the herpes family that is responsible for chickenpox (varicella), the primary infection, and herpes zoster (shingles), a reactivation of the virus occurring at any age but with an increasing incidence in adulthood. Varicella is an acute highly infectious disease that is transmitted by droplet spread, by direct personal contact with vesicle fluid or indirectly via fomites. The primary infection (chickenpox) is characterised by fever, malaise and a pruritic rash that develops into crops of vesicles which crust over before healing. The incubation period is 10–21 days (commonly 14–15 days). The disease is infectious 48 hours before the rash appears and lasts until the vesicles crust over. Chickenpox is a common disease of childhood (when it usually causes a mild infection), such that over 85% of the UK adult population are seropositive for VZV immunoglobulin G (IgG) antibody. Direct and indirect contact with chickenpox in pregnancy is common and leads to clinical infection in the mother in one in 2000 pregnancies in the UK.[1,2] Infection is only seen in those with no history of chickenpox and in those with no detectable VZV antibodies. Higher proportions of adults from tropical and subtropical areas are susceptible to VZV infection.[3]

Herpes zoster is a reactivation of the virus, which resides in dorsal root ganglion cells, and usually appears clinically as a localised vesicular eruption in a single dermatome. Although more common in the elderly and in immunosuppressed patients, herpes zoster is occasionally seen during pregnancy. Herpes zoster in pregnancy does not result in intrauterine infection or infection of the neonate. In the largest reported study[4] involving 366 cases of herpes zoster in pregnancy, no cases of fetal varicella syndrome or neonatal herpes zoster were reported, and there was no evidence of persistent VZV antibodies at one year of age. Direct contact with a case of herpes zoster can result in chickenpox, but not herpes zoster, in the susceptible host.

Primary VZV infection in pregnancy can be associated with an adverse outcome in three possible ways, as discussed below.

Maternal chickenpox

Chickenpox can be more severe in normal adults than in children. There is anecdotal evidence that pregnancy increases the risks of disease-associated complications, particularly in the later stages of pregnancy. Pneumonia occurs in approximately 10% of adult cases, although rates of between 2% and 35% have been reported in pregnant patients. In two maternal reports,[5,6] severe chickenpox with pneumonitis occurred in 7% and 9%, respectively, and required mechanical ventilation. A 2% mortality was observed in both studies. In the period 1985 to 1996, eight indirect maternal deaths and one late maternal death were reported in the UK in association with maternal varicella pneumonia.[7–10]

Fetal varicella syndrome

Fetal varicella syndrome, previously referred to as congenital varicella syndrome, occurs when the fetus is infected during the viraemic phase of maternal chickenpox before 20 weeks of gestation. The syndrome, first described in 1947,[11] is associated not with fetal chickenpox *per se* but with a subsequent herpes zoster reactivation *in utero* that occurs in a minority of the infected fetuses. VZV reactivation within infected dorsal root ganglia results in herpes zoster occurring at single or multiple sites, involving internal and external tissues and includes one or more of the following:

- skin scarring in a dermatomal distribution and growth restriction
- eye defects (microphthalmia, chorioretinitis, cataracts)
- hypoplasia of the limbs
- neurological abnormalities (microcephaly, cortical atrophy, mental retardation and dysfunction of bowel and bladder sphincters).

The risk of fetal varicella syndrome is estimated to be 0.4% in the first 12 weeks of gestation and approximately 2% between 13 and 20 weeks.[4] The syndrome does not occur if the primary maternal infection occurs after 20 weeks of gestation,[4,12–14] The mortality in affected cases is high. The risk of spontaneous miscarriage after first-trimester varicella is not increased.[15] Prenatal diagnosis of fetal varicella syndrome is essentially by ultrasound rather than by virological screening of the fetus. Polyhydramnios, hyperechogenic foci in the liver and hydrops fetalis have been described.[16] Ultrasonography carried out five weeks or later after the primary infection may demonstrate structural changes. Cordocentesis and amniocentesis for VZV antibodies[17] or molecular methods for the detection of viral DNA are of limited value.

Varicella of the newborn

Varicella of the newborn, previously referred to as congenital varicella, occurs when varicella infects the fetus around the time of delivery. This terminology therefore excludes horizontally acquired infection of the neonate. Transplacental passage of the virus appears to increase as gestation advances. Maternal infection during the last month of pregnancy is associated with perinatal infection in 20–60% of cases.[4–6,18] Neonatal infection rates, at approximately 60%, were similar whether the maternal infection occurred 0 or 28 days before delivery. However, the asymptomatic subclinical rate of 40% was higher in neonates of mothers with a rash 15–28 days before delivery, compared with only 8% in those neonates of mothers with a rash 0–7 days before delivery.[18] When the onset of maternal infection is five days before to two days after delivery, it may lead to more severe infection, with a historical reported mortality of 20–30%.[6,19] It is likely that the increased severity is due to a high viral load from maternal viraemia without the attenuating effects of passively acquired maternal antibodies. The use of hyperimmune gammaglobulin (varicella-zoster immunoglobulin, VZIG, which has a titre of VZV antibody eight-fold higher than normal immunoglobulin), given to babies born to mothers with varicella during the delivery period, also appears to reduce the morbidity of this disease. Similarly, babies born to mothers with clinical varicella during pregnancy and up to one week of delivery have detectable VZV antibody at birth, which persists. These infants are at risk of herpes zoster in the first few months of life as their first postnatal experience of VZV infection. Although these infants cannot be included in the definition of fetal varicella syndrome, the evidence is consistent with primary infection *in utero* and the failure of the immature immune system to maintain viral latency. Herpes zoster in these infants is usually benign.[20]

Immunoprophylaxis

A previous history of exposure to chickenpox or shingles should be ascertained from all pregnant women when a pregnancy is confirmed. The VZV status of all pregnant women who do not give a convincing history of previous chickenpox, by VZV antibody detection (available through local microbiology services or the Public Health Laboratory Service) should be determined. This programme would be beneficial to the virus laboratory by reducing the number of urgent VZV determinations after a chickenpox or shingles contact, and to the patient by reducing delays in the procurement of VZIG. It is likely that only a minority of patients will require this screening service and testing can thus be incorporated within the antibody screening programme at booking. Immunoprophylaxis will only be required by those susceptible patients in contact with varicella who are found to be VZV antibody-negative.

Live attenuated varicella vaccine is part of the national immunisation programme for children in a number of countries and has been shown to be safe and effective in preventing chickenpox in adults,[21] but it is not yet licensed for general use in the UK.

There may be a case for immunising all susceptible women prior to pregnancy[22] and also for immunising healthcare workers in regular contact with pregnant women. It is worthwhile to ask those patients who have lived overseas, particularly in the USA or Japan, whether they have received the varicella vaccine. Pending the availability of live attenuated varicella vaccine for primary prevention in the UK, the use of VZIG is the preferred post-exposure strategy for susceptible pregnant women. There is some evidence that VZIG may reduce the severity of chickenpox in both neonates[18] and pregnant women,[23,24] and reduce the number of cases of fetal varicella syndrome in babies born to mothers given VZIG when compared with those without immunoprophylaxis.[4] However, administration of VZIG to susceptible pregnant women has not been shown to wholly prevent maternal viraemia, fetal infection, fetal varicella syndrome or varicella of the newborn. The use of VZIG after VZV exposure[23] appears to result in subclinical infection in 25% of pregnant patients, a mild case of chickenpox in a further 32%, and severe infection (no protective effect) in a further 16%. The other 27% of patients remained uninfected. Analysis of differences between attack rates in the household setting indicate that the UK VZIG product prepared by Bio Products Ltd UK appears to have a protective efficacy of approximately 40% against clinical chickenpox,[23] although severe maternal varicella and varicella of the newborn may still occur despite prophylaxis given appropriately. As VZIG is a product obtained from human volunteers with high titres of VZV antibodies, its use carries the infection risks associated with human-derived blood products, although purified immunoglobulins carry a substantially lower risk than whole blood.

At the present time, all immunoglobulin products are sourced from outside the UK, to avoid the theoretical risk of prion contamination. VZIG should be given to susceptible patients (i.e. VZV antibody-negative) as soon as possible after a recent contact with either chickenpox or shingles, although there is some evidence that clinical outcome is not compromised if it is administered up to ten days after exposure.[23] However, as the protective benefit of VZIG is incomplete, patients should seek prompt medical treatment over the following 28 days should vesicles appear.

Antiviral treatment with aciclovir during pregnancy

Aciclovir has been the mainstay of treatment for severe varicella and herpes zoster infections but concerns relating to its anti-nucleoside action have prevented formal studies in pregnancy. Aciclovir has, however, been used in pregnancy since 1984 for the treatment of serious herpes simplex and VZV infections. The Acyclovir in Pregnancy Registry was created and a six-year report[25] was published in 1992. This report concluded that, although aciclovir was used in 312 patients, case numbers were too low to represent a sample of sufficient size. Nevertheless, the data showed no increase in the number of fetal defects when compared with that expected in the general population. No consistent pattern of abnormality was reported, providing some qualified reassurance to pregnant women exposed to the drug. The Registry closed in June 1998 with over 1000 exposures to women with either herpes simplex or varicella infection in pregnancy, with no change in the reported adverse data. There is no longer a requirement to enter patients onto the Registry unless adverse events are suspected (GlaxoSmithKline Medical Information Department 0800 413828).

Aciclovir has been used successfully in the treatment of varicella pneumonitis during pregnancy.[26] Of the 21 cases treated (12 cases in the second trimester and nine in the third trimester of pregnancy, with 12 patients requiring mechanical ventilation), only three patients (14%) died of overwhelming infection. None of the children born developed varicella. Oral aciclovir treatment has been recommended after peer review in the UK for the management of chickenpox in the adult,[27] when used within 24 hours of rash development. These recommendations have been incorporated in the recommendations[2] for management of pregnant women with chickenpox who are over 20 weeks of gestation.

Management of a woman with suspected varicella contact in pregnancy

It is important to elucidate, from the contact history, the following, in respect of the certainty of the infection:

- the likelihood of a true infectious contact (vesicular rash or development of rash within 48 hours of contact)
- the degree of exposure (household, face-to-face for five minutes, or contact indoors, e.g. same hospital two- to four-bed bay for more than 15 minutes).

All pregnant women in contact with a case of chickenpox or shingles should see their general practitioner or midwife for assessment of the need for passive protection with VZIG, and to receive information about early notification of any subsequent vesicular eruption, so that the need for further assessment and future antiviral therapy can be planned.

If the pregnant woman has a previous history of varicella, it is reasonable to assume that she is immune to primary VZV infection. However, if there is any doubt, the presence of pre-existing VZV IgG should be checked. Antibodies detected within ten days of contact must have been acquired before contact.

If the pregnant woman (of any gestational age) has had a significant contact and no previous history of varicella, her VZV IgG in serum should be assessed (using a 5–10 ml sample of clotted blood). The virology laboratory may be able to use serum stored from antenatal booking blood samples, thus saving time and expense. A sensitive method of detection should be used, such as enzyme-linked immunoassay or indirect immuno-fluorescence tests. The complement fixation test for VZV antibodies should not be used in this context. In one UK study[28] of pregnant women who reported no previous history of chickenpox, 89% were positive for VZV antibodies. It is therefore highly desirable to test those pregnant patients who are in contact with varicella and have a doubtful or negative history of previous chickenpox for VZV antibodies, before the administration of VZIG. Laboratories are able to turn around a VZV IgG results in one to two days if the sample is marked 'urgent – chickenpox contact in pregnancy – VZV IgG antibodies please'. The need for these urgent investigations could be removed by the routine screening for varicella antibodies at booking for those women without a history of previous chickenpox.

If antibodies are detected and the sample of blood taken is within ten days of the contact, the patient can be regarded as immune. In this context, VZIG is not required. If the pregnant woman (of any gestational age) is not immune to VZV, she should be given VZIG as soon as possible after a chickenpox or herpes zoster contact, although there is evidence of efficacy if given within ten days of the contact. When there are restrictions in the availability of VZIG, the preparation is made available only to women at less than 20 weeks of gestation and to those within three weeks of delivery. The dose of VZIG is 1000 mg, given as an intramuscular injection, as a stat dose (divided to gluteal and deltoid muscles). The preparation (which must not be given by the intravenous route) is available through the microbiology laboratories providing VZV antibody screening or directly from the Public Health Laboratory Service (Communicable Disease Surveillance Centre, London. Telephone: 020 8200 6868).

Detection of rising antibody titres and the presence of VZV immunoglobulin M (IgM) in maternal serum indicates primary VZV infection. Rising antibody levels of

VZV IgG antibody are also seen during herpes zoster, while VZV IgM is usually absent.

If the pregnant woman develops chickenpox and shows serological evidence of infection in the first 20 weeks of pregnancy there is a 0.4% risk (0–12 weeks of gestation) and a 2% risk (13–20 weeks of gestation) of fetal varicella syndrome developing in her child. Varicella in pregnancy *per se* is not an indication for termination. Referral to a specialist centre for detailed ultrasound examination and follow-up should be arranged after a further six weeks in all those who do become infected in the first 20 weeks of gestation. Neonatal ophthalmic examination should be organised at birth.

If there is no previous history of varicella and the contact occurs after 20 weeks, there is no risk of fetal varicella syndrome, but the risk of complications following clinical varicella (e.g. pneumonitis, haemorrhage and bacterial superinfection) remains, particularly towards the end of pregnancy. The fetus is unaffected by maternal herpes zoster unless the mother is immunosuppressed and there is evidence of maternal viraemia and dissemination of the virus.

Management of a pregnant woman with chickenpox in the community

There is no benefit when VZV hyperimmune globulin is used during chickenpox. VZIG is therefore reserved exclusively for use after a varicella contact.

It has been recommended[2] that the uncomplicated patient at between 20 and 40 weeks of gestation, presenting within 24 hours of the chickenpox rash, should receive oral aciclovir 800 mg five times daily for seven days after counselling. Full informed consent must be obtained prior to treatment.

Oral aciclovir therapy should be offered (rather than recommended) to uncomplicated patients at less than 20 weeks of gestation, with full informed consent.

These recommendations are in line with the guidelines already published[27] that all non-pregnant adults be treated with oral aciclovir (at 800 mg three times daily for seven days) if they present on the first day of the rash. The use of oral aciclovir in pregnancy is not a licensed indication but its administration may be expected to reduce the severity and duration of the illness, based on data in children, adolescents and adults. However, there are no formal studies in pregnancy *per se* to confirm this benefit. There are theoretical concerns about teratogenesis when aciclovir is used in the first trimester, although there are no data to support an increase in congenital defects.

The uncomplicated patient at between 20 and 40 weeks of gestation presenting more than 24 hours after the rash should be closely observed. There is no benefit in administering oral aciclovir therapy under these conditions, as there is no evidence that this would alter the natural history of the infection.

All patients should be monitored every 24–48 hours for disease progression, focusing on chest symptoms, the extent and character of the rash and systemic features.

Which pregnant patients with chickenpox should be referred for hospital assessment?

The following patients should be referred:

- all patients with chickenpox after 36 weeks of gestation who are not eligible for oral aciclovir therapy and who cannot be closely observed
- all patients with clinical deterioration, e.g. toxicity, continued cropping at day six and/or renewed fever after day six, and where social conditions at home are unfavourable for recovery.

The following patients must be referred:

- all patients of any gestational age with chickenpox and with risk factors for varicella pneumonitis, e.g. history of smoking, chronic lung disease and/or having received oral steroids within the previous three months, who develop respiratory symptoms such as a dry cough or mild exertional dyspnoea from one to six days after onset of the rash
- all patients with the clinical features of varicella pneumonitis or other serious sequelae, e.g. productive cough, tachypnoea, dyspnoea at rest, lung crepitations, systemic toxicity, dense rash, bleeding and bruising, neurological symptoms other than headache and significant immunosuppression.

When should intravenous aciclovir be used in a pregnant patient with chickenpox?

Intravenous aciclovir should be administered in cases, particularly in those at more than 36 weeks of gestation, with the features of clinical progression, e.g. continued cropping of the rash beyond day six, reappearance of fever after day six, evidence of thrombocytopenia or elevated liver aminotransaminases, and secondary skin sepsis.

In all cases where there is direct evidence of varicella pneumonitis, encephalitis and/or bleeding, intravenous aciclovir must be used. There should be a low threshold for using high-dose intravenous aciclovir (10 mg/kg eight-hourly) in patients at more than 36 weeks of gestation, and in those with risk factors for varicella pneumonitis and other sequelae of infection, as therapeutic resolution of established multisystem disease is not always successful and death can occur early in the course of the infection (mortality in ventilated patients is approximately 37%).

Is there a place for the early conclusion of the pregnancy during severe chickenpox?

In the third trimester of pregnancy, obstetric complications during chickenpox may lead to fetal distress. Caesarean section and other interventions during the viraemic period are likely to be extremely hazardous. These are associated with a high risk of varicella of the newborn and of intrauterine and wound bleeding. Such bleeding is associated with profound thrombocytopenia, hepatitis and disseminated intravascular coagulation, all of which are seen during severe varicella. If possible, the pregnancy should be allowed to continue for as long as possible under cover of antiviral and other supportive treatments (preferably to day five after appearance of the rash). This will allow immune recovery and protection of the fetus by maternal antibodies, which are generated within two to four days of the rash.

Do pregnant patients with herpes zoster require antiviral treatment?

As herpes zoster is usually mild in women of childbearing age and viraemia is uncommon unless complicated by immunosuppressive disease or therapy, antiviral treatment is usually unnecessary. This does, however, depend on the site and extent of the rash and the presence of moderate or severe pain or other complications. When these complications are present, oral aciclovir at 800 mg three times daily should be given, with full informed consent, for seven days and commenced within 72 hours of rash presentation. Only aciclovir has been used to any extent in pregnancy. There are no published data on the safety of either valaciclovir or famciclovir in pregnancy. Consequently, these antiviral prodrugs, which are used in the treatment of herpes zoster, have not been recommended in pregnancy.

Otherwise, the management of the herpes zoster rash should be conservative with topical lotions, e.g. calamine lotion, and mild analgesics if acute pain is a problem. Ophthalmic zoster is occasionally very serious and all cases should be referred to an ophthalmologist. When appropriate, the use of topical aciclovir in the eye can be extremely beneficial and prevent complications. Oral aciclovir at 800 mg five times daily for seven days should be used as an adjunct to topical ophthalmic therapy.

Management and treatment of the neonate with varicella

Where maternal infection occurs from five days before or two days after delivery there is a 20–30% risk of mortality following varicella of the newborn. Thus, where possible, delivery should be delayed until five days after the onset of maternal illness to allow for the passive transfer of antibodies that appear within three days of rash development.

VZIG is indicated for neonates whose mothers have the signs and symptoms of varicella within the period five days before and two days after delivery. The availability of VZIG for the neonate is extended to seven days before to seven days after delivery as a practical solution to the problem of determining when maternal vesiculation commenced. The neonate should be given VZIG (250 mg intramuscularly stat) as soon as possible after birth. The aim of using VZIG in a neonate whose mother had varicella within one week of delivery is to provide passive antibodies that will attenuate neonatal infection, as there is little evidence that infection can be prevented.

If varicella of the newborn occurs, treatment with aciclovir is indicated even if the disease initially appears mild. Intravenous aciclovir is given at a dose of 10 mg/kg eight-hourly for ten days. VZIG has no clinical benefits for neonates who have developed chickenpox.

Maternal herpes zoster at term does not constitute a risk to the newborn child as the baby is protected by adequate amounts of transplacentally acquired maternal antibodies. VZIG is not required in these infants.

Infection control aspects

Pregnant women with varicella and herpes zoster should be isolated from all other pregnant women and neonates. Visiting should be restricted to those with a history of previous chickenpox.

Hospitalisation with facilities for patient isolation and consultation with a specialist in infectious diseases is indicated when any patient with chickenpox is admitted. The following symptoms raise the possibility of severe varicella:

- cough and shortness of breath
- lesions appear dense, with or without bruising and haemorrhage
- new lesions continue to develop or fever reappears, six days after the onset of lesions.

All reasonable steps should be taken to isolate and prevent individuals with VZV infection, including healthcare professionals, from direct contact with susceptible pregnant women attending hospitals or general practitioner surgeries. To this end, screening pregnant women without a history of chickenpox during the antenatal period is highly desirable and may be a cost-effective and disease-preventive strategy. Patients with chickenpox should be seen at home or at the end of the clinic to avoid further transmission to 'at risk' patients.

Staff who are thought (or known by previous testing) to be 'non-immune' should avoid contact with varicella patients. However, those patients who are exposed in this way should be tested for varicella antibodies and, if found to be susceptible, should be warned that they may develop varicella. As the incubation period is 10–21 days, the healthcare worker may pose a risk to susceptible patients and colleagues, during the period 8–21 days after contact with a case. It may be necessary for exposed healthcare workers to take approved sick leave during this period and to consider varicella vaccination (at a later date) to provide future protection if previous contact exposures do not result in VZV seroconversion. VZIG is not available to healthcare workers in contact with varicella unless they themselves are considered at 'high risk' of infection with serious sequelae.

On occasion, a sibling has varicella or herpes zoster around the time the mother and newborn baby are due for discharge from hospital. If the mother is immune to varicella there is little risk to the newborn, as the baby will have maternal antibodies sufficient to give protection against varicella. However, cases of chickenpox have occasionally occurred in such infants exposed to chickenpox within the first two months of life. The data suggest that maternal antibodies may not be protective to all infants exposed in the early neonatal period. If the mother is found to be susceptible, the newborn up to seven days of age should be given VZIG (250 mg intramuscularly stat). The mother will not be eligible for VZIG immunoprophylaxis but aciclovir prophylaxis (800 mg four times daily for one week, commencing eight days after contact) may be considered and may provide some useful protection against infection.[29,30] This may also effect a reduction in transmission to the newborn during the neonatal period. However, aciclovir therapy is not recommended by the manufacturers during breastfeeding, due to lack of supporting data, but no adverse consequences have been reported when used in this context.

Horizontal transmission of varicella in maternity wards is unusual: most mothers are immune, their babies are protected by maternally derived antibodies, exposure times are brief and intimate exposure with other babies is uncommon. However, some babies are not protected by maternal antibodies, due to low birthweight (less than 1000 g) and low gestational age (less than 28 weeks), which may not provide opportunities for sufficient antibody transfer, and where maternal history of varicella is negative or uncertain. Routine practice is to administer VZIG to all exposed infants 'at risk' unless VZV antibody testing of neonatal and/or maternal samples can be offered rapidly. Testing is preferred to the indiscriminate use of VZIG as this is costly and unnecessary for many infants, and it allows the sensible isolation and cohorting of infants. Aciclovir therapy should be given to any breakthrough cases.

Conclusions

Maternal chickenpox poses difficulties for the mother, her fetus or newborn, and her carers. The outcome of the pregnancy can be altered by serious complications that increase morbidity and mortality of the pregnant mother over the nonpregnant female. Chickenpox in the first 20 weeks of pregnancy may lead to fetal varicella syndrome, and around delivery to varicella of the newborn, both with significant morbidity and mortality to the infected child.

When maternal contact with a case of chickenpox occurs, assessment of previously acquired immunity or susceptibility is urgently required, as is attention to the early administration of VZIG. If protection against chickenpox fails or is not possible, the early recognition of chickenpox is vital if aciclovir is to be administered within 24 hours of rash onset. The use of this antiviral has been recommended after peer review, when infection begins in the pregnant mother over 20 weeks of gestation. When infection is acquired below 20 weeks of gestation, aciclovir therapy may be offered, rather than recommended, with full counselling.

The management of maternal chickenpox requires careful assessment of the risks of serious disease, and early hospitalisation is advised when risk factors are identified. These factors are a history of smoking, chronic chest disease, immunosuppression received within the previous three months, and the clinical features of chest symptoms and signs, bleeding, severe dense rash and systemic toxicity.

Careful management of a mother with chickenpox around the time of delivery can prevent infection of the neonate and reduce complications for the mother. These management measures include the early use of aciclovir therapy, continuing the pregnancy for as long as possible to allow the passage of mother's antibodies to the fetus, and the use of VZIG in the neonate. If managed appropriately, the morbidity and mortality of chickenpox can be reduced for mother and baby.

Herpes zoster is an infrequent problem for pregnant women. This is because the incidence and severity of complications increase after childbearing age. When complications are suspected, oral aciclovir should be used. Topical aciclovir drops in the eyes are usually added when herpes zoster on the face affects the orbit. The use of valaciclovir or famciclovir in herpes zoster during pregnancy has not been approved.

References

1. Gershon, AA, Raker A, Steinburg S, Topf-Olstein B, Drusin LM. Antibody to varicella-zoster virus in parturient women and their offspring during the first year of the life. *Pediatrics* 1976;**58**:692–6.
2. Nathwani D, MacLean A, Conway A, Carrington D. Varicella infections in pregnancy and the newborn. *J Infection* 1998;**36** Suppl 1:59–71.
3. Sinha DP, Chickenpox – a disease predominantly affecting adults in rural West Bengal, India. *Int J Epidemiol* 1976;**5**:367–74.
4. Enders G, Miller E, Cradock-Watson J, Bolley I, Ridehalgh M. Consequences of varicella and herpes zoster in pregnancy: prospective study of 1739 cases. *Lancet* 1994;**343**:1548–51.
5. Paryani SG, Arvin AM. Intrauterine infection with varicella-zoster virus after maternal varicella. *N Engl J Med* 1986;**314**:1542–6.
6. Meyer JD. Congenital varicella in term infants: risk reconsidered. *J Infect Dis* 1974;**129**:215–17.
7. Department of Health. *Report on Confidential Enquiries into Maternal Deaths in the United Kingdom 1985–87*. London: HMSO; 1991.
8. Department of Health. *Report on Confidential Enquiries into Maternal Deaths in the United Kingdom 1988–90*. London: HMSO; 1994.
9. Hibbard BM, Anderson MM, Drife JO, Tighe JR, Garden G, Willats S, *et al. Department of Health. Report on Confidential Enquiries into Maternal Deaths in the United Kingdom 1991–93*. London: HMSO; 1996.
10. Drife J, Lewis G, editors. *Why Mothers Die. Report on Confidential Enquiries into Maternal Deaths in the United Kingdom 1994–96*. London: The Stationery Office; 1998.
11. Laforet EG, Lynch CL. Multiple congenital defects following maternal varicella. *N Engl J Med* 1947;**236**:534–7.
12. Preblud SR, Cochi S1, Orenstein WA. Varicella-zoster infection in pregnancy [letter]. *N Engl J Med* 1986;**315**:1416–17.
13. Pastuszak AL, Levy M, Schick B, Zuber C, Feldkamp M, Gladstone J, *et al*. Outcome after maternal varicella infection in the first 20 weeks of pregnancy. *N Engl J Med* 1994;**330**:901–5.
14. Jones KL, Johnson KA, Chambers CD. Offspring of women infected with varicella during pregnancy: a prospective study. *Teratology* 1994;**49**:29–32.
15. Siegel M, Fuerst HT, Peress NS. Comparative fetal mortality in maternal virus diseases. *N Engl J Med* 1966;**274**:768–71.
16. Pretorius DH, Hayward I, Jones KL, Stamm E. Sonographic evaluation of pregnancies with maternal varicella infection. *J Ultrasound Med* 1992;**11**:459–63.
17. Lecuru F, Taurelle R, Bernard JP, Parrat S, Lafay-pillet MC, Rozenberg F, *et al*. Varicella zoster virus infection during pregnancy: the limits of prenatal diagnosis. *Eur J Obstet Gynecol Reprod Biol* 1994;**56**:67–8.
18. Miller E, Cradock-Watson JE, Ridehalgh MKS. Outcome in newborn babies given anti-varicella zoster immunoglobulin after perinatal maternal infection with varicella zoster virus. *Lancet* 1989;**ii**:371–3.
19. DeNicola LK, Hanshaw JB. Congenital and neonatal varicella. *J Pediatr* 1979;**94**:175–6.
20. Brunell PA, Kotchmer GS. Zoster in infancy: failure to maintain virus latency following intrauterine infection. *J Pediatr* 1981;**98**:71–3.
21. Gershon AA, Steinberg SP. Live attenuated varicella vaccine: protection in healthy adults compared with leukemic children. National Institute of Allergy and Infectious Diseases Varicella Vaccine Collaborative Study Group. *J Infect Dis* 1990;**158**:661–6.
22. Seidman DS, Stevenson DK, Arvin AM. Varicella vaccine in pregnancy. *BMJ* 1996;**313**:701–2.
23. Miller E, Marshall R, Vurdien J. Epidemiology, outcome and control of varicella-zoster infection. *Rev Med Microbiol* 1993;**4**:222–30.
24. Enders G. Management of varicella zoster contact and infection in pregnancy using a standardized varicella-zoster ELISA test. *Postgrad Med J* 1985;**61** Suppl 4:23–30.
25. Andrews EB, Yankaskas BC, Cordero JF, Schoeffler K, Hampp S. Acyclovir in pregnancy registry: six years' experience. The Acyclovir in Pregnancy Registry Advisory Committee. *Obstet Gynecol* 1992;**79**:7–13.
26. Smego RA, Asperilla MO. Use of acyclovir for varicella pneumonia during pregnancy. *Obstet Gynecol* 1991;**78**:1112–16.
27. Wilkins EGL, Leen CLS, McKendrick MW, Carrington D. Management of chickenpox in the adult. A review prepared for the UK Advisory Group on Chickenpox on behalf of the British Society for the Study of Infection. *J Infect* 1998;**36** Suppl 1: 49–58.

28.   Evans EB, Pollock TM, Cradock-Watson JE, Ridehalgh MK. Human anti-chickenpox immunoglobulin in the prevention of chickenpox. *Lancet* 1980;**i**:354–6.

29.   Asano Y, Yoshikawa T, Suga S, Kobayashi T, Yazaki T, Ozaki T, *et al.* Post-exposure prophylaxis of varicella in family contact by oral aciclovir. *Pediatrics* 1993;**92**:219–22.

30.   Lin TY, Huang YC, Ning HC, Hsueh C. Oral acyclovir prophylaxis of varicella after intimate contact. *Pediatr Infect Dis J* 1997;**16**:1162–5.

Chapter 20

The management of herpes simplex virus infection in pregnancy

Naomi Low-Beer and J Richard Smith

Introduction

Genital infection with the herpes simplex virus (HSV) is a common condition in women of reproductive age. Genital herpes in pregnancy, particularly a primary infection acquired at or near the time of delivery, is associated with a significant risk of transmission to the neonate.[1] Since the severe consequences of neonatal herpes infection are well established, obstetricians need to be aware of interventions that may reduce the risk of perinatal transmission. A survey of Fellows and Members of the Royal College of Obstetricians and Gynaecologists, published in 1995, found that only 31% of those surveyed had a formal policy governing the management of herpes in pregnancy and that there was a wide variation in practice.[2] More recently, the availability of assays that can distinguish between antibodies to HSV type 1 (HSV-1) and type 2 (HSV-2) has added to the range of management options.[3]

In order to facilitate the development of recommendations for management of genital herpes in pregnancy, a literature search was performed using Medline (1983–2000). The key words were 'genital-herpes', 'neonatal-herpes', 'herpes simplex virus', and 'pregnancy complications-infectious'. Reference lists of the articles identified were hand searched for additional articles.

Herpes simplex infections

HSV is a double-stranded DNA virus. There are two viral types, HSV-1 and HSV-2. The majority of orolabial infections are caused by HSV-1 and these infections are usually acquired during childhood through direct physical contact. Genital herpes is a sexually transmitted infection and is most commonly caused by HSV-2. However, an increasing prevalence of genital HSV-1 infections has been described in studies from many countries, including the UK, USA and Scandinavia.[4-7]

Genital herpes

Epidemiology

According to national surveillance data from the Public Health Laboratory Service, genital herpes is the most common ulcerative sexually transmitted infection in the UK. Between 1989 and 1998, diagnoses of first-episode genital herpes in women at genitourinary clinics increased from 25 to 37 per 100 000 in England and Wales. The incidence was higher in London, compared with elsewhere in England and Wales, and higher in women than in men (ratio 1.4:1). However, the extent of asymptomatic infection has been difficult to quantify. Until recently, serological assays for detecting antibodies to HSV were unable to distinguish accurately between antibodies to HSV-1 and to HSV-2. The development of reliable type-specific serological tests has now enabled the extent of undiagnosed and asymptomatic infection to be determined.

Epidemiological surveys of herpes serology have been carried out in several populations throughout the world. The prevalence of HSV-2 infection varies markedly, being high in developing countries and the USA and lower in Europe. Irrespective of geographical location, these studies show that the prevalence of both HSV-1 and HSV-2 antibodies increases with age and that HSV-2 antibodies are more common in women than in men.[3] Among the general population in the USA, around 26% of women and 18% of men are HSV-2 seropositive.[8] In London, surveys of patients attending genitourinary clinics and blood donors indicate that 25% and 12%, respectively, are HSV-2 seropositive.[9] The prevalence of HSV-2 is lower elsewhere in England and Wales.[7] These surveys suggest that, at most, only one-third of those infected have had their infection previously diagnosed.[8,9] Contrary to earlier studies, recent data from large prospective cohort studies of HSV acquisition in pregnant women[1] and in nonpregnant adults,[10] suggest that previous HSV-1 infection does not protect against HSV-2 acquisition.

Clinical features and natural history

Initial genital infection with HSV-1 or HSV-2 (primary genital herpes) may result in symptomatic disease at the site of viral entry, i.e. the genital area, although most primary infections are asymptomatic and thus unrecognised.[10] As with other acute viral illnesses, systemic symptoms may occur. Following primary infection, the virus remains latent within the local sensory ganglia. Viral reactivation occurs when replication of HSV in the ganglia is triggered and the virus returns to the skin or mucosal surfaces via the nerve axons. This may result in symptomatic lesions or asymptomatic viral shedding. There is now good evidence that the majority of those with subclinical HSV-2 infection intermittently shed virus from the genital tract.[11] The frequency of subclinical viral shedding makes control of this chronic infection more difficult – genital herpes infections are commonly acquired from partners who are asymptomatic and who may have no clinical history of genital herpes.[12]

First-episode genital herpes, defined as the first clinical episode of genital herpes, may occur at the same time as primary infection, although it commonly occurs some time later.[10] It may be difficult to distinguish clinically between primary genital herpes and a non-primary first episode, although the presence of systemic symptoms is suggestive of the former.[13,14] Women with symptomatic primary genital herpes infection usually present with vesicles on the external genitalia, with possible involvement of the cervix, occurring between two and 14 days following exposure to the infectious virus. The initial vesicles rupture and subsequently appear as shallow ulcers, causing pain, dysuria and vaginal discharge. Inguinal lymphadenopathy occurs as a result of viral replication in the lymph nodes. Viraemia may cause transient systemic symptoms, such as fever, malaise and myalgia, which may occasionally be the only presenting symptoms of herpes infection. Without antiviral therapy, the lesions of primary genital herpes usually resolve within three weeks, although subclinical viral shedding may continue after the lesions have healed. Local complications include secondary bacterial infection, labial adhesions, and autonomic neuropathy, which can cause urinary retention. Occasionally the viraemia is complicated by meningitis and/or encephalitis. Very rarely, a disseminated HSV infection occurs, which is a life-threatening condition affecting multiple organs.[15]

Both recurrent episodes of HSV and non-primary first episodes are usually associated with little or no systemic manifestations. The genital lesions, which are usually smaller in size and fewer in number, tend to resolve more rapidly than in primary genital herpes infection, and the duration of viral shedding is shorter. While genital infection with HSV-1 is clinically indistinguishable from HSV-2, it is less likely to cause clinically recurrent disease, and subclinical viral shedding occurs less frequently.[16,17]

Genital herpes and pregnancy

During pregnancy, the incidence of primary genital herpes is not thought to be increased and the risk of acquiring this infection is relatively small. A prospective study from the USA by Brown *et al.*[1] of 7046 pregnant women susceptible to infection with HSV (HSV-1, HSV-2 or both) found that 2% of these women acquired infection during pregnancy. In 60% of cases, the herpes infection was subclinical, which was consistent with the high frequency of unrecognised HSV infection found in other studies.

Complications associated with HSV infection in pregnant women may be pregnancy-related or maternal. The most important pregnancy-related complication is neonatal herpes, which is discussed below. Isolated case reports have associated *in utero* infection during the first trimester with a variety of anomalies, such as microcephaly and chorioretinitis. An association of first-episode genital herpes with preterm labour, intrauterine growth restriction and spontaneous abortion has been demonstrated in some studies.[18–20] However, these studies were based on use of cultures and serological tests performed at the time of labour. In the large prospective controlled study of HSV acquisition during pregnancy by Brown *et al.*,[1] there was no increase in pregnancy-related morbidity among the 94 women infected prior to labour. Maternal complications are generally similar to those occurring in the nonpregnant state. However, the incidence of disseminated HSV, although rare, is probably increased.[21] In most reported cases, this condition occurs in the second or third trimester. It may present as encephalitis without hepatic involvement, hepatitis with or without central nervous system findings, or disseminated skin lesions. Where the liver is involved, rapidly progressive hepatic necrosis and severe coagulopathy are common and the mortality is high.[21,22]

All immunocompromised women are at increased risk of severe frequent recurrent episodes of genital HSV, which may not respond to standard antiviral therapy. Pregnant women with HIV-1 infection are more likely to be co-infected with HSV-2 and are more prone to HSV reactivation in labour.[23] As co-infection with HSV and HIV results in increased replication of both viruses,[24] there are concerns that genital reactivation of HSV may increase the risk of perinatal transmission of both HIV and HSV.[23] The interrelationship of HSV and HIV infection during pregnancy is an area in need of further study.

Neonatal herpes

Epidemiology

Neonatal herpes is a serious infection with a high morbidity and mortality. Active surveillance by the British Paediatric Surveillance Unit suggests that neonatal herpes in the UK is rare, with an incidence of 1.65 per 100 000 live births.[25] In the USA, while some researchers have estimated incidence rates of between 20 per 100 000 and 50 per 100 000 live births,[26] the evidence to support this is weak. A thorough review of the literature suggests that the true incidence is around 7 per 100 000 (95% CI 3–13 per 100 000 live births).[27]

Transmission

Almost all cases of neonatal herpes occur as a result of direct contact with infected maternal secretions, although cases of postnatal transmission have been described.[25] Neonatal HSV infection usually occurs where there is primary maternal HSV infection during late pregnancy, so that the baby is delivered before the development of protective maternal antibodies.[1,18] Most of these maternal infections are asymptomatic or unrecognised.[1,25]

The timing of maternal HSV infection is crucial to the risk of perinatal transmission. It had been suggested that HSV infection acquired at any time during the third trimester was associated with a significant risk of neonatal herpes infection because of the persistence of viral shedding after healing of the genital lesions.[20] However, the large prospective study by Brown et al.[1] from the USA demonstrated a significant risk of neonatal herpes only when maternal HSV infection was acquired at or just before the onset of labour. In this study of 7046 pregnant women susceptible to infection with either HSV-1 or HSV-2, although the timing of maternal infection was relatively uniform throughout pregnancy, there were four cases of neonatal herpes among nine women who acquired infection shortly before the onset of labour but no cases among the women who acquired infection prior to this.

This study also highlighted the importance of primary rather than recurrent genital HSV as a risk factor for neonatal herpes – there were no infected babies born to women who had acquired HSV-2 antibodies prior to pregnancy. Where a baby delivered vaginally is exposed to symptomatic or asymptomatic recurrent genital HSV at the time of labour, studies have demonstrated rates of perinatal transmission of between 0% and 3%;[28,29] the corresponding risk associated with first-episode genital HSV at the time of delivery, calculated from five studies, was 19/46 or 41% (95% CI 26–56%).[1,20,28,30,31] In one of these studies,[31] the risk of transmission was associated with duration of rupture of the membranes, the risk increasing considerably after the membranes had been ruptured for more than four hours.

Clinical features of neonatal herpes

Neonatal herpes can be caused by HSV-1 or HSV-2. Infection may be localised to the skin, eyes or mouth, or cause encephalitis or disseminated infection. With antiviral treatment, death is rare among babies with localised infection, in comparison with encephalitis or disseminated infection.[18] Infection with HSV-2 has a poorer prognosis than HSV-1.[18,32]

Diagnosis of herpes infections

Symptomatic herpes infections are confirmed by direct detection of HSV. Virus culture and typing is the 'gold standard' method for detecting HSV in clinical specimens. The quality of samples is critical and specimens from ulcerated lesions should be sampled by swabbing the base of the ulcer, while vesicular lesions should be de-roofed and the fluid sampled.[33] The polymerase chain reaction (PCR) is the diagnostic method of choice for cases of neonatal herpes where there is neurological disease in the absence of mucocutaneous lesions. In these cases, samples of cerebrospinal fluid obtained at lumbar puncture can be analysed by PCR. Studies[4,11,34] have demonstrated the greater sensitivity of PCR compared with viral culture in the detection of genital HSV (both from lesions and asymptomatic viral shedding) and PCR is likely to be more widely used in the diagnosis of genital HSV in the future.

Type-specific HSV antibody testing has been used to survey the prevalence of HSV infections and, more recently, the incidence of HSV infections in different populations.[3] However, reliable type-specific HSV antibody kits have only recently become commercially available and their use for patient management has not been fully assessed. Type-specific immune responses may take 8–12 weeks to develop following primary infection. Therefore, for a patient with a first-episode genital lesion, from which HSV is cultured, a negative HSV-2 antibody test would confirm recent acquisition of infection (primary HSV infection), whereas a positive HSV-2 antibody test would suggest reactivation of past herpes infection (a non-primary first-episode infection). As HSV-1 may cause genital herpes infections, interpretation of serology results may sometimes be difficult. Potential clinical uses of HSV serology include the diagnosis of recurrent genital ulceration of unknown cause, counselling patients with initial episodes of disease and the diagnosis of asymptomatic partners of patients with HSV-2 infection. However, as genital HSV infection is a chronic sexually transmitted disease, identification of HSV-2 infection in these individuals, particularly those in the latter group, may cause adverse psychological sequelae. It is therefore recommended that genitourinary clinics should have protocols for the use of HSV serology in clinical practice.[33] The clinical utility of HSV serology in pregnant women is discussed below.

Table 20.1. Levels of evidence (as devised by Scottish Intercollegiate Guidelines Network)

Level	Definition
Ia	Evidence obtained from a meta-analysis of randomised controlled trials
Ib	Evidence obtained from at least one randomised controlled trial
IIa	Evidence obtained from at least one well-designed controlled study without randomisation
IIb	Evidence obtained from at least one other type of well-designed quasi-experimental study
III	Evidence obtained from well-designed non-experimental descriptive studies, such as comparative studies, correlation studies and case–control studies
IV	Evidence obtained from expert committee reports or opinions and/or clinical experience of respected authorities

Management of genital herpes in pregnancy

While it is not possible to make definitive recommendations about the management of first-episode genital herpes in pregnancy on the basis of the published literature, Table 20.2 offers some guidelines based on a review of the best available evidence to date. (Definitions of the levels of evidence are listed in Table 20.1.) All pregnant women with first-episode genital herpes should be referred to genitourinary physicians, who will advise on management and arrange for the woman to be screened for other sexually transmitted infections.

Table 20.2. Considerations for the management of pregnant women with first-episode genital herpes

Recommendations	Evidence level
Presentation in any trimester	
1. Referral to genitourinary medicine physicians should be made.	IV
2. Management of the woman should be in line with her clinical condition and will often involve a five-day course of oral aciclovir in standard doses.	IV
3. Type-specific serology may aid management by differentiating primary from non-primary first-episode HSV infections.	IV
4. Daily suppressive aciclovir in the last four weeks of pregnancy may prevent HSV recurrences at term and thus the need for delivery by caesarean section.	Ib
Presentation in the first or second trimester	
1. Providing that delivery does not ensue, the pregnancy should be managed expectantly and vaginal delivery anticipated.	III
Presentation in the third trimester	
1. Caesarean section should be performed for women who have genital HSV lesions at the time of delivery.	III
2. Elective caesarean section at term may be considered for all women, particularly those who develop genital HSV lesions within six weeks of their expected date of delivery, because of the risk of viral shedding in labour.	III
3. If women opt for vaginal delivery, aciclovir treatment of the mother and baby may be indicated.	IV
4. The paediatrician should be informed as soon as possible to ensure appropriate neonatal care.	IV

Management of first-episode genital herpes

Women presenting with suspected first-episode genital herpes in pregnancy should have samples taken for viral culture in order to confirm the diagnosis. Type-specific antibody testing may be useful in distinguishing a primary infection (higher risk of perinatal transmission) from a non-primary first-episode infection (lower risk of perinatal transmission). Decisions regarding management of these women should be made in conjunction with the genitourinary physician and the patient herself. For women presenting in the third trimester of pregnancy, a paediatrician should also be involved. Symptomatic treatment includes saline bathing and simple analgesia. Topical local anaesthetic gels may also be used. Guidelines from the American College of Obstetricians and Gynecologists (ACOG) recommend that a course of the antiviral drug aciclovir should be prescribed for women with first-episode genital HSV infection during pregnancy.[35] The recommended dosing regimen is the same as for nonpregnant adults: 200 mg five times a day for five days. An extended course of treatment for up to 14 days may sometimes be indicated and higher doses may be required for immunocompromised women. Where there are severe systemic complications of HSV or where a first-episode infection is associated with imminent delivery, women should be treated with intravenous aciclovir. In nonpregnant adults, treatment of first-episode genital herpes is known to reduce the duration and severity of symptoms and decrease the duration of viral shedding. Three small pharmacokinetic studies[36–38] of aciclovir use in the later stages of pregnancy have demonstrated similar values to those obtained in studies of nonpregnant adults. When given orally or intravenously, aciclovir crosses the placenta and concentrates in the amniotic fluid, with no preferential accumulation in the fetus. Use of aciclovir in pregnancy has not been associated with embryotoxic or fetotoxic effects in animal studies and the drug is well tolerated by term and preterm infants who receive parenteral therapy. Prospective data from 1207 pregnancies reported to the Aciclovir Pregnancy Registry between 1984 and 1998 (including 739 where exposure occurred in the first trimester) have demonstrated no evidence of teratogenicity.[39] The Aciclovir Pregnancy Registry has since been discontinued. However, aciclovir is not licensed for use in pregnancy and the responsibility for prescribing rests with the doctor. Detailed discussion with the woman and her partner of the risks and benefits of aciclovir treatment should take place and the results of these discussions should be carefully documented in the case notes.

In nonpregnant adults, the aciclovir prodrugs valaciclovir and famciclovir provide significantly better bioavailability than oral aciclovir itself and they therefore require a less frequent dosing regimen. However, there are only limited data on the use of such alternative antiviral agents in pregnancy[38] and their use for treatment of genital herpes in pregnancy is not justified at the present time. Women inadvertently given these drugs should be registered prospectively with the relevant company.

Women with first-episode herpes infection during the first or second trimesters should be reassured that there is no evidence of associated birth defects and that this infection is not considered an indication for termination of pregnancy. HSV infection during the first or second trimester is not an indication for subsequent delivery by caesarean section. Should these women develop recurrent episodes later in pregnancy, they should be managed accordingly (see below).

For women who develop uncomplicated first-episode genital herpes at any time in the third trimester, some obstetricians have advocated elective delivery by caesarean section at 38 weeks, particularly if symptoms began within six weeks of the estimated date of delivery, because of the risk of continued viral shedding during labour.[20] However, many clinicians may opt for a more conservative approach in light of the prospective study by Brown *et al.*[1] demonstrating a significant risk of neonatal herpes and adverse pregnancy outcome only where infection occurred at or near the time of labour. When first-episode genital herpes occurring in the third trimester is associated with established labour (which may be premature), there is a strong case for treatment with intravenous aciclovir and delivery by caesarean section on the basis that this will minimise maternal viraemia and reduce exposure of the fetus to the virus.

All women with first-episode genital herpes lesions at the onset of labour should be advised that there is a significant risk of neonatal herpes infection and that delivery by caesarean section is advisable. However, for women who nevertheless choose to opt for vaginal delivery, or where vaginal delivery occurs inadvertently, it seems appropriate that mother and baby should be treated with intravenous aciclovir. Use of fetal scalp electrode monitoring should be avoided, as there have been case reports linking their use with the development of neonatal herpes. Where the membranes have been ruptured for more than four hours, there are insufficient data regarding mode of delivery and the decision is a matter for individual judgement.

Management of recurrent episodes of genital herpes

Table 20.3 lists considerations for the management of pregnant women with recurrent genital herpes. Most cases of recurrent herpes in pregnancy may be treated effectively with saline bathing and simple analgesia. Antiviral treatment is not usually indicated.

ACOG recommends that caesarean section for recurrent herpes infection should be performed only if active lesions are present at the onset of labour.[35] The majority of UK obstetricians surveyed by Brocklehurst *et al.*[2] agreed with this view. However, a cost–benefit analysis derived from American data has suggested that, if all women with an episode of recurrent genital herpes at the onset of labour were to undergo caesarean section, 1583 (range 632–6340) caesarean sections would be performed to prevent one case of HSV-related mortality or morbidity, at a cost of $2.5 million per case averted.[26] Moreover, in The Netherlands, caesarean sections have not been routinely performed for this indication since 1987. Over this period of time there has been a substantial reduction in the number of caesarean sections performed with no increase in the incidence of neonatal herpes.[40]

Table 20.3. Considerations for the management of pregnant women with recurrent genital herpes

Recommendations	Evidence level
1. Sequential cultures during late gestation to predict viral shedding at term are not indicated.	III
2. Recurrent genital herpes is not an indication for delivery by caesarean section unless genital HSV lesions are present at the onset of labour.	III
3. For women with genital lesions at the onset of labour:	
(a) Current practice in the UK and USA is for delivery by caesarean section.	III
(b) The risks to the baby from vaginal delivery are small and should be set against the risks to the mother of caesarean section.	

Suppressive aciclovir to prevent HSV reactivation at term

In nonpregnant adults with frequent symptomatic HSV recurrences, daily suppressive oral aciclovir used prophylactically has been shown to reduce the number of recurrences significantly. This has led some researchers to propose the use of suppressive aciclovir for pregnant women with a history of HSV infection (acquired either before or during the current pregnancy), in order to reduce the incidence of recurrent HSV lesions at the onset of labour, thereby reducing the incidence of caesarean delivery.[30,36,41] There is evidence from one double-blind placebo-controlled trial[42] that women who experience their first genital herpes outbreak while they are pregnant may benefit from aciclovir suppression. In this study, 46 women who presented with their first episode of genital HSV during their current pregnancy were randomised at 36 weeks of gestation to receive either daily suppressive aciclovir or placebo until delivery. No infants in either group developed neonatal herpes. None of the 21 women treated with aciclovir and nine of the 25 women (36%) treated with placebo had clinical evidence of recurrent genital herpes at delivery (OR 0.04; 95% CI 0.002–0.745). This study, although limited by its failure to differentiate between primary and non-primary first episodes, and between HSV-1 and HSV-2 infections, did demonstrate that use of suppressive aciclovir was associated with a significant reduction in caesarean delivery. Based on these data, ACOG recommends that daily prophylactic aciclovir during the last four weeks of pregnancy should be considered for women who have experienced a first-episode HSV infection during their current pregnancy. The recommended dosing regimen is 400 mg aciclovir twice daily.[35]

There are fewer data to support the use of suppressive aciclovir in women with a history of recurrent rather than first-episode herpes infection during pregnancy. Stray-Pedersen,[43] in a small uncontrolled series, claimed to show benefit. A randomised placebo-controlled trial by Brocklehurst et al.[44] also demonstrated a significant decrease in clinical recurrences at the time of delivery in women receiving aciclovir after 36 weeks of gestation, but the sample size was inadequate to demonstrate a significant reduction in the number of caesarean deliveries performed for active infection. Furthermore, suppressive aciclovir failed to prevent asymptomatic viral shedding in all women. Similarly, in a small uncontrolled study by Haddad et al.,[37] suppressive aciclovir given to pregnant women after 37 weeks of gestation failed to prevent asymptomatic viral shedding in one of five pregnant women who had therapeutic plasma levels of aciclovir.

Use of viral cultures to detect asymptomatic viral shedding

Guidelines from the American Academy of Pediatrics in 1980 advised that all women with a history of genital herpes should have weekly viral cultures taken from the cervix and external genitalia during the last six weeks of pregnancy with the aim of detecting recurrent episodes, both symptomatic and asymptomatic. Positive cultures near term were an indication for delivery by caesarean section.[45] However, Arvin et al.[30] showed that antenatal swabbing did not predict the shedding of virus at the onset of labour and this policy was abandoned by the Infectious Disease Society for Obstetrics and Gynecology in 1988.

Prevention of acquisition of maternal infection

Table 20.4 lists considerations for the prevention of acquisition of herpes infection in pregnant women, taken from the national guidelines for the management of genital herpes.[33] The greatest risk of neonatal herpes occurs when a pregnant woman acquires herpes infection at or near the time of delivery, and current strategies to prevent such maternal infections rely on history-taking and examination. As many of these infections are subclinical, this approach is likely to have little, if any, impact on the prevention of neonatal herpes.

Antenatal serum screening for herpes antibodies

Almost all neonatal infections (100% of HSV-2 infections and 75% of HSV-1) infections occur as a result of first-episode maternal infection during late pregnancy, when delivery occurs before the onset of maternal antibodies.[1] As reliable type-specific HSV antibody assays are now available, it has been proposed that serological testing for HSV in the latter half of pregnancy could identify women who are susceptible to HSV infection, so that serological testing of their partners and appropriate counselling as to the risk of acquiring genital herpes could be undertaken. However, routine HSV screening in pregnancy could have a profound impact on cost, intrapartum care and psychological stress. A detailed cost–benefit analysis using a decision analysis model in the USA concluded that screening for maternal type-specific herpes simplex virus antibodies could not be recommended to prevent neonatal herpes.[46] Such an analysis has not been performed in the UK. However, in order to evaluate the use of antenatal serological screening of women and their partners at the Chelsea and Westminster Hospital in London, a preliminary study was performed to evaluate the level of concern and knowledge about genital herpes among pregnant women and their attitudes towards serum screening for herpes in pregnancy.[47] In this study, 100 women who were randomly selected at their first antenatal clinic visit completed a questionnaire concerning their understanding of genital herpes and its transmission. The women then read an information sheet that stated the current incidence, mortality and morbidity of neonatal herpes in the UK. Finally, the women were asked whether they would consider being serologically tested for HSV and whether they would encourage their partners to be tested.

Table 20.4. Considerations for the prevention of acquisition of genital herpes infection in pregnancy

Recommendations	Evidence level
1. All women should be asked at their first antenatal visit if they or their partner have ever had genital herpes.	IV
2. Female partners of men with genital herpes, who themselves give no history of genital herpes, should be strongly advised not to have sex at the time of lesional recurrence. Use of condoms throughout pregnancy may diminish the risk of acquisition.	IV
3. Pregnant women should be advised of the risk of acquiring HSV-1 as a result of orogenital contact.	IV
4. Identifying susceptible women by means of type-specific antibody testing has not been evaluated in the UK in terms of costs and benefits.	IV

The majority (80%) were aware that genital herpes is a sexually transmitted disease and 60% were aware that it can be transmitted to the baby in pregnancy. Only 34% thought that genital herpes is always symptomatic and 56% thought they would know whether their partners had ever been infected. Eighty percent of the women surveyed said they would consider serological testing and 76% said they would encourage their partner to be tested. This study demonstrated that this population of women had a good understanding of the nature of genital herpes and its transmission and that, despite an awareness of the low incidence of neonatal herpes in the UK, most would accept antenatal screening. The views of the male partners of these women were not addressed in this study.

Ethical, psychological and cost implications of serum screening

Considerable distress may be caused to couples where a pregnant woman and/or her male partner are found unsuspectingly to be HSV-2 antibody seropositive. Furthermore, measures to reduce the risk of an HSV-2 seronegative woman acquiring primary herpes from her infected male partner may be unacceptable to some couples. Regular genital self-examination and condom use or abstinence from sexual intercourse may exacerbate the psychosexual problems associated with a diagnosis of HSV. Counselling would be essential for all couples prior to testing, for newly diagnosed cases of HSV and for discordant couples where the woman is HSV-2 seronegative. The acceptability of serum screening in pregnancy is likely to vary both between and within different populations according to socio-cultural differences and the local epidemiology of adult and neonatal infection.

If serum screening for HSV in pregnant women is to be introduced in antenatal clinics, it must be cost-effective and successful in reducing the incidence of neonatal disease. The practice of taking antenatal viral cultures from women with a history of genital herpes was abandoned precisely because neither of these criteria was fulfilled.[30] The appropriateness of such programmes will ultimately depend on the prevalence of adult and neonatal HSV infection, patient attitudes and the availability of resources, including laboratory facilities and counselling staff. Although serum screening was acceptable to the majority of the women surveyed in the Chelsea and Westminster study, in practice, health providers are unlikely to consider such a programme to be justified at present in the UK, given the current very low incidence of neonatal herpes.

Management of the neonate

Early recognition and treatment of neonatal HSV infection are important to reduce the mortality and the incidence of serious neurological sequelae in surviving children.[18] Any neonate with suspected herpes infection and any neonate whose mother had genital herpes lesions at delivery should have swabs taken for viral culture from the eyes, oropharynx and any mucocutaneous lesions. The taking of cerebrospinal fluid and other samples may also be appropriate. Routine viral culture is not recommended for babies born to asymptomatic mothers with a history of genital herpes, although parents should be advised to report early signs of infection (e.g. lethargy, poor feeding or lesions).

Neonates with suspected herpes infection (with or without central nervous system signs or symptoms) should have a lumbar puncture in order to obtain specimens of cerebrospinal fluid for PCR and/or culture. They should be treated with intravenous aciclovir. Many paediatricians would also recommend aciclovir treatment for babies born to mothers with first-episode herpes lesions at delivery, although evidence for this intervention is lacking and prophylactic treatment may only delay the onset of infection. Aciclovir therapy can be discontinued if the swabs are negative and the baby is well.

Summary

Although the incidence of neonatal herpes simplex infection is very low in the UK at the present time, this is a serious condition with high morbidity and mortality. Most cases occur as a result of primary genital HSV infection in the mother at the time of delivery. However, both primary infections and HSV reactivations are commonly asymptomatic or unrecognised. Severe persistent genital herpes ulceration may occur in those with immunosuppression due to HIV infection.

For all pregnant women with first-episode genital HSV infection, management decisions should be made in conjunction with genitourinary physicians and the patient herself. Type-specific HSV serology may aid further management by differentiating between a primary and a non-primary first episode. Treatment with a course of aciclovir is often indicated, and daily aciclovir prophylaxis in the last four weeks of pregnancy may prevent recurrences at term and thus the need for caesarean section. Elective caesarean section at term may be considered for all women presenting with first-episode genital herpes in the third trimester, particularly if the onset of symptoms is within six weeks of their expected date of delivery, because of the risk of viral shedding during labour. However, the greatest risk of neonatal herpes occurs where there are first-episode genital lesions at the onset of labour and for these women delivery by caesarean section should be advised. However, the benefits of caesarean delivery may be compromised if membranes have already ruptured and the fetus already exposed *in utero*.

Recurrent genital HSV infection is generally associated with relatively minor symptoms and antiviral treatment is not usually required. In the absence of genital lesions at the time of delivery, a history of recurrent genital herpes is not an indication for elective caesarean section. Where active genital lesions of recurrent HSV infection are present at the onset of labour, delivery by caesarean section should be considered, although the risks of neonatal herpes are very small.

Acknowledgements

This chapter is an updated and modified version of a review that originally appeared in the *British Journal of Obstetrics and Gynaecology* (Smith JR, Cowan FM, Munday P. *Br J Obstet Gynaecol* 1998;**105**:255–60). FM Cowan, P Munday and the Pregnancy Subgroup of the Herpes Simplex Advisory Panel, of which JR Smith was Chairman, contributed to the original paper.

References

1. Brown ZA, Selke S, Zeh J, Kopelman J, Maslow A, Ashley RL, *et al.* The acquisition of herpes simplex virus during pregnancy. *N Engl J Med* 1997;**337**:509–15.
2. Brocklehurst P, Carney O, Ross E, Mindel A. The management of recurrent genital herpes infection in pregnancy: a postal survey of obstetric practice. *Br J Obstet Gynaecol* 1995;**102**:791–7.
3. Cowan FM. Testing for type-specific antibody to herpes simplex virus – implications for clinical practice. *J Antimicrob Chemother* 2000;**45** Suppl T3:9–13.
4. Wald A, Corey L, Cone R, Hobson A, Davis G, Zeh J. Frequent genital herpes simplex virus 2 shedding in immunocompetent women. Effect of acyclovir treatment. *J Clin Invest* 1997;**99**:1092–7.
5. Lowhagen GB, Tunback P, Andersson K, Bergstrom T, Johannisson G. First episodes of genital herpes in a Swedish STD population: a study of epidemiology and transmission by the use of herpes simplex virus (HSV) typing and specific serology. *Sex Transm Infect* 2000;**76**:179–82.
6. Nilsen A, Myrmel H. Changing trends in genital herpes simplex virus infection in Bergen, Norway. *Acta Obstet Gynecol Scand* 2000;**79**:693–6.
7. Vyse AJ, Gay NJ, Slomka MJ, Gopal R, Gibbs T, Morgan-Capner P, *et al.* The burden of infection with HSV-1 and HSV-2 in England and Wales: implications for the changing epidemiology of genital herpes. *Sex Transm Infect* 2000;**76**:183–7.
8. Fleming DT, McQuillan GM, Johnson RE, Nahmias AJ, Aral SO, Lee FK, *et al.* Herpes simplex virus type 2 in the United States 1976 to 1994. *N Engl J Med* 1997;**337**:1105–11.
9. Cowan FM, Johnson AM, Ashley R, Corey L, Mindel A. Antibody to herpes simplex virus type 2 as serological marker of sexual lifestyle in populations. *BMJ* 1994;**309**:1325–9.
10. Langenberg AG, Corey L, Ashley RL, Leong WP, Straus SE. A prospective study of new infections with herpes simplex virus type 1 and type 2. Chiron HSV Vaccine Study Group. *N Engl J Med* 1999;**341**:1432–8.
11. Wald A, Zeh J, Selke S, Warren T, Ryncarz AJ, Ashley R, *et al.* Reactivation of genital herpes simplex virus type 2 infection in asymptomatic seropositive persons. *N Engl J Med* 2000;**342**:844–50.
12. Corey L, Handsfield HH. Genital herpes and public health: addressing a global problem. *JAMA* 2000;**283**:791–4.
13. Diamond C, Selke S, Ashley R, Benedetti J, Corey L. Clinical course of patients with serologic evidence of recurrent genital herpes presenting with signs and symptoms of first episode disease. *Sex Transm Dis* 1999;**26**:221–5.
14. Hensleigh PA, Andrews WW, Brown Z, Greenspoon J, Yasukawa L, Prober CG. Genital herpes during pregnancy: inability to distinguish primary and recurrent infections clinically. *Obstet Gynecol* 1997;**89**:891–5.
15. Corey L, Spear PG. Infections with herpes simplex viruses (1). *N Engl J Med* 1986;**314**:686–91.
16. Benedetti J, Corey L, Ashley R. Recurrence rates in genital herpes after symptomatic first-episode infection. *Ann Intern Med* 1994;**121**:847–54.
17. Koelle DM, Benedetti J, Langenberg A, Corey L. Asymptomatic reactivation of herpes simplex virus in women after the first episode of genital herpes. *Ann Intern Med* 1992;**116**:433–7.
18. Whitley R, Arvin A, Prober C, Corey L, Burchett S, Plotkin S, *et al.* Predictors of morbidity and mortality in neonates with herpes simplex virus infections. The National Institute of Allergy and Infectious Diseases Collaborative Antiviral Study Group. *N Engl J Med* 1991;**324**:450–4.
19. Brown ZA, Benedetti J, Selke S, Ashley R, Watts DH, Corey L. Asymptomatic maternal shedding of herpes simplex virus at the onset of labor: relationship to preterm labor. *Obstet Gynecol* 1996;**87**:483–8.
20. Brown ZA, Vontver LA, Benedetti J, Critchlow CW, Sells CJ, Berry S, *et al.* Effects on infants of a first episode of genital herpes during pregnancy. *N Engl J Med* 1987;**317**:1246–51.
21. Young EJ, Chafizadeh E, Oliveira VL, Genta RM. Disseminated herpesvirus infection during pregnancy. *Clin Infect Dis* 1996;**22**:51–8.
22. Kang AH, Graves CR. Herpes simplex hepatitis in pregnancy: a case report and review of the literature. *Obstet Gynecol Surv* 1999;**54**:463–8.
23. Hitti J, Watts DH, Burchett SK, Schacker T, Selke S, Brown ZA, *et al.* Herpes simplex virus seropositivity and reactivation at delivery among pregnant women infected with human immunodeficiency virus-1. *Am J Obstet Gynecol* 1997;**177**:450–4.
24. Heng MC, Heng SY, Allen SG. Co-infection and synergy of human immunodeficiency virus-1 and herpes simplex virus-1. *Lancet* 1994;**343**:255–8.
25. Tookey P, Peckham CS. Neonatal herpes simplex virus infection in the British Isles. *Paediatr Perinat Epidemiol* 1996;**10**:432–42.

26. Randolph AG, Washington AE, Prober CG. Cesarean delivery for women presenting with genital herpes lesions. Efficacy risks and costs. *JAMA* 1993;**270**:77–82.

27. Chuang TY. Neonatal herpes: incidence prevention and consequences. *Am J Prev Med* 1988;**4**:47–53.

28. Brown ZA, Benedetti J, Ashley R, Burchett S, Selke S, Berry S, *et al.* Neonatal herpes simplex virus infection in relation to asymptomatic maternal infection at the time of labor. *N Engl J Med* 1991;**324**:1247–52.

29. Prober CG, Sullender WM, Yasukawa LL, Au DS, Yeager AS, Arvin AM. Low risk of herpes simplex virus infections in neonates exposed to the virus at the time of vaginal delivery to mothers with recurrent genital herpes simplex virus infections. *N Engl J Med* 1987;**316**:240–4.

30. Arvin AM, Hensleigh PA, Prober CG, Au DS, Yasukawa LL, Wittek AE, *et al.* Failure of antepartum maternal cultures to predict the infant's risk of exposure to herpes simplex virus at delivery. *N Engl J Med* 1986;**315**:796–800.

31. Nahmias AJ, Josey WE, Naib ZM, Freeman MG, Fernandez RJ, Wheeler JH. Perinatal risk associated with maternal genital herpes simplex virus infection. *Am J Obstet Gynecol* 1971;**110**:825–37.

32. Corey L, Whitley RJ, Stone EF, Mohan K. Difference between herpes simplex virus type 1 and type 2 neonatal encephalitis in neurological outcome. *Lancet* 1988;**i**:1–4.

33. Anonymous. National guideline for the management of genital herpes. Clinical Effectiveness Group (Association of Genitourinary Medicine and the Medical Society for the Study of Venereal Diseases). *Sex Transm Infect* 1999;**75** Suppl 1:S24–8.

34. Ryncarz AJ, Goddard J, Wald A, Huang ML, Roizman B, Corey L. Development of a high-throughput quantitative assay for detecting herpes simplex virus DNA in clinical samples. *J Clin Microbiol* 1999;**37**:1941–7.

35. Preboth M. ACOG practice bulletin on management of herpes in pregnancy. American College of Obstetricians and Gynecologists. *Am Fam Physician* 2000;**61**:556–61.

36. Frenkel LM, Brown ZA, Bryson YJ, Corey L, Unadkat JD, Hensleigh PA, *et al.* Pharmacokinetics of acyclovir in the term human pregnancy and neonate. *Am J Obstet Gynecol* 1991;**164**:569–76.

37. Haddad J, Langer B, Astruc D, Messer J, Lokiec F. Oral acyclovir and recurrent genital herpes during late pregnancy. *Obstet Gynecol* 1993;**82**:102–4.

38. Kimberlin DF, Weller S, Whitley RJ, Andrews WW, Hauth JC, Lakeman F, *et al.* Pharmacokinetics of oral valacyclovir and acyclovir in late pregnancy. *Am J Obstet Gynecol* 1998;**179**:846–51.

39. Reiff-Eldridge R, Heffner CR, Ephross SA, Tennis PS, White AD, Andrews EB. Monitoring pregnancy outcomes after prenatal drug exposure through prospective pregnancy registries: a pharmaceutical company commitment. *Am J Obstet Gynecol* 2000;**182**:159–63.

40. van Everdingen JJ, Peeters MF, ten Have P. Neonatal herpes policy in The Netherlands. Five years after a consensus conference. *J Perinat Med* 1993;**21**:371–5.

41. Brown ZA, Baker DA. Acyclovir therapy during pregnancy. *Obstet Gynecol* 1989;**73**:526–531.

42. Scott LL, Sanchez PJ, Jackson GL, Zeray F, Wendel GD Jr. Acyclovir suppression to prevent cesarean delivery after first-episode genital herpes. *Obstet Gynecol* 1996;**87**:69–73.

43. Stray-Pedersen B. Acyclovir in late pregnancy to prevent neonatal herpes simplex [letter]. *Lancet* 1990;**336**:756.

44. Brocklehurst P, Kinghorn G, Carney O, Helsen K, Ross E, Ellis E, *et al.* A randomised placebo controlled trial of suppressive acyclovir in late pregnancy in women with recurrent genital herpes infection. *Br J Obstet Gynaecol* 1998;**105**:275–80.

45. Prober CG, Corey L, Brown ZA, Hensleigh PA, Frenkel LM, Bryson YJ, *et al.* The management of pregnancies complicated by genital infections with herpes simplex virus. *Clin Infect Dis* 1992;**15**:1031–8.

46. Rouse DJ, Stringer JS. An appraisal of screening for maternal type-specific herpes simplex virus antibodies to prevent neonatal herpes. *Am J Obstet Gynecol* 2000;**183**:400–6.

47. Vonau B, Low-Beer N, Barton SE, Smith JR. Antenatal serum screening for genital herpes: a study of knowledge and attitudes of women at a central London hospital. *Br J Obstet Gynaecol* 1997;**104**:347–9.

Chapter 21

Viruses and pregnancy I

Discussion

Discussion following Professor Fox's paper

Carrington: You have related the size of the placenta in viral infections to damage and so on, but is there a correlation between placental size and weight, and known congenital viral infection?

Fox: No.

Carrington: None at all?

Fox: Some placentas are unusually large, because they are oedematous. That is a feature of parvovirus B19 and some cases of cytomegalovirus, as well as toxoplasmosis, I might add. That is because of the oedema and the anaemia and so on.
In some cases of villitis the placenta is of somewhat reduced weight, but I do not want to dwell on placental weight, because that is another irrelevance.

Carrington: You were referring presumably to structural defects that are observable. Do you have any idea of the number of infected cells within the placenta that might have a cellular dysfunction as opposed to a structural dysfunction?

Fox: No. However, I must stress to you another failure of conceptual thinking here, which is widespread – although not in your case. The syncytiotrophoblast of the placental villi is a syncytium extending over the entire villus population and is therefore a single cell. You cannot quantitate the number of cells if you have syncytiotrophoblastic infection: the whole syncytium is in continuity, as you can show by microinjection studies. It is a true syncytium. That is where infection is seen most clearly, in the syncytiotrophoblast. You cannot therefore talk about the number of cells that are involved.

Discussion following Professor Griffiths' paper

Carrington: Was the quantitative polymerase chain reaction (PCR) testing on amniotic fluid or urine?

Griffiths: In the results from Italy,[1] the quantitative PCR tested amniotic fluid, while tests in our laboratory were on either urine or whole blood.

Carrington: Is there a particular recommendation that you would make on that? Do you feel that perhaps both would be worthwhile investigations?

Griffiths: Specifically looking at pregnancy, you would want to measure the viral load in amniotic fluid. In a placebo-controlled trial, measuring viral load in the blood would also be a further aim to try to identify which women were at risk of transmission.

As I see it at the moment, the ethics of running a placebo-controlled trial are that two-thirds of women will not transmit and so, arguably, will be given drug unnecessarily. If you could show in your natural history study that you could focus on women who had a 60% or 70% risk of intrauterine transmission, then you would be targeting the critical population who would need an intervention.

Hay: For how long do you need to treat the infants with intravenous ganciclovir?

Griffiths: If you look at the curve of viral load after birth, you would want to treat them certainly for six months and preferably for 12 months of life to try to reduce virus replication. However, you cannot do this with the drug we have at the moment, ganciclovir. This is primarily because of the need for intravenous access, but also because it is actually quite toxic and you do not want to do too much harm. What is remarkable is that they have had any effect at all with the six-week intervention. However, when safe orally bioavailable compounds are developed, I think six months' or 12 months' therapy will be given in the next trial from the Collaborative Antiviral Study Group. I hope that the groups at the Royal Free Hospital and St George's Hospital will be involved in that trial, so UK children will be included.

Peckham: We are re-analysing and looking at the data we gathered some time ago. The children are now being followed and examined to the age of five years. It has emerged quite clearly, when trying to see whether they had primary or recurrent infections, that among those with quite clear-cut seroconversion there was no damage at all. Most of the children with damage were from women who actually booked late, where we presumed it was a primary infection.

If one were trying to design a trial, there could be problems in deciding who should be treated. It is interesting that in none of the seroconversions was there evidence of damage.

Griffiths: Yes. Of course, the trial could only address the people who were eligible for study – that is a very good point. The trial in itself would not be designed to solve all known problems to do with cytomegalovirus (CMV), but rather to ask the question: is inhibiting CMV during pregnancy (in the group to whom you have access) valuable? However, I take the point that this strategy would not necessarily cover all of the women at risk of CMV – only a vaccine would do that.

Carrington: It seems that amniotic fluid, again, is the fluid of choice here. Why is fetal blood such a poor sample for CMV PCR?

Griffiths: That is an interesting question. The Italian group looked at fetal blood and gave up halfway through because it was poorly predictive and of low sensitivity. The amniotic fluid has this delay of requiring the fetal kidneys to become infected before excreting virus into the fluid. You would think that fetal blood would be the better sample but the results do not support that. I do not have an explanation for that.

Discussion following Dr Carrington's paper

Brink: Why did you choose 20 weeks as your cut-off for using aciclovir? There are clearly maternal benefits, but what about using it in the second trimester for potential fetal benefits, bearing in mind that there is the highest chance of fetal varicella syndrome at this time?

Carrington: The data in chickenpox are somewhat limited in relation to aciclovir use in pregnancy, particularly at the higher dose. It was the view of the UK Advisory Group on Chickenpox that there were insufficient data to say that it was safe, but no data to say that it would cause an adverse event. There were no data to suggest that aciclovir could impact on fetal varicella syndrome. The final recommendation of the Advisory Group was therefore regarded as a compromise. We thought that physicians would comply with a recommendation to treat at over 20 weeks of gestation, after organogenesis had substantially taken place, and where there would not be too much concern about its use. There is a slight misgiving about not recommending this treatment earlier in pregnancy, because clearly aciclovir use would be recommended for all adults.

Our view was that we would not achieve full compliance with a recommendation for treatment under 20 weeks of gestation, and it is clearly not licensed for that indication. We therefore had to tread carefully. Maternal infections are worse in the second half of the pregnancy and so we were targeting the major group at risk, particularly those in the last month of the pregnancy.

Brink: I was thinking particularly of the potential effect on fetal varicella syndrome, rather than maternal benefit.

Carrington: It may well be that, if we concentrate on the use of varicella immunoglobulin after contact, we may reduce the incidence of fetal varicella syndrome. There is some evidence for this. However, where a mother has chickenpox, there is clearly potential for benefit with antiviral therapy.

If the syndrome is a herpes zoster reactivation, for how long do you actually treat the baby? The reactivation may take some time to develop in its clinical course after maternal viraemia. You may therefore have to give the mother antiviral therapy throughout the rest of the pregnancy, if that was going to be preventive. Do you agree?

Brink: Yes, unless you are looking at minimising maternal viraemia by using aciclovir, and so actually preventing fetal involvement.

Carrington: You mean trying to stop the fetus becoming infected?

Brink: Yes.

Carrington: That has not been well thought out to date. Perhaps it is food for thought. It is important that guidelines are based on some sort of evidence.

Griffiths: I had the same concern. I know the logic on which it is based, i.e. not to treat women at less than 20 weeks of gestation. When the International Herpes Management Forum reviewed this, the logic was that aciclovir should be given to all adults with chickenpox, unless they happened to be in the early stage of pregnancy. It seemed that you were penalising the most vulnerable people if you put it that way round. We eventually settled on advising women that the drug was not licensed in pregnancy and that there was no evidence that it reduced fetal varicella syndrome but that we would nevertheless recommend it. There never will be such a trial because you cannot in practice do such a trial under those circumstances. However, based on the pathogenesis, you have to go forward and make a prediction of what may happen. It is just a question of stopping viraemic spread to the fetus.

Carrington: Yes, that is logical. The difficulty here is perhaps on the medico-legal side. I am not quite sure how we would get general consensus for use, even if we recommended it.

Miller: That is the nub of the question: the aciclovir in pregnancy registry shows about a 3% birth defect rate in the first trimester, which is considered compatible with the background rate of abnormality in any pregnancy. However, the potential problem from a medico-legal perspective is how to distinguish between an attributable and a chance effect. It is also important to remember that the risk of fetal varicella syndrome itself is only 1–2%, so the potential benefit from giving aciclovir to protect the fetus is small.

In relation to whether varicella-zoster immunoglobulin (VZIG) has any significant effect, the number of women who receive this prophylactic treatment as a result of presenting in pregnancy with a history of contact is about 600 a year, although a further 2000–3000 pregnant women get varicella without being given VZIG. This is because the majority of infections in pregnancy do not occur under circumstances where a contact is reported. Therefore, I do not think that VZIG is having any significant effect overall on the incidence of fetal varicella syndrome. Indeed, the one case in the Pastuszak study[2] where there was clear fetal varicella syndrome occurred in a woman who had been given VZIG prophylaxis after infection.

The idea that perhaps you reduce the risk to the fetus by reducing the viraemia is not necessarily established. It may be some fetal consequences that determine whether or not that particular infection in that fetus results in herpes zoster. In our study[3] we showed that when maternal varicella occurred despite VZIG prophylaxis, the risk of the fetus being infected was reduced. Under these circumstances it seems reasonable to assume this would therefore reduce the risk of fetal varicella syndrome. However, if the fetus gets infected under these circumstances it does not necessarily follow that because the degree of viraemia may be less the fetus is less likely to develop fetal varicella syndrome.

Discussion following Mr Smith's paper

Soothill: I thought the evidence was that viral shedding often occurred even when no lesions could be seen, and perhaps vice versa, although not as clearly. If you are to recommend inspection, it has to be only if you are prepared to do a caesarean section if you see anything, otherwise there is little point in doing the inspection. Do you really feel that you should leave that as a recommendation – performing vaginal examination for lesions?

Smith: I was keen to get the group's view on what people thought. I quite agree with you. Much of this stems from the fact that those guidelines were published two years ago, when we decided to recommend a caesarean section in the event of there being sores – active ulceration – present. If you take that away, then you remove the requirement to do anything – I quite agree with you. That is the nub of this. The evidence to support caesarean section in recurrence is thin.

Brocklehurst: This is a difficult issue. We are cavalier about performing caesarean sections when there is absolutely no clinical indication and yet, when it comes to genital herpes, everybody seems to want to stop doing caesarean sections. I am not entirely sure why that is.

The risk of transmission, if it exists, is very low. It is not 0%, because you showed that it has occurred. The data from the British Paediatric Surveillance Unit study[4] showed that some babies with neonatal herpes infection had been born to mothers with recurrent herpes, who had symptomatic lesions at the time of delivery. So the risk is present.

I still recommend caesarean delivery for women who have recurrences at the time of labour. Even considering the small number of women who have a history of recurrent genital herpes, the number who have a recurrence when they go into labour is tiny. I tend to err on the side of caution.

When it comes to whether I accept my own data about aciclovir as being definite evidence of effectiveness, I do not – and I do not prescribe aciclovir for these women. However, we did show a statistically significant decrease in the incidence of recurrent episodes from 36 weeks of gestation until delivery. What we did not show was any difference in the caesarean section rate, but the trial was underpowered because we recruited very poorly. It ended up being an underpowered, small study, where we were not necessarily expecting such a large difference in the recurrence rate. As I still tend to recommend the occasional caesarean section, I tend not to use aciclovir.

MacLean: We have to take into account the fact that many of these women know a great deal about their herpes. Because of the prodromal symptoms, they know whether they are infected. Women are now asking for caesarean sections without medical reasons. If you have someone who comes in to hospital in early labour saying they believe they have a recurrence and they want a caesarean section, then it would be foolish to ignore their request. On the other hand, if the patient comes in and wants guidance then you can direct them along the lines you have discussed, which is that the risk of infection is very small, provided they understand that their baby should be kept under observation for 48 hours. That, perhaps, is a better option.

Soothill: If you are going to hold that line, should you not then apply that to all babies? Many people who are shedding the virus will not know about it. Where would you stop?

MacLean: I agree that there will be many patients who have asymptomatic shedding, and there is no way you will be able to anticipate them. If a patient comes in believing that she has a lesion at that time, it is difficult to ignore. To tell a patient that we are going to insist that she has a vaginal delivery, even though she has an open lesion, is perhaps asking for trouble.

Soothill: I was asking about the patient who was seeking guidance.

MacLean: You have to say that the risk of the baby being infected is very small. One of the problems, as we are all aware, is that babies do not stay long enough in hospital now to have any sort of observation. We are dependent on the midwife who visits the mother and baby at home being able to recognise that something is wrong.

Smith: The sense I am getting is that we should leave it to clinical judgement. It is interesting because the Dutch have stopped doing caesarean sections for herpes, and they have not noticed any increase in neonatal infection.

Brocklehurst: Are they monitoring?

Smith: Yes. But the point is taken that there is a small risk. You cannot say that there is zero risk.

Carrington: I would like to make one further point. Most of the data in the USA are based on herpes simplex virus (HSV) 2, and the prevalence of HSV-2 is not the same in this country. In terms of the isolation between types 1 and 2, it is 50:50 for heterosexuals. The whole nature of the epidemiology of this disease, and its consequences, is very different in the UK and therefore perhaps requires a different approach.

Griffiths: Some would say that the difference between the UK and the USA is that the British have not yet discovered sex, and that is our problem. The prevalence of HSV-2 antibodies is much lower in the UK.

Also, where the woman has a history of recurrent genital herpes with symptoms at term, avoid instrumental delivery, particularly fetal scalp electrodes.

General discussion

Miller: We did not quite resolve the issue about the referral of patients who have varicella-zoster virus infection in pregnancy. The recommendation that they should be referred to specialist centres is quite a major one. If that were a recommendation from this group, it would significantly impact on the advice and practice of most of us in this room.

Jauniaux: We should have a fetal infection clinic attached to fetal medicine, so that people in other hospitals, or GPs, know that they can refer patients to a group with the facilities not only for fetal-medicine diagnosis but also virology, microbiology and, eventually, counselling for the patient. Perhaps it could be a recommendation that, in each regional centre, there should be access to a unit, or to a session of a clinic once a week, that can deal specifically with these problems.

Carrington: Do you not think that that might be a research recommendation, rather than a general one?

Jauniaux: No, it is practical – there is no research involved at all. The evidence is there.

Miller: The difference is whether all patients should be referred to a specialist centre, or whether that service should be available only for those who wish further follow-up or counselling.

Jauniaux: The service has to be available before the patient can be referred to it. It is a question of the specialist in fetal medicine in each centre sitting down with a virologist and a microbiologist and agreeing on how to run such a clinic.

MacLean: One of the concerns in the recommendations was that fetal medicine units are not always associated with infectious diseases units. Certainly, there is a problem when patients at an isolation unit need ventilation and have to be transferred to an intensive therapy unit at another hospital. Most obstetricians are appalled at the idea that a patient covered with vesicles is going to be sitting in an antenatal clinic waiting to be seen – probably by a senior house officer who is not really able to make the diagnosis. It depends very much on your set-up and your access to infectious-diseases physicians.

References

1. Lazzarotto T, Varani S, Guerra B, Nicolosi A, Lanari M, Landini MP. Prenatal indicators of congenital cytomegalovirus infection. *J Pediatr* 2000;**137**:90–5.
2. Pastuszak AL, Levy M, Schick B, Zuber C, Feldkamp M, Gladstone J, *et al.* Outcome after maternal varicella infection in the first 20 weeks of pregnancy. *N Engl J Med* 1994;**330**:901–5.
3. Enders G, Miller E, Cradock-Watson J, Bolley I, Ridehalgh M. Consequences of varicella and herpes zoster in pregnancy: prospective study of 1739 cases. *Lancet* 1994;**343**:1548–51.
4. Tookey P, Peckham CS. Neonatal herpes simplex virus infection in the British Isles. *Paediatr Perinat Epidemiol* 1996;**10**:432–42.

SECTION 6

VIRUSES AND PREGNANCY II

Chapter 22

HIV and pregnancy

James McIntyre

Introduction

Human immunodeficiency virus (HIV) type-1 infection has become an important and common complication of pregnancy in many settings. With more than 34 million people infected worldwide, it is estimated that two million HIV-infected women become pregnant each year, with over 600 000 of their children infected.[1] Almost 4 million children are thought to have died from AIDS since the start of the epidemic, while most of the 1.3 million children living today with HIV infection will die before they become teenagers. Almost all of these children were infected from their mothers. Ninety percent of all these infections occur in sub-Saharan Africa but mother-to-child transmission has increased rapidly in Asia and South America.[1,2] Infant and child mortality in southern Africa has risen by 50% as a result of AIDS and will rise further in the future.[3]

In contrast to the growing problem of mother-to-child transmission in developing countries, perinatal HIV infection has been reduced dramatically in more developed countries, where access to voluntary counselling and testing, anti-retroviral treatment and infant formula are available. The annual incidence of perinatally acquired AIDS in the United States increased steadily from 1984, reached a peak in 1992, and declined by 67% between 1992 and 1997, corresponding to the increased use of zidovudine in pregnancy over this time.[4]

Management of HIV-positive women in pregnancy must consider the appropriate treatment for the mother's stage of illness and interventions to reduce the risk of transmission of HIV.

Mother-to-child transmission of HIV

The rate of mother-to-child transmission of HIV in the absence of any treatment intervention varies from 14% to 48% in different settings.[5,6] This difference is most likely to be due to the higher rates of postpartum transmission through breast milk in Africa, but may also reflect strain differences and obstetric factors.

Transmission can occur *in utero*, intrapartum or postpartum. In non-breastfed infants, up to 75% of transmission is thought to occur in late pregnancy and in the period covering the labour and delivery. Transmission is influenced by a number of factors: maternal, obstetric and infant.[7-9] The maternal plasma viral load appears to be the most important correlate, although there appears to be no absolute cut-off for transmission, which can occur at low levels of viral load. A strong association between viral load and risk of transmission was seen in Thailand, for both *in utero* and intrapartum transmission. In this study,[10,11] transmitting mothers had 4.3-fold higher median plasma HIV RNA levels at delivery than did nontransmitters ($P < 0.001$). The level of virus shed in cervicovaginal secretions may be an independent risk factor for perinatal HIV-1 transmission. In Thailand, the perinatal transmission rate was 28.7% among women with quantifiable HIV-1 in cervicovaginal lavage (CVL) specimens and high plasma virus levels (greater than 10 000 copies/ml) but only 1% among women without quantifiable CVL HIV-1 and with low plasma virus levels ($P < 0.001$). A one-log increase in plasma HIV-1 increased the transmission odds 1.8 and 6.1 times (95% CI 0.9–3.5 and 2.4–15.4) for women with and without quantifiable CVL HIV-1, respectively ($P = 0.03$).[12]

In the earlier PACTG076 trial,[13] the Ariel trial[14] and in other trials in the USA, a weaker association was seen with maternal viral load, raising the possibility of a post-exposure protective effect of the anti-retroviral treatment in the child. This is supported by the reduction in transmission seen in a retrospective study of children who received only postnatal zidovudine.[15] In this study, transmission was decreased to 9.3% (95% CI 4.1–17.5%) if treatment was started within 48 hours of birth. A small study in Brazil[16] has demonstrated a transmission rate of 5.4% in infants treated with zidovudine whose mothers had not received treatment.

Other factors which have been associated with an increased risk of transmission include advanced clinical HIV disease, impaired maternal immunocompetence, maternal nutritional status, resistant viral strains, vaginal delivery, prolonged rupture of membranes, invasive obstetric procedures, the presence of maternal ulcerative genital infection, recreational drug use during pregnancy, high rates of unprotected sexual intercourse during pregnancy, being a first-born twin, prematurity, low birthweight and breastfeeding.[7,17-20] It has been suggested, but not conclusively proven, that some clades or viral subtypes may be more likely to be transmitted from mother to child than others: in particular, Clade C, the most common clade in southern Africa, may have a higher rate of transmission.[21] Viral co-receptor usage (CRCX4 or CCR5) has also been suggested as a potential factor in transmission.[22,23]

Prevention of mother-to-child transmission of HIV

Since 1994, the successful results of trials of anti-retroviral treatment in pregnancy have led to rapid policy changes and implementation. The use of anti-retroviral treatment during pregnancy has resulted in a dramatic decline in the number of perinatal infections in the USA and Europe. Transmission rates in the USA and France declined by between one-half and two-thirds within the first three years of routine use of zidovudine in pregnancy.[24,25] Transmission rates in Los Angeles dropped from 30% to 10% and in North Carolina from 21% to 8.5%.[26] Further reductions have been seen, with transmission rates of less than 5% now recorded. The long-course anti-retroviral regimens remain costly and not feasible for most developing countries. Following the successful short-course zidovudine trial in Thailand, the World Health Organization and other United Nations agencies endorsed and recommended the use of short-course regimens in developing countries.[27] The results from peripartum nevirapine trials have added further evidence that ultra-short course treatments could be employed.

Two other interventions have been demonstrated to reduce the risk of mother-to-child transmission: elective caesarean section and the avoidance of breastfeeding.[28,29] Both of these have implementation problems in under-resourced areas.

Long-course zidovudine regimens

The first trial to demonstrate the efficacy of anti-retroviral treatment in reducing mother-to-child transmission was the Pediatric AIDS Clinical Trials Group (PACTG) trial PACTG076.[30] Zidovudine given orally after 14 weeks of gestation, intravenously during labour and for six weeks to the neonate in a non-breastfed population was shown to reduce mother-to-child transmission of HIV-1 significantly. The study demonstrated a rate of mother-to-child transmission of 25.5% in the placebo group and 8.3% in the zidovudine group, representing a 67.5% reduction in transmission risk. The drug was well tolerated in the short term in the pregnant women and the neonates. The effect of zidovudine in reducing transmission appears to be partly through the reduction of maternal viral load, although transmission occurred at a wide range of viral loads in the PACTG076 study.[13] An additional level of protection through post-exposure prophylaxis in the infant is also hypothesised, as zidovudine readily crosses the placenta. A study in France[31] showed that HIV-positive women who received this zidovudine regimen and underwent elective caesarean section had a transmission rate of 0.8%.

The use of very high doses of zidovudine has been implicated in the development of tumours in mice, but there has been no evidence of teratogenicity or short-term adverse effects in the human fetus or newborn. No late deaths and no malignancies have been shown with follow-up to age five years of uninfected children who were exposed to *in utero* zidovudine, and no differences could be detected in any parameters of growth, cognitive and developmental function assessed by the Bailey Scales of Infant Development, immunological function, cardiac function or ophthalmological function[32-34] Concern has been expressed about the possibility of selecting resistant viral variants during the use of zidovudine monotherapy in pregnancy. Some resistant strains of virus have been reported after zidovudine treatment to prevent transmission.[35] Although resistance appears to be uncommon, there has been concern about the efficacy of zidovudine monotherapy in the management of any subsequent pregnancy. Retrospective analysis of specimens from the PACTG076 study showed no development of high-level resistance and that low-level resistance was not associated with an increased risk of transmission. A prospective Swiss study[36] showed that 9.6% of treated mothers had a codon T215F mutation, although none of these women transmitted the virus to their children. However, in the Women and Infants Transmission Study Group,[37] maternal zidovudine-resistant virus was predictive of transmission, independent of viral load, in mothers with moderately advanced HIV-1 disease, many of whom had been treated with zidovudine before pregnancy.

Long-course zidovudine treatment has become the minimum standard of care in the USA, Europe and other developed country settings. The Thailand Perinatal Prevention

Trial[38] was a multicentre, randomised, four-arm, double-blind equivalence trial to compare the safety and efficacy of maternal zidovudine treatment starting at 28 weeks of gestation (300 mg twice a day; 300 mg every three hours orally during labour) and six weeks of infant treatment (2 mg/kg every six hours) (LL for long-long, the PACTG076-like reference arm) with maternal zidovudine starting at 35 weeks and/or infant zidovudine shortened to three days (long-short, short-long, short-short). Infants were formula fed. Following the first safety interim analysis, SS was stopped, and enrolment continued in LL, SL and LS. The final accrual was 1437 women. Transmission rates at six months were 6.7% (95% CI 3.7–9.7%) in LL, 5.7% (95% CI 3.2–8.3%) in LS, 8.4% (95% CI 5.3–11.5%) in SL and 10.6% (95% CI 6.5–14.5%) in SS. The investigators concluded that the LS and LL regimens appear safe, easy to comply with and equally efficacious. Both are simpler to implement and much less costly than the original PACTG076 regimen. While six weeks of zidovudine treatment in infants may not add benefit when mothers receive long treatment, it may prevent some infections when mothers receive shorter treatment.

Long-course combination treatment

In settings where anti-retroviral drug therapy is available for continuing treatment, many pregnant women will receive combination anti-retroviral therapy throughout pregnancy. Experience with HAART (highly active anti-retroviral therapy) or dual combination therapy during pregnancy is limited, but suggests that transmission rates of less than 5% can be achieved.[39] An increased rate of preterm delivery was reported in a retrospective Swiss study[40] of 30 infected pregnant women receiving combination anti-retroviral viral therapy with and without protease inhibitors. A larger study[41] of 462 infected pregnant women in clinical trial sites in the USA showed no difference in the incidence of preterm delivery and low birthweight by type of maternal anti-retroviral therapy.

Short-course zidovudine regimens

Unfortunately, the use of long-course zidovudine regimens is not feasible for most women at risk in the developing world, due to the expense of the treatment and the logistics of laboratory monitoring, intravenous infusions during delivery and treatment to the newborn for six weeks. In addition, the treatment needs to be introduced early in pregnancy, while most women in resource-poor settings only attend for antenatal care late in pregnancy. Lack of access to counselling and testing in these settings further limits the use of anti-retroviral therapy in pregnancy. Women in developing countries have higher rates of anaemia, which may be exacerbated by prolonged anti-retroviral treatment, and may differ in disease status from those in developed countries.

Shorter drug regimens in pregnancy would be more feasible in resource-poor settings. Several randomised controlled trials have shown a reduction of between 37% and 50% in transmission with the use of anti-retrovirals in late pregnancy and labour, with or without postpartum treatment.

A trial in Thailand[10] was the first to show a significant effect of short-regimen zidovudine treatment in preventing transmission. The Bangkok Perinatal AZT study[10] was a randomised placebo-controlled trial to evaluate the safety and efficacy of a short regimen of oral zidovudine administered during late pregnancy and labour to reduce the risk of perinatal HIV transmission. The regimen was 300 mg zidovudine orally twice daily from 36 weeks of gestation until the onset of labour and 300 mg every three hours from the onset of labour until delivery. All women were advised not to breastfeed and were provided with infant formula, and these results are directly applicable only to formula-fed infants. Transmission in the treatment group was 9.4% (95% CI 5.2–13.5%) and 18.9% (95% CI 13.2–24.2%) in the placebo group, representing a 50% reduction in transmission risk (95% CI 15.4–70.6%).

A second randomised trial[42] of this zidovudine regimen was conducted in 260 women in Côte d'Ivoire. In this trial population, over 95% of the infants were breastfed by their mothers and there was a 37% reduction in transmission at three months of age: 19 of 115 babies in the zidovudine group were HIV infected compared with 30 of 115 in the placebo group. There were similar transmission rates at three months, showing that breastfeeding had produced no substantial narrowing of the difference between the two groups.

A further trial[43] of short-course zidovudine conducted in Burkina Faso and Côte d'Ivoire in over 350 women compared placebo with oral zidovudine, started between 36 and 38 weeks of gestation at 300 mg twice daily, followed by a single loading dose of 600 mg at the onset of labour and oral zidovudine 300 mg twice a day to the mother for seven days after delivery. In this trial, over 85% of infants were breastfed for longer than three months. The efficacy of zidovudine was estimated at 38% (95% CI 5–60%) at six months of age of the infants.

A pooled analysis[44] of these two West African studies has demonstrated that there was an increase in transmission rates to 24 months in both arms, due to breast milk transmission. The postnatal transmission risk was 9.4% in the zidovudine group and 8.6% in the placebo group among the 494 children at risk (95% CI for the difference: −4.6–5.5%). By month 24, cumulative HIV infections in the placebo group were 30.1% and 22.1% in the zidovudine group, showing that in this breastfeeding population an oral short course of zidovudine significantly reduced overall maternal transmission at 24 months of age.

Other short-course anti-retroviral regimens

The UNAIDS Perinatal Transmission (PETRA) study,[45] conducted in five African sites, investigated different regimens of a combination of zidovudine and lamivudine in over 1700 women. Interim early efficacy results at six weeks of age of the infant have been reported. This trial compared the effectiveness of three different drug regimens with placebo. Arm A received zidovudine and lamivudine from 36 weeks of gestation, during labour and for one week postpartum to mother and child. Arm B received zidovudine and lamivudine from the onset of labour and for one week postpartum to mother and child. Arm C received zidovudine and lamivudine during labour only. The risk of transmission by six weeks of age in Arm A was 8.6%, in Arm B 10.8%, Arm C 17.7% and in the placebo group 17.2%.[45,46] Follow-up data to 18 months showed no difference between the arms in HIV infection and deaths, and further analysis is needed to distinguish the effect of HIV infection and other causes of mortality in this study.[47]

A French study[48] has raised concerns about the safety of zidovudine and lamivudine administration in pregnancy, which may argue for caution in the use of this combination regimen. In this cohort of around 200 infants whose mothers had received nucleoside analogues, eight children had mitochondrial dysfunction. Five, of whom two died, presented with delayed neurological symptoms and three were symptom-free but had severe biological or neurological abnormalities. Four of these children had been exposed to combined zidovudine and lamivudine, and four to zidovudine alone. No child was infected with HIV-1. All children had abnormally low absolute or relative activities of respiratory-chain complexes I, IV, or both, months or years after the end of anti-retroviral treatment. These results remain controversial and a large-scale look-back investigation in the USA[49] has not confirmed any cases of mitochondrial dysfunction in more than 20 000 children who had received perinatal zidovudine or lamivudine. One study[50] has described the rapid development of resistance to lamivudine when combined with zidovudine in pregnancy, which may also limit the use of short-course combination treatments where lamivudine is a treatment option for children.

A phase II trial[51] of other nucleoside analogues, didanosine and stavudine, given to mothers from 36 weeks of gestation and in labour and to children for six weeks, demonstrated a significant reduction of mother-to-child transmission to 3.6% in the overall study population ($n = 197$). Statistically comparable transmission rates were 4.2% in the stavudine arm, 1.9% for didanosine, 2.0% for didanosine and stavudine combined and 3% in the zidovudine arms. The small numbers in this study do not allow for definitive comparisons between the treatments but the use of other nucleoside analogues does look promising.

Ultra-short-course regimens

Anti-retroviral treatment in labour or postpartum would provide a feasible and more cost-effective approach. Nevirapine is a potent inhibitor of HIV-1 reverse transcriptase and has several properties that make it a valuable option for use during labour and in the early intrapartum period.[52,53] These include the rapid absorption of nevirapine, good crossing of the placenta and a long half-life. The drug is highly lipophilic and has wide distribution throughout the body.[54] In addition, studies in chimpanzees have shown a prophylactic effect.[55] These properties led to the investigation of intrapartum and postpartum nevirapine for the prevention of mother-to-child transmission in the HIVNET 012 study.[56] The results provide evidence for a short and affordable anti-retroviral treatment with a significant reduction in mother-to-child transmission.

The HIVNET 012 trial in Uganda investigated the use of one 200 mg dose of nevirapine administered orally to women at the onset of labour and one dose of 2 mg/kg to the baby within 72 hours, compared with intrapartum zidovudine and one week of zidovudine treatment to the child. Almost all babies were breastfed. In the nevirapine treatment group, the transmission rate at 14–16 weeks was 13.1% compared with 25.1% in the comparison group. The efficacy of nevirapine was 47% (95% CI 20–64%). Adverse effects were similar in the two regimens, both of which were well tolerated.[57] Transmission rates for all infants at 12 months were 15.7% in the nevirapine arm and 24.1% in the zidovudine arm, representing an absolute reduction of 8.4% and a relative risk reduction of 39% at 12 months.[58]

The South African Intrapartum Nevirapine Trial (SAINT) investigated intrapartum and postpartum nevirapine compared with the Arm B regimen from the PETRA study. Mother-to-child transmission rates by Kaplan-Meier estimates were 11.9% (95% CI 9.1–14.6%) and 8.6% (95% CI 6.2–10.9%) for nevirapine and zidovudine/lamivudine arms respectively at four weeks and 14.1 % (95% CI 11.0-17.0%) and 10.8 % (95% CI 8.1–13.5%) for nevirapine and zidovudine/lamivudine respectively at eight weeks. There were no significant differences between arms ($P > 0.10$) and no significant drug-related adverse events.[59,60]

A small study in Uganda[61] has demonstrated the development of nevirapine-resistant virus in three of fourteen women who received only one intrapartum dose of nevirapine. In the HIVNET 012 study, nevirapine resistance mutations were detected at six weeks postpartum in seven (23%) of thirty women whose infants were HIV-1 infected. The K103N nevirapine resistance mutation was detected in all seven women and, in addition, one woman had the Y181C mutation and another had both the Y181C and V106A mutations. Nevirapine resistance mutations were also detected in three of the seven infected infants. The K103N mutation was detected in one infant and the Y181C mutation was detected in two infants. The maternal and infant HIV-1 genotypes were different for each mother–infant pair. Follow-up of these mothers and children showed that the resistant mutations had disappeared by 13–18 months. The persistence of mutations could be much shorter than this, however, as a full range of specimens at other time points was not available to the investigators.[62] The clinical significance of this transient selection of resistant virus is uncertain but generally believed not to be a reason to avoid the use of single-dose nevirapine regimens for the prevention of mother-to-child transmission.

Choice of anti-retroviral regimen

The use of anti-retrovirals is one strategy to combat the problem of mother-to-child transmission and should be considered along with appropriate obstetric management and an informed decision by the mother on the risks and benefits of breastfeeding versus replacement feeding. There is a spectrum of anti-retroviral treatment available in pregnancy, with varying efficacy in reducing mother-to-child transmission. The choice of the most appropriate regimen for an individual patient or a health service will depend upon the clinical needs of the patient, the service setting, the circumstances and the available finance.

The major advantages for developing countries of a nevirapine regimen over the other treatments described above lie in the ease of administration and the very short course of treatment, which result in a significant reduction in costs. There are many advantages to an intrapartum and postpartum dosing regimen for the prevention of mother-to-child transmission. Exposure to the anti-retroviral is reduced for both mother and child, the logistics of administration are much easier and the regimen is available to women diagnosed at a later stage of pregnancy. In situations where many women may deliver outside the health service, the maternal dose of nevirapine can be supplied to women for them to keep with them and take at home at the onset of labour (as in the HIVNET 012 study), which reduces the risk of missing the labour treatment. A one-dose regimen for the child minimises the burden on health services and dispensaries and can be given before discharge from hospital or on a return visit, in a supervised manner.

Caesarean section

Several prospective follow-up studies have suggested that caesarean section is protective for mother-to-child transmission. Two reports published in 1999 provide more conclusive evidence of this. In the European Collaborative Group's randomised mode of delivery trial,[63] elective caesarean section was compared with vaginal delivery. In this trial, eligible women were between 34 and 36 weeks of gestation, with a confirmed diagnosis of HIV-1 infection, and with no indication for caesarean delivery or a contraindication to this mode of delivery. Women were randomly assigned elective caesarean section or vaginal delivery at 38 weeks of gestation. The transmission rate in the elective caesarean section group was 1.8% compared with 10.5% in the vaginal delivery group. In this European setting, there were few postpartum complications and no serious adverse events in either group.

The second report is from a large meta-analysis conducted by the International Perinatal HIV Group.[64] This meta-analysis included data from 8533 mother–infant pairs from fifteen prospective cohort studies. After adjustment for anti-retroviral therapy, maternal stage of disease and infant birthweight, the likelihood of transmission of HIV-1 was 50% lower with elective caesarean section than with other modes of delivery (OR 0.43; 95% CI 0.33–0.56). A reduction of 87% was seen with long-course zidovudine treatment and elective caesarean section compared with no treatment and other modes of delivery (OR 0.13; 95% CI 0.09–0.19).

The meta-analysis supports the findings of Mandelbrot et al.[31] in a French study where the transmission rate with long-course zidovudine and elective caesarean section was less than 1%. Postpartum complications of caesarean section are rare in developed country settings. More work is needed in developing countries, where infectious complications are more common. While elective caesarean section remains a useful tool, it seems unlikely that it will be an option for most developing country health services, where HIV seroprevalence rates are often over 20%.

Infant feeding

Infant feeding remains a major concern in the prevention of mother-to-child transmission of HIV. Breastfeeding has been associated with a doubling of transmission rates[65] but alternative feeding options may be difficult or impossible to implement in many high-prevalence settings. Transmission through breast milk may occur early or late in infant life. A Malawi study[66] showed a relatively high risk of HIV transmission during the early breastfeeding period (0.7% and 0.6% per month for months 1–5 and 6–11 respectively) and a lower but continued risk later (0.3% and 0.2% per month for months 12–17 and 18–23 respectively). The cumulative risk of postnatal transmission in this study was 3.5%, 7.0%, 8.9% and 20.3% after 5, 11, 17 and 23 months of breastfeeding, respectively. A pooled analysis[67] of eight cohort studies demonstrated that the risk of late postnatal transmission (after age four months) was 3.2% per year of breastfeeding.

A randomised trial[29] of breastfeeding versus formula feeding undertaken in Nairobi, Kenya, also showed that most transmission through breastfeeding occurred early, with 75% of attributable infection occurring in the first six months. In this study, breast milk transmission was responsible for 44% of all infections. There was a high mortality rate up to 24 months in both the formula-fed and breastfed groups in this study (20% and 24% respectively), although HIV survival was higher in the formula-fed group.

It has been suggested[68,69] that mixed feeding may be more likely to facilitate HIV transmission than exclusive breastfeeding, presumably through an effect on the infant gastrointestinal tract. More research is required before a policy recommendation for exclusive breastfeeding by HIV-infected women can be made.

Care of the mother during pregnancy and beyond

The care of an HIV-infected woman during pregnancy should be tailored to her individual clinical condition. Where anti-retroviral treatment is available, current guidelines recommend starting with appropriate therapy if clinically indicated, which should not be deferred because of the pregnancy.[70] The primary factor in deciding treatment options should be the woman's clinical, immunological and virological status. As many of the anti-retrovirals have not been tested exhaustively for use in pregnancy, their benefits need to be balanced against the possible complications, and these should be discussed with the patient.

Even where anti-retroviral treatment is not available, the management of pregnant women infected with HIV should include screening for and treatment of concurrent sexually transmitted diseases, diagnosis and management of any other opportunistic infections and consideration of prophylaxis with co-trimoxazole where the CD4 count is below $200/mm^3$.[7] HIV-infected women are more likely to have cervical dysplasia and a cervical smear should be part of the antenatal or postnatal management. All HIV-positive women should have access to information about contraception and the provision of an appropriate method, including tubal ligation if desired. The management of an HIV-positive woman in pregnancy should be seen as an integral part of her long-term continuing clinical treatment.

References

1. UNAIDS. *Report on the Global HIV/AIDS Epidemic – June 2000*. Geneva; 2000.
2. UNAIDS. *Report on the Global HIV/AIDS Epidemic – June 1998*. Geneva; 1998.
3. Stanecki KA, Way PO. Focus on HIV/AIDS in the developing world. In: *World Population Profile: 1998*. Washington DC: US Government Printing Office; 1999. US Bureau of the Census Report WP/98.
4. Lindegren ML, Byers RH Jr, Thomas P, Davis SF, Caldwell B, Rogers M, *et al*. Trends in perinatal transmission of HIV/AIDS in the United States. *JAMA* 1999;**282**:531–8.
5. Fowler MG. Update: transmission of HIV-1 from mother to child. *Curr Opin Obstet Gynecol* 1997;**9**:343–8.
6. Wiktor SZ, Ekpini E, Nduati RW. Prevention of mother-to-child transmission of HIV-1 in Africa. AIDS 1997;**11** Suppl B:S79–87.
7. McIntyre JA. HIV in Pregnancy: a Review. Geneva: World Health Organization; 1999. Occasional paper no 2.
8. Newell ML. Mechanisms and timing of mother-to-child transmission of HIV-1. *AIDS* 1998;**12**:831–7.
9. Fowler MG, Simonds RJ, Roongpisuthipong A. Update on perinatal HIV transmission. *Pediatr Clin North Am* 2000;**47**:21–38.
10. Shaffer N, Chuachoowong R, Mock PA, Bhadrakom C, Siriwasin W, Young NL, *et al*. Short-course zidovudine for perinatal HIV-1 transmission in Bangkok, Thailand: a randomised controlled trial. Bangkok Collaborative Perinatal HIV Transmission Study Group. *Lancet* 1999;**353**:773–80.

11. Mock PA, Shaffer N, Bhadrakom C, Siriwasin W, Chotpitayasunondh T, Chearskul S, et al. Maternal viral load and timing of mother-to-child HIV transmission, Bangkok, Thailand. Bangkok Collaborative Perinatal HIV Transmission Study Group. AIDS 1999;13:407–14.

12. Chuachoowong R, Shaffer N, VanCott TC, Chaisilwattana P, Siriwasin W, Waranawat N, et al. Lack of association between human immunodeficiency virus type 1 antibody in cervicovaginal lavage fluid and plasma and perinatal transmission, in Thailand. J Infect Dis 2000;181:1957–63.

13. Sperling RS, Shapiro DE, Coombs RW, Todd JA, Herman SA, McSherry GD, et al. Maternal viral load, zidovudine treatment, and the risk of transmission of human immunodeficiency virus type 1 from mother to infant. Pediatric AIDS Clinical Trials Group Protocol 076 Study Group. N Engl J Med 1996;335:1621–9.

14. Cao Y, Krogstad P, Korber BT, Koup RA, Muldoon M, Macken C, et al. Maternal HIV-1 viral load and vertical transmission of infection: the Ariel Project for the prevention of HIV transmission from mother to infant. Nat Med 1997;3:549–52.

15. Wade NA, Birkhead GS, Warren BL, Charbonneau TT, French PT, Wang L et al. Abbreviated regimens of zidovudine prophylaxis and perinatal transmission of the human immunodeficiency virus. N Engl J Med 1998;339:1409–14.

16. Duarte G, Mussi-Pinhata MM, Cervi MC, Kato CM, Paschoini MC, Quintana SM. Can isolated postpartum zidovudine prophylaxis reduce perinatal HIV transmission? XVI FIGO World Congress of Gynecology and Obstetrics, 3–8 September 2000, Washington DC, USA. Abstract P4.12.01.

17. Peckham C, Newell ML. Mother-to-child transmission of HIV infection: nutrition/HIV interactions. Nutr Rev 2000;58 (2 Pt 2):S38–45.

18. O'Shea S, Newell ML, Dunn DT, Garcia-Rodriguez MC, Bates I, Mullen J, et al. Maternal viral load, CD4 cell count and vertical transmission of HIV-1. J Med Virol 1998;54:113–17.

19. Pitt J, Brambilla D, Reichelderfer P, Landay A, McIntosh K, Burns D, et al. Maternal immunologic and virologic risk factors for infant human immunodeficiency virus type 1 infection: findings from the Women and Infants Transmission Study. J Infect Dis 1997;175:567–75.

20. Chen F, Pau AK, Piscitelli SC. Update on preventing vertical transmission of HIV type 1. Am J Health Syst Pharm 2000;57:1616–23.

21. Renjifo B, Essex M, Mwakagile D, Hunter D, Msamanga G, Spiegelman D, et al. Differences in vertical transmission between HIV phenotypes. Second Conference on Global Strategies for the Prevention of HIV Transmission from Mothers to Infants, 1–5 September 1999, Montreal, Canada. Abstract 099.

22. Paul MO, Abrams EO, Bakshi S. Mother-to-child transmission of HIV-1: evaluation of HIV-1 co-receptor usage. 6th Conference on Retroviruses and Opportunistic Infections, 31 January – 4 February 1999, Chicago, USA. Abstract 2312000.

23. Pollack H, Rochford G, Monard S, Borkowsky W. Absence of expression of the chemokine receptors CCR5 and CXCR4 on human placental term trophoblasts. 6th Conference on Retroviruses and Opportunistic Infections, 31 January – 4 February 1999, Chicago, USA. Abstract 2292000.

24. Simonds RJ, Steketee R, Nesheim S, Matheson P, Palumbo P, Alger L, et al. Impact of zidovudine use on risk and risk factors for perinatal transmission of HIV. Perinatal AIDS Collaborative Transmission Studies. AIDS 1998;12:301–8.

25. Mayaux MJ, Teglas JP, Mandelbrot L, Berrebi A, Gallais H, Matheron S, et al. Acceptability and impact of zidovudine for prevention of mother-to-child human immunodeficiency virus-1 transmission in France. J Pediatr 1997;131:857–62.

26. Fiscus SA, Adimora AA, Schoenbach VJ, Lim W, McKinney R, Rupar D, et al. Perinatal HIV infection and the effect of zidovudine therapy on transmission in rural and urban counties. JAMA 1996;275:1483–8.

27. World Health Organization. Recommendations on the safe and effective use of short-course ZDV for the prevention of mother-to-child transmission of HIV. Wkly Epidemiol Rec 1998;73:313–20.

28. Brocklehurst P. Interventions aimed at decreasing the risk of mother-to-child transmission of HIV infection. Cochrane Database Syst Rev 2000;2:CD000102.

29. Nduati R, John G, Mbori-Ngacha D, Richardson B, Overbaugh J, Mwatha A, et al. Effect of breastfeeding and formula feeding on transmission of HIV-1: a randomized clinical trial. JAMA 2000;283:1167–74.

30. Connor EM, Sperling RS, Gelber R, Kiselev P, Scott G, O'Sullivan MJ, et al. Reduction of maternal-infant transmission of human immunodeficiency virus type 1 with zidovudine treatment. Pediatric AIDS Clinical Trials Group Protocol 076 Study Group. N Engl J Med 1994;331:1173–80.

31. Mandelbrot L, Le Chenadec J, Berrebi A, Bongain A, Benifla JL, Delfraissy JF, et al. Perinatal HIV-1 transmission: interaction between zidovudine prophylaxis and mode of delivery in the French Perinatal Cohort. JAMA 1998;280:55–60.

32. Sperling RS, Shapiro DE, McSherry GD, Britto P, Cunningham BE, Culnane M, et al. Safety of the

maternal-infant zidovudine regimen utilized in the Pediatric AIDS Clinical Trial Group 076 Study. *AIDS* 1998;**12**:1805–13.

33. Hanson IC, Antonelli TA, Sperling RS, Oleske JM, Cooper E, Culnane M, *et al*. Lack of tumors in infants with perinatal HIV-1 exposure and fetal/neonatal exposure to zidovudine. *J Acquir Immune Defic Syndr Hum Retrovirol* 1999;**20**:463–7.

34. Culnane M, Fowler M, Lee SS, McSherry G, Brady M, O'Donnell K, *et al*. Lack of long-term effects of *in utero* exposure to zidovudine among uninfected children born to HIV-infected women. Pediatric AIDS Clinical Trials Group Protocol 219/076 Teams. *JAMA* 1999;**281**:151–7.

35. Srinivas RV, Holden WT, Su T, Flynn PM. Development of zidovudine-resistant HIV genotypes following postnatal prophylaxis in a perinatally infected infant. *AIDS* 1996;**10**:795–6.

36. Kully C, Yerly S, Erb P, Kind C, Krautheim A, Perrin L, *et al*. Codon 215 mutations in human immunodeficiency virus-infected pregnant women. Swiss Collaborative 'HIV and Pregnancy' Study. *J Infect Dis* 1999;**179**:705–8

37. Welles SL, Pitt J, Colgrove R, McIntosh K, Chung PH, Colson A, *et al*. HIV-1 genotypic zidovudine drug resistance and the risk of maternal–infant transmission in the women and infants transmission study. The Women and Infants Transmission Study Group. *AIDS* 2000;**14**:263–71.

38. Lallemant M, Jourdain G, Le Coeur S, Kim S, Karnchanamayul V, Hansudewechakul R, *et al*. Perinatal HIV prevention trial (PHPT), Thailand: simplified and shortened zidovudine prophylaxis regimen as efficacious as PACTG076. XIII International AIDS Conference, 9–14 July 2000, Durban, South Africa. Abstract LbOr032000.

39. Silverman NS, Watts DH, Hitti J, Money DM, Livingston E, Axelrod J, *et al*. Initial multicenter experience with double nucleoside therapy for human immunodeficiency virus infection during pregnancy. *Infect Dis Obstet Gynecol* 1998;**6**:237–43.

40. Lorenzi P, Spicher VM, Laubereau B, Hirschel B, Kind C, Rudin C, *et al*. Anti-retroviral therapies in pregnancy: maternal, fetal and neonatal effects. Swiss HIV Cohort Study, the Swiss Collaborative HIV and Pregnancy Study, and the Swiss Neonatal HIV Study. *AIDS* 1998;**12**:F241–7.

41. Shapiro D, Tuomala R, Samelson R, *et al*. Antepartum anti-retroviral therapy and pregnancy outcomes in 462 HIV-infected women in 1998–1999 (PACTG 367). 7th Conference on Retroviruses and Opportunistic Infections, 30 January – 2 February 2000, San Francisco, USA. Abstract 664.

42. Wiktor SZ, Ekpini E, Karon JM, Nkengasong J, Maurice C, Severin ST, *et al*. Short-course oral zidovudine for prevention of mother-to-child transmission of HIV-1 in Abidjan, Cote d'Ivoire: a randomised trial. *Lancet* 1999;**353**:781–5.

43. Dabis F, Msellati P, Meda N, Welffens-Ekra C, You B, Manigart O, *et al*. 6-month efficacy, tolerance, and acceptability of a short regimen of oral zidovudine to reduce vertical transmission of HIV in breastfed children in Cote d'Ivoire and Burkina Faso: a double-blind placebo-controlled multicentre trial. DITRAME Study Group. Diminution de la Transmission Mère-Enfant. *Lancet* 1999;**353**:786–92.

44. Wiktor SZ, Leroy V, Ekpini ER, Alioum A, Karon J, Msellati P, *et al*. 24-month efficacy of short-course maternal zidovudine for the prevention of mother-to-child HIV-1 transmission in a breast feeding population: a pooled analysis of two randomized clinical trials in West Africa. XIII International AIDS Conference, 9–14 July 2000, Durban, South Africa. Abstract TuOrB3542000.

45. Saba J. The PETRA Trial Study Group. Interim analysis of early efficacy of various short-term ZDV/3TC combination regimens in preventing mother-to-child transmission of HIV-1: the PETRA trial. 6th Conference on Retroviruses and Opportunistic Infections, 31 January – 4 February 1999, Chicago, USA. Abstract S7:212.

46. Saba J. PETRA Study Group. Current status of the PETRA Study. Second Conference on Global Strategies for the Prevention of HIV Transmission from Mothers to Infants, 1–5 September 1999, Montreal, Canada.

47. Gray G. PETRA Trial Group. The PETRA Study: early and late efficacy of three short ZDV/3TC combination regimens to prevent mother-to-child transmission of HIV-1. XIII International AIDS Conference, 9–14 July 2000, Durban, South Africa. Abstract LbOr052000.

48. Blanche S, Tardieu M, Rustin P, Slama A, Barret B, Firtion G, *et al*. Persistent mitochondrial dysfunction and perinatal exposure to anti-retroviral nucleoside analogues. *Lancet* 1999;**354**:1084–9.

49. Smith ME, U. S. Nucleoside Safety Review Working Group. Ongoing nucleoside safety review of HIV-exposed children in U. S. studies. Second Conference on Global Strategies for the Prevention of HIV Transmission from Mothers to Infants, 1–5 September 1999, Montreal, Canada. Abstract 096.

50. Clarke JR, Braganza R, Mirza A, Stainsby C, Ait-Khaled M, Wright A, *et al*. Rapid development of genotypic resistance to lamivudine when combined with zidovudine in pregnancy. *J Med Virol* 1999;**59**:364–8.

51. Gray G, McIntyre J, Jivkov B, Schorn M, Lala S, Reynolds L, *et al*. Preliminary efficacy, safety, tolerability, and pharmacokinetics of short course regimens of nucleoside analogues for the prevention

of mother-to-child transmission (MTCT) of HIV. XIII International AIDS Conference, 9–14 July 2000, Durban, South Africa. Abstract TuOrB3552000.

52. Mirochnick M, Fenton T, Gagnier P, Pav J, Gwynne M, Siminski S, et al. Pharmacokinetics of nevirapine in human immunodeficiency virus type 1-infected pregnant women and their neonates. Pediatric AIDS Clinical Trials Group Protocol 250 Team. *J Infect Dis* 1998;**178**:368–74.

53. Merluzzi VJ, Hargrave KD, Labadia M, Grozinger K, Skoog M, Wu JC, et al. Inhibition of HIV-1 replication by a nonnucleoside reverse transcriptase inhibitor. *Science* 1990;**250**:1411–3.

54. Havlir D, Cheeseman SH, McLaughlin M, Murphy R, Erice A, Spector SA, et al. High-dose nevirapine: safety, pharmacokinetics, and antiviral effect in patients with human immunodeficiency virus infection. *J Infect Dis* 1995;**171**:537–45.

55. De Cock KM, Fowler MG, Mercier E, de Vincenzi I, Saba J, Hoff E, et al. Prevention of mother-to-child HIV transmission in resource-poor countries: translating research into policy and practice. *JAMA* 2000;**283**:1175–82.

56. Musoke P, Guay LA, Bagenda D, Mirochnick M, Nakabiito C, Fleming T, et al. A phase I/II study of the safety and pharmacokinetics of nevirapine in HIV-1-infected pregnant Ugandan women and their neonates (HIVNET 006). *AIDS* 1999;**13**:479–86.

57. Guay LA, Musoke P, Fleming T, Bagenda D, Allen M, Nakabiito C, et al. Intrapartum and neonatal single-dose nevirapine compared with zidovudine for prevention of mother-to-child transmission of HIV-1 in Kampala, Uganda: HIVNET 012 randomised trial. *Lancet* 1999;**354**:795–802.

58. Owor M, Deseyve M, Duefield C, Musisi M, Fleming T, Musoke P, et al. The one year safety and efficacy data of the HIVNET 012 trial. XIII International AIDS Conference, 9–14 July 2000, Durban, South Africa. Abstract LbOr01.

59. Moodley D, SAINT Study Team. Evaluation of efficacy of two simple regimens for the prevention of mother to child transmission (MTCT) of HIV infection: nevirapine vs lamivudine and zidovudine used in a randomised clinical trial (the SAINT study). XIII International AIDS Conference, 9–14 July 2000, Durban, South Africa. Abstract LbOr022000.

60. McIntyre J, SAINT Study Team. Evaluation of safety of two simple regimens for the prevention of mother to child transmission (MTCT) of HIV infection: nevirapine vs lamivudine and zidovudine used in a randomised clinical trial (the SAINT study). XIII International AIDS Conference, 9–14 July 2000, Durban, South Africa. Abstract TuOrB3562000.

61. Becker-Pergola G, Guay L, Mmiro F, Musoke P, Fung S, Jackson J, et al. Selection of the K103N nevirapine resistance mutation in Ugandan women receiving NVP prophylaxis to prevent HIV-1 vertical transmission (HIVNET-006). 7th Conference on Retroviruses and Opportunistic Infections, 30 January – 2 February 2000, San Francisco, USA.

62. Jackson JB, Mracna M, Guay L, Dileanis JA, Musoke P, Mmiro F, et al. Selection of nevirapine (NVP) resistance mutations in Ugandan women and infants receiving NVP prophylaxis to prevent HIV-1 vertical transmission (HIVNET 012). XIII International AIDS Conference, 9–14 July 2000, Durban, South Africa. Abstract LbOr0132000.

63. Elective caesarean-section versus vaginal delivery in prevention of vertical HIV-1 transmission: a randomised clinical trial. The European Mode of Delivery Collaboration. *Lancet* 1999;**353**:1035–9.

64. The mode of delivery and the risk of vertical transmission of human immunodeficiency virus type 1 – a meta-analysis of 15 prospective cohort studies. The International Perinatal HIV Group. *N Engl J Med* 1999;**340**:977–87.

65. Mofenson LM, McIntyre JA. Advances and research directions in the prevention of mother-to-child HIV-1 transmission. *Lancet* 2000;**355**:2237–44.

66. Miotti PG, Taha TE, Kumwenda NI, Broadhead R, Mtimavalye LA, Van der Hoeven L, et al. HIV transmission through breastfeeding: a study in Malawi. *JAMA* 1999;**282**:744–9.

67. Leroy V, Newell ML, Dabis F, Peckham C, Van de Perre P, Bulterys M, et al. International multicentre pooled analysis of late postnatal mother-to-child transmission of HIV-1 infection. Ghent International Working Group on Mother-to-Child Transmission of HIV. *Lancet* 1998;**352**:597–600.

68. Tess BH, Rodrigues LC, Newell ML, Dunn DT, Lago TD. Infant feeding and risk of mother-to-child transmission of HIV-1 in Sao Paulo State, Brazil. Sao Paulo Collaborative Study for Vertical Transmission of HIV-1. *J Acquir Immune Defic Syndr Hum Retrovirol* 1998;**19**:189–94.

69. Coutsoudis A, Pillay K, Spooner E, Kuhn L, Coovadia HM. Influence of infant-feeding patterns on early mother-to-child transmission of HIV-1 in Durban, South Africa: a prospective cohort study. South African Vitamin A Study Group. *Lancet* 1999;**354**:471–6.

70. US Public Health Service. US Public Health Service Task Force Recommendations for the Use of Anti-retroviral Drugs in Pregnant Women Infected with HIV-1 for Maternal Health and for Reducing Perinatal HIV-1 Transmission in the United States. 25 February 2000. Available on The HIV/AIDS Treatment Information Service web site at www.hivatis.org.

Chapter 23

Hepatitis C virus and pregnancy

Peter Simmonds

Epidemiology of hepatitis C virus in pregnancy

Hepatitis C virus (HCV) infection is detected in between 1% and 2% of pregnant women,[1] of whom the majority will be persistently infected and potentially a source of infection for their children. In Western Europe, Australia and North America, most HCV-infected individuals have a history of percutaneous exposure to the virus, and the majority are (or have been) intravenous drug users. The seroconversion rate of intravenous drug users has been estimated at 20% per year and thus long-term drug users are almost invariably HCV-infected. Drug use was uncommon before the 1960s and so those infected by this route are more likely to be younger than patients infected through transfusion and are also more likely to be infected with genotypes other than type 1b. Past drug use is therefore the most common source of infection in women during pregnancy. Most HCV-positive women who are pregnant are therefore in early stages of infection, which is typically asymptomatic. Most will have underlying chronic hepatitis and a small proportion will have developed cirrhosis.

Other risk factors for HCV infection are less common in antenatal groups. Parenteral routes of HCV infection include exposure to non-virally inactivated blood products (as in the well-known outbreak among recipients of anti-D immunoglobulin in Ireland in 1977[2]), haemodialysis and past needle-stick injuries in healthcare workers. Tattooing and acupuncture may also be responsible for some percutaneous exposure and, in countries of high prevalence, the use of unsterilised needles for cultural rituals, medical treatment or vaccination programmes may result in HCV infection.

For many women infected with HCV, previous parenteral exposure cannot be identified. However, there appears to be only a low risk of infection associated with sexual contact with an HCV carrier. HIV/HCV co-infection may increase the risk for sexual transmission of HCV. This is probably secondary to the increased viral load associated with immunosuppression. In this setting, barrier methods of protection are clearly appropriate.

HCV disease outcome in pregnancy

Until recently, there was no evidence that pregnancy influences the course of chronic HCV infection. Indeed, at the 1999 EASL International Consensus Conference on Hepatitis C, it was recommended that women should be counselled that pregnancy is unlikely to influence the severity of liver disease or long-term prognosis.[3] However, a case–control study[4] published in 2000 demonstrated a significant worsening of liver biopsy appearance, particularly the necroinflammatory score between biopsies collected over a period in which the subjects had been pregnant. The authors suggested that the postpartum immune rebound may exacerbate liver deterioration through an immunopathologic mechanism. In those with advanced liver disease, there are the additional complications of coagulopathies and thrombocytopenia in pregnancy associated with significant hepatic dysfunction. Portal hypertension may also predispose towards oesophageal haemorrhage. There is no evidence that HCV alters the course of pregnancy or increases the risk of congenital abnormalities, spontaneous abortion or prematurity. This is consistent with the evidence that mother-to-child transmission occurs in the perinatal period rather than *in utero*.

Currently available treatment for HCV infection comprises α- or lymphoblastoid interferon, usually in combination with ribavirin.[5,6] Frequencies of response range from 30% to 70% for the HCV genotypes likely to be found in antenatal groups (types 1 and 3a). Viral clearance or reduction in viral load may reduce the likelihood of mother-to-child transmission. However, both interferon and ribavirin are known to affect fetal development adversely and are contraindicated in pregnancy. The use of antiviral treatment as a method for preventing transmission (as has proven so effective for HIV-1) therefore awaits the development of new antiviral agents.

Mother-to-child transmission of HCV

Early studies documented a low but detectable rate (5–15%) of mother-to-child transmission of HCV[7-9] and these estimates have since been confirmed in larger studies in many different centres.[1,10] HCV RNA viral load in the mother during pregnancy increases the risk of mother-to-child transmission,[1,11-13] and most (although not all) reports also describe an increased frequency of transmission in women co-infected with HIV-1.[8,12,14,15] The association with HIV is generally considered to result from the greater circulating viral load in HIV-seropositive individuals.

Diagnosis of HCV transmission is generally made by polymerase chain reaction (PCR) for HCV RNA sequences in plasma. Maternal antibody to HCV can be detected in all samples from neonates collected around the time of birth; it subsequently declines in titre in those who are HCV uninfected, with most children being negative by one year.[10] Although it is likely that titration of antibody to HCV may provide earlier evidence for HCV infection in the infant, PCR testing at three months provides the earliest and most conclusive evidence of both infection and lack of infection.[10] Transmission of HCV is now recognised to occur predominantly or exclusively in the perinatal period and thus PCR assay of infant samples collected at birth are unhelpful in diagnosis, particularly as there is a likelihood of contamination with maternal blood in some samples. An algorithm describing the samples and tests required for accurate determination of infant HCV status has been prepared by the Public Health Laboratory Service (PHLS) Hepatitis and Blood-borne Virus Advisory Committee and distributed to PHLS laboratories in England and Wales. A draft of the provisional recommendations resulting from this exercise is provided in Figure 23.1. More effective identification of women with HCV infection during pregnancy, more standardised diagnostic testing and the active follow-up of children of HCV-infected women will provide much more accurate data on the risk factors for transmission and the natural history of HCV infection in children. Several prospective studies are underway in the UK and elsewhere.[10]

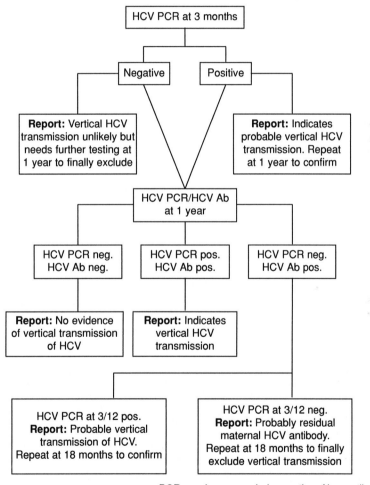

PCR = polymerase chain reaction; Ab = antibody

Fig. 23.1. Algorithm for diagnosis of hepatitis C virus (HCV) infection in infants (*to be finalised by the Public Health Laboratory Service*)

Assisted conception

At present, there is no agreed advice in the UK concerning assisted reproduction techniques for infertile couples in which one partner is infected with HCV. As described above, transmission of HCV by sexual contact is rare and inefficient. In contrast to HIV-1, only low levels of HCV RNA have been found in semen[16-18] and there is no evidence so far that transmission has been documented after intrauterine insemination attempts[19] or after *in vitro* fertilisation. Some authors have investigated the possibility of processing sperm to remove potentially infective HCV virions present in seminal plasma.[17,18] For example, in a study[18] published in 2000, cells isolated by Percoll selection were invariably negative, in contrast to a frequency of detection of HCV RNA of 5% in unprocessed sperm samples.

Prevention of mother-to-child transmission

The potential teratogenicity of currently available antiviral treatments for HCV infection (interferon and ribavirin) have prevented the use of these agents in pregnancy. Considerable efforts are underway to develop methods for therapeutic immunisation that may be safe in pregnancy (e.g. the stimulation of the immune response in chronically infected carriers of HCV to induce virus clearance[20]). Planned therapies include immunisation with DNA vaccines expressing cytotoxic T cell-reactive epitopes, and the *ex vivo* stimulation of cytotoxic T cells by peptide antigens and their reintroduction into the patient. It is hoped that stimulating immune responses may assist in the clearance of persistent infection either alone or in combination with other antiviral therapies. However, the availability of therapeutic immunisation to prevent mother-to-child transmission remains only a future possibility at present.

Attempts to produce vaccines that prevent primary infection are also at an early stage. There is currently no equivalent of the recombinant hepatitis B virus (HBV) surface antigen vaccine that has proved so effective at preventing perinatal transmission of HBV. Problems with the development of a protective vaccine include the great genetic variability of HCV[21] and the likelihood that a multivalent vaccine will be required to protect from variants of HCV that may be quite antigenically distinct from each other (as is the case for poliovirus vaccines). Furthermore, in chimpanzees, which are the only animal model currently available for vaccine development, the immune response provoked by repeated immunisation with recombinant envelope proteins of HCV is so poor that it fails to prevent infection from challenge with the homologous virus strain.

In the absence of maternal treatment to reduce viral load, or effective vaccination for neonates, interest has been centred on obstetric variables that may increase the likelihood of transmission. In particular, there are many possible interventions that reduce or prevent exposure of the fetus to maternal blood, such as avoidance of invasive procedures (e.g. chorionic villus biopsy that damages the integrity of the placental membrane) and fetal blood sampling. Interventions may also be effective at the time of birth, such as the avoidance of the use of scalp electrodes. However, the effectiveness of these measures has not been demonstrated.

An effective preventive measure for HIV-1 transmission that reduces blood contact during delivery is elective caesarean section, before rupture of membranes.[22,23] However, there is at present little conclusive evidence that caesarean section also reduces the frequency of HCV transmission,[12] although it is unclear in many studies whether procedures were elective or emergency. However, in 2000, Gibb *et al.*[10] reported an absence of HCV transmission in 31 women who had undergone elective caesarean delivery without rupture of membranes, which was significantly different from the 6–7% frequency of transmission observed in those with normal vaginal delivery or emergency caesarean delivery. This finding is consistent with a previous report describing an association between HCV transmission and length of time between rupture of membranes and delivery.[24] In view of the potential importance of elective caesarean section in preventing mother-to-child transmission of HCV, these conclusions require to be backed up by greater numbers, and results from other centres.

Finally, there has been considerable uncertainty about the advice to be given to mothers on the safety of breastfeeding, particularly as it has been identified as an important risk factor for the transmission of HIV-1. Although there have been sporadic reports of the detection of HCV RNA in breast milk from HCV-infected mothers,[25-27] levels are undetectable in the great majority of individuals.[24,28,29] Furthermore, apart from one study that attempted to show a correlation between detection of HCV RNA in breast milk and transmission,[27] no other evidence that links breastfeeding with an increased frequency of infant infection has been obtained.[10,24,29,30]

Summary

HCV transmission from mother to child occurs in approximately one in 20 births. Prevention of transmission is problematic in the absence of suitable antivirals (during pregnancy) or vaccines. HCV infection is transmitted at birth and detection of infant infection becomes reliable only after three months. The outcome of HCV infection in children is currently uncertain, although it is likely that a proportion will progress to severe liver disease.

References

1. Thomas SL, Newell ML, Peckham CS, Ades AE, Hall AJ. A review of hepatitis C virus (HCV) vertical transmission: risks of transmission to infants born to mothers with and without HCV viraemia or human immunodeficiency virus infection. *Int J Epidemiol* 1998;**27**:108–17.

2. Power JP, Lawlor E, Davidson F, Holmes EC, Yap PL, Simmonds P. Molecular epidemiology of an outbreak of infection with hepatitis C virus in recipients of anti-D immunoglobulin. *Lancet* 1995;**345**:1211–13.

3. European Association for the Study of the Liver. EASL International Consensus Conference on Hepatitis C. Paris, 26–28 February 1999, Consensus Statement. *J Hepatol* 1999;**30**:956–61.

4. Fontaine H, Nalpas B, Carnot F, Brechot C, Pol S. Effect of pregnancy on chronic hepatitis C: a case–control study. *Lancet* 2000;**356**:1328–9.

5. Braconier JH, Paulsen O, Engman K, Widell A. Combined alpha-interferon and ribavirin treatment in chronic hepatitis C: a pilot study. *Scand J Infect Dis* 1995;**27**:325–9.

6. Chemello L, Cavalletto L, Bernardinello E, Guido M, Pontisso P, Alberti A. The effect of interferon alfa and ribavirin combination therapy in naive patients with chronic hepatitis C. *J Hepatol* 1995;**23**:8–12.

7. Novati R, Thiers V, Monforte AD, Maisonneuve P, Principi N, Conti M, *et al.* Mother-to-child transmission of hepatitis C virus detected by nested polymerase chain reaction. *J Infect Dis* 1992;**165**:720–3.
8. Lam JPH, McOmish F, Burns SM, Yap PL, Mok JYQ, Simmonds P. Infrequent vertical transmission of hepatitis C virus. *J Infect Dis* 1993;**167**:572–6.
9. Wejstal R, Widell A, Mansson AS, Hermodsson S, Norkrans G. Mother-to-infant transmission of hepatitis C virus. *Ann Intern Med* 1992;**117**:887–90.
10. Gibb DM, Goodall RL, Dunn DT, Healy M, Neave P, Cafferkey M, *et al.* Mother-to-child transmission of hepatitis C virus: evidence for preventable peripartum transmission. *Lancet* 2000;**356**:904–7.
11. Ohto H, Terazawa S, Sasaki N, Hino K, Ishiwata C, Kako M, *et al.* Transmission of hepatitis C virus from mothers to infants. *N Engl J Med* 1994;**330**:744–50.
12. Zanetti AR, Tanzi E, Newell ML. Mother-to-infant transmission of hepatitis C virus. *J Hepatol* 1999;**31** Suppl 1:96–100.
13. Thomas DL, Villano SA, Riester KA, Hershow R, Mofenson LM, Landesman SH, *et al.* Perinatal transmission of hepatitis C virus from human immunodeficiency virus type 1-infected mothers. *J Infect Dis* 1998;**177**:1480–8.
14. Zanetti AR, Tanzi E, Romano L, Zuin G, Minola E, Vecchi L, *et al.* A prospective study on mother-to-infant transmission of hepatitis C virus. *Intervirology* 1998;**41**:208–12.
15. Manzini P, Saracco G, Cerchier A, Riva C, Musso A, Ricotti E, *et al.* Human immunodeficiency virus infection as risk factor for mother-to-child hepatitis C virus transmission; persistence of anti-hepatitis C virus in children is associated with the mother's anti-hepatitis C virus immunoblotting pattern. *Hepatology* 1995;**21**:328–32.
16. Debono E, Halfon P, Bourliere M, Gerolami-Santandrea V, Gastaldi M, Castellani P, *et al.* Absence of hepatitis C genome in semen of infected men by polymerase chain reaction, branched DNA and *in situ* hybridization. *Liver* 2000;**20**:257–61.
17. McKee TA, Avery S, Majid A, Brinsden PR. Risks for transmission of hepatitis C virus during artificial insemination. *Fertil Steril* 1996;**66**:161–3.
18. Levy R, Tardy JC, Bourlet T, Cordonier H, Mion F, Lornage J, *et al.* Transmission risk of hepatitis C virus in assisted reproductive techniques. *Hum Reprod* 2000;**15**:810–16.
19. Semprini AE, Persico T, Thiers V, Oneta M, Tuveri R, Serafini P, *et al.* Absence of hepatitis C virus and detection of hepatitis G virus/GB virus C RNA sequences in the semen of infected men. *J Infect Dis* 1998;**177**:848–54.
20. Houghton M. Strategies and prospects for vaccination against the hepatitis C viruses. *Curr Top Microbiol Immunol* 2000;**242**:327–39.
21. Simmonds P, Holmes EC, Cha TA, Chan S-W, McOmish F, Irvine B, *et al.* Classification of hepatitis C virus into six major genotypes and a series of subtypes by phylogenetic analysis of the NS-5 region. *J Gen Virol* 1993;**74**:2391–9.
22. The European Mode of Delivery Collaboration. Elective caesarean-section versus vaginal delivery in prevention of vertical HIV-1 transmission: a randomised clinical trial. *Lancet* 1999;**353**:1035–9.
23. The International Perinatal HIV Group. The mode of delivery and the risk of vertical transmission of human immunodeficiency virus type 1 – a meta-analysis of 15 prospective cohort studies. *N Engl J Med* 1999;**340**:977–87.
24. Spencer JD, Latt N, Beeby PJ, Collins E, Saunders JB, McCaughan GW, *et al.* Transmission of hepatitis C virus to infants of human immunodeficiency virus-negative intravenous drug-using mothers: rate of infection and assessment of risk factors for transmission. *J Viral Hepat* 1997;**4**:395–409.
25. Ogasawara S, Kage M, Kosai K, Shimamatsu K, Kojiro M. Hepatitis C virus RNA in saliva and breastmilk of hepatitis C carrier mothers. *Lancet* 1993;**341**:561.
26. Zimmermann R, Perucchini D, Fauchere JC, Joller Jemelka H, Geyer M, Huch R, *et al.* Hepatitis C virus in breast milk. *Lancet* 1995;**345**:928.
27. Ruiz-Extremera A, Salmeron J, Torres C, De Rueda PM, Gimenez F, Robles C, *et al.* Follow-up of transmission of hepatitis C to babies of human immunodeficiency virus-negative women: the role of breast-feeding in transmission. *Pediatr Infect Dis J* 2000;**19**:511–16.
28. Kage M, Ogasawara S, Kosai KI, Nakashima E, Shimamatsu K, Kojiro M, *et al.* Hepatitis C virus RNA present in saliva but absent in breast-milk of the hepatitis C carrier mother. *J Gastroenterol Hepatol* 1997;**12**:518–21.
29. Polywka S, Schroter M, Feucht HH, Zollner B, Laufs R. Low risk of vertical transmission of hepatitis C virus by breast milk. *Clin Infect Dis* 1999;**29**:1327–9.
30. Kumar RM, Shahul S. Role of breast-feeding in transmission of hepatitis C virus to infants of HCV-infected mothers. *J Hepatol* 1998;**29**:191–7.

Chapter 24

Parvovirus B19 infection in pregnancy

Sherif A Abdel-Fattah and Peter W Soothill

Introduction

Parvovirus B19 is a recently discovered virus that is known to be the cause of erythema infectiosum, or fifth disease, which commonly affects primary-school children. The organism is also responsible for arthralgias in adults. The virus is of interest to obstetricians and gynaecologists because infected mothers can transmit the organism to the fetus, causing non-immune fetal hydrops and death.

Virology

Parvoviruses are small (20–25 nm) single-stranded DNA viruses that require rapidly dividing cells for replication. They are non-enveloped and structurally simple, being able to code from only a few proteins. Parvovirus B19 is a member of the genus *Parvovirus* in family Parvoviridae and it is the only strain of that family that is pathogenic to humans. The mammalian parvoviruses are highly species-specific. The B19 strain does not infect other animals, and strains of parvovirus that infect animals do not infect humans. Thus, replication of parvovirus B19 has been demonstrated only in human progenitor cells.[1]

The virus binds to an antigen of the P system blood group known as P antigen or globoside. The P blood group consists of two common antigens, P_1 and P, and a third rarer P^k antigen. The P antigen is present not only on the surface of erythrocytes and erythroblasts but also on megakaryocytes, endothelial cells, placental cells, and fetal liver and heart cells.[2] The few individuals who lack the P antigen on red cells and erythrocyte precursors are resistant to infection by parvovirus B19. A study published in 1994 found no serological evidence of previous parvovirus infection in 17 individuals without the P antigen, compared with 47–71% in controls.[3]

Epidemiology

Human parvovirus B19 was first discovered in 1975 in sera from healthy blood donors during screening of blood units for hepatitis B surface antigen.[4] The route of transmission is mainly through respiratory droplets and epidemics typically occur on three- to five-year cycles. Outbreaks tend to occur during the spring, although they may develop at any time of the year and isolated infections are not uncommon. The risk of becoming infected may be occupation-related, with individuals working in school catering, daycare centres, and school teachers having the highest infection rates.[5]

Following the initial infection, immunoglobulin M (IgM) antibodies appear three to four days after the onset of the clinical illness and persist in the blood for three to four months. Immunoglobulin G (IgG) antibodies appear 7–14 days following the clinical symptoms and persist for years.[6,7] The immunoglobulin pattern of previous infection by parvovirus B19 (IgG-positive, IgM-negative) confers immunity and has not been reported to be associated with adverse perinatal outcome. About 50% of women of childbearing age have serological evidence of past exposure and, therefore, immunity to parvovirus B19. Several studies in different countries have demonstrated IgG seropositivity ranging between 40% and 81%.[8-11] Consequently, about 50% of adults are susceptible to infection. The overall risk of infection in the general population for these susceptible seronegative individuals is about 1%, although the risk can be as high as 13.5% during epidemics.[11] The risk of infection in susceptible people following household exposure to a B19-infected person is about 50%, while the risk following school exposures during outbreaks is 20–30%.[5,11,12]

Clinical manifestations

The most common clinical presentation of infection by parvovirus B19 is erythema infectiosum, which is a relatively mild influenza-like disease accompanied by a maculopapular rash and low-grade fever. The condition is most common in primary-school children and is characterised by diffuse erythema of the cheeks, hence the name 'slapped-cheek disease'. The incubation period is 4–20 days. Viraemia occurs 6–8 days after exposure and persists for 4–7 days, during which time the person is infective. The rash appears 16 days after the initial exposure, or 8 days after the viraemia. The patient is no longer infectious when the rash appears. The erythematous macular rash typically develops on the chin and cheeks and then spreads to the trunk and limbs. It persists for about 10 days then fades.[1,6] In adults, the most common symptom is symmetric arthralgia, typically involving the proximal interphalangeal joints and the knees, and may last for several weeks. However, infection in adults is usually asymptomatic in spite of serological evidence of recent infection. Alternatively, patients may recall only flu-like symptoms, with sore throat and mild fever.[13,14]

Parvovirus B19 replicates in the upper respiratory tract but it also has a special affinity for the erythroid system, as it replicates in the erythroid precursor cells in the bone marrow, causing red blood cell hypoplasia. The haematological features are self-limiting, clinically inapparent and last for 7–10 days. Renewed production of reticulocytes then gradually begins and the bone marrow usually recovers fully within the following two to three weeks. The virus may occasionally hit all cell lines, causing pancytopenia.[15] The resulting anaemia is only of minor clinical significance in children or healthy adults but it can cause severe aplastic-anaemia crisis in patients with sickle-cell disease and other haemolytic anaemias where erythrocyte turnover is rapid, such as hereditary spherocytosis, thalassaemia or chronic haemolytic anaemia.[16–18] The viral infection can also cause severe chronic anaemia in immunocompromised patients, such as those with HIV or who have undergone organ transplantation.[19]

Fetal infection

Transplacental transmission of infection

Parvovirus B19 was identified as a fetal pathogen in 1984, when two separate reports described cases of hydrops fetalis associated with confirmed congenital infections.[20,21] Several cases have been reported since. Earlier studies suggested high rates (65–75%) of fetal transmission following maternal infection.[22] This was proved to be inaccurate when a large study[23] of 190 women demonstrated that the majority (84%) of serologically proven infected pregnant women will go to term and deliver normal healthy babies. The rate of transplacental transmission was 33% and the risk of fetal loss was 9%.[23] Other prospective studies with more accurate diagnostic tools, such as polymerase chain reaction (PCR), have reported fetal loss rates as low as 3.4%.[8,24] It appears that the risk of fetal death is much higher when infection occurs before 20 weeks of gestation.[23,25] Fetal death can still occur with infection in later gestation, although less frequently.[26] It is important to note, however, that the true rates of fetal infection and risks of death are difficult to assess precisely in view of the high percentage of asymptomatic maternal infections.

Fetal hydrops

Hydrops is the most common presentation for fetuses with congenital parvovirus infection. Hydrops usually develops three to eight weeks after maternal infection, although it has been reported as late as 12 weeks following the initial infection and was even described to appear after 18 weeks in one report.[25] The affected fetus may show a combination of the ultrasonographic signs of hydrops such as ascites, subcutaneous oedema, pleural effusion, pericardial effusion, scalp oedema and polyhydramnios (Figure 24.1). The main mechanism of hydropic development is severe anaemia due to the infection and lysis of erythroid progenitor cells in the liver and bone marrow. Anaemia leads to excessive, compensatory extrahepatic erythropoiesis and further hepatic erythropoiesis, which may result in portal hypertension and hypoproteinaemia with consequent ascites. However, there are reports of hydrops developing in cases with relatively mild fetal anaemia, suggesting that other mechanisms may also be involved.[1] Viral myocarditis with subsequent heart failure is one possible mechanism, particularly since viral infection of fetal myocardial cells has been reported in postmortem examinations.[27,28]

It is estimated that fetal parvovirus B19 infection is currently responsible for 8–10% of cases of non-immune hydrops fetalis. The risk of developing hydrops is highest when maternal infection occurs between 12 and 18 weeks of gestation.[23,25] This may be

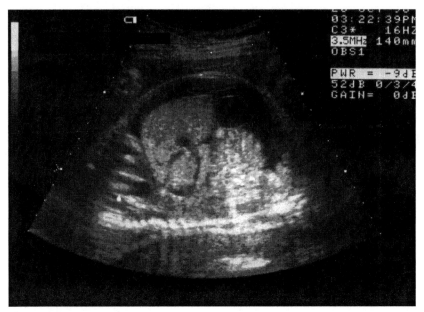

Fig. 24.1.   Ultrasonography of fetal ascites

secondary to the rapidly increasing red cell mass and the short half-life of the fetal red cells. One study[29] suggested that the risk of fetal hydrops and death may be greater in women with asymptomatic infections but this was not the case in other studies.[25] Fetal deaths in the third trimester due to proven parvovirus infections have been described, although without hydropic development. A Swedish study, published in 2000, examined placental and fetal tissues from 93 cases of intrauterine fetal deaths in the third trimester over a seven-year period for evidence of parvovirus infection using PCR techniques. The authors found B19 DNA in seven (7.5%) of these cases and none with hydrops. As there were no other possible explanations for these fetal deaths, it was concluded that parvovirus B19 infection was the most likely cause in these cases.[26]

There are also reports of hydrops fetalis due to congenital parvovirus infection developing in the first trimester of pregnancy.[30,31] Fetal anaemia at that early stage is unusual because bone marrow erythroid precursors are not sufficiently functional before 16 weeks of gestation, and the liver is the primary site for haematopoiesis. It is suggested that fetal hydrops, in some of these cases, may be due to heart failure secondary to myocarditis, rather than due to anaemia.[31]

Congenital malformation

Parvovirus B19 is unlikely to be associated with congenital malformations in humans, although other parvoviruses are known to cause characteristic congenital anomalies in animals, such as cerebellar agenesis, microcephaly and heart defects. Only a few cases of congenital anomalies in parvovirus-infected human fetuses have been reported in the literature. The anomalies described included eye abnormalities,[32] facial and limb anomalies[33] and hydrocephalus.[34] However, the association between these anomalies and the viral infection was not proven and no similar anomalies were identified in any of the other larger series of investigations into parvovirus infection in pregnancy that followed.[35,36]

Diagnosis

Serological and immunological tests

Unlike most viruses, human parvovirus B19 cannot be cultured in traditional tissue culture cell lines, although replication in erythroid precursor cell lines has been successful. Parvovirus culture is therefore impractical in the diagnostic setting. In addition, testing for specific IgM antibodies in the fetus is not reliable because antibodies usually appear in the fetal circulation in detectable amounts only after 22 weeks of gestation. The low detection rate of fetal IgM in earlier gestations is probably due to the immature immune system of the fetus. In several reports, fetal antibody tests were negative despite proven active fetal infection both clinically and by other diagnostic tests.[35,36]

More reliable tests include detection of B19 DNA in maternal or fetal serum or tissues by dot-blot analysis or *in situ* hybridisation.[37,38] The virus can also be identified by the characteristic intranuclear inclusions demonstrated on histological samples or by direct visualisation of viral particles in infected tissues or serum using electron microscopy. More recently, viral DNA amplification using PCR in maternal and fetal serum or tissues and in the placenta has proved to be the most sensitive and accurate diagnostic test.[39–41] One study concluded that while virological and serological tests are complementary for maternal investigation, the detection of B19 DNA in the fetal blood is the most useful diagnostic test.[35]

Fetal haematology

As already discussed, the main effect of parvovirus infection is fetal anaemia. The most common presentation of such fetuses is by non-immune hydrops diagnosed on ultrasound scan, with or without a history of maternal exposure to parvovirus. Therefore, fetal blood sampling by cordocentesis should be undertaken and the typical findings are of severe fetal anaemia often associated with thrombocytopenia, negative Coombs test and low reticulocyte count. Parvovirus particles can be seen by electron microscopy in fetal blood. In addition, B19 DNA testing by PCR is invariably positive and fetal parvovirus-specific IgM might be detected. Bilirubin levels are normal, as the fetal anaemia is not due to antibody-mediated haemolysis. The liver enzymes might be elevated, reflecting hepatic dysfunction due to direct liver affection by the virus.[42,43]

Maternal serum alpha-fetoprotein

In the 1980s, some studies observed an elevation in maternal serum alpha-fetoprotein (α-FP) in women infected by parvovirus B19. This elevation is probably due to infection of the fetal liver or the placenta, which are the major sources of α-FP in pregnancy. This elevation of α-FP was noted to occur as early as four weeks prior to the development of fetal hydrops. It was then suggested that maternal serum α-FP can serve as a diagnostic and prognostic tool to monitor the fetal infection.[44,45] More recent reports, however, described cases where the maternal serum α-FP was normal despite severe fetal infection.[46] This test is clearly too non-specific to be of any real value in the management of parvovirus-infected pregnancies, particularly with the current level of understanding of the pathophysiology of congenital fetal B19 infection and with the recent advances in diagnostic techniques.

Management

Women with suspected parvovirus infection during pregnancy present either following contact with a known infected case, or with an unexpected diagnosis of fetal hydrops during a routine ultrasound scan. The management protocol will obviously depend on the presentation.

Patients presenting following contact with an infected case

A detailed history of the timing of contact and any maternal symptoms suggestive of recent parvovirus infection should be taken. Some women might describe flu-like symptoms but this is not always the case. The next step will be maternal serological testing for parvovirus B19 antibodies. If the mother is IgG-positive and IgM-negative, this indicates past infection and confers immunity and the woman can then be reassured. If neither antibody is detected, the mother is susceptible to infection. There is unfortunately no vaccine currently available against the virus and susceptible women are advised to avoid contact with known or suspected cases. Further testing can be undertaken three to four weeks later for evidence of seroconversion. The presence of maternal IgM antibodies with or without IgG will indicate recent infection and the possibility of fetal infection.[1]

A detailed ultrasound examination of the fetus should be undertaken, looking for fetal hydrops or other signs suggestive of fetal anaemia. Fetal hydrops indicates severe fetal anaemia.[47] In recent years, several non-invasive methods for the prediction of earlier stages of fetal anaemia have been assessed, with a view to initiating treatment for fetuses at risk before the anaemia becomes too severe. In particular, the fetal middle cerebral artery bloodflow velocity Doppler studies seem to be encouraging in this respect. The concept that Doppler bloodflow velocity evaluation is useful to identify anaemic fetuses is mainly based on, firstly, the assumption of decreased blood viscosity due to the decreased fetal red blood cell count and, secondly, the increased cardiac output due to the hyperdynamic circulation normally associated with anaemia. Both factors are expected to result in an increase in the peak blood velocity measurable by Doppler.[48,49] The studies demonstrating good predictive values for the increased fetal middle cerebral artery bloodflow velocity for the prediction of fetal anaemia have been undertaken in cases of rhesus alloimmunisation.[49-51] The pathophysiology of anaemia in these cases (haemolysis) is different from that in cases of parvovirus (destruction of erythroid progenitor cells) but the effects of anaemia on blood viscosity and cardiac output should be the same. Therefore, Doppler blood velocity studies are almost certainly equally useful for detection of fetal anaemia in cases of fetal parvovirus infection, although this has never been specifically studied.

The first sign of fetal hydrops due to anaemia is typically the development of fetal ascites[52] but some cases of B19-related fetal hydrops present with pleural or pericardial effusions without ascites. This is particularly noted in severely affected fetuses in the first trimester (Figure 24.2). The cause of fetal hydrops in these cases is probably heart failure secondary to severe viral myocarditis, rather than fetal anaemia.[31] In cases with no hydrops or other signs suggestive of fetal anaemia, follow-up is necessary for the development of these signs. Fetal hydrops usually develops within three to eight weeks following the initial maternal infection although this may take up to 12 weeks. Therefore, these patients should have weekly ultrasound scans for at least 12 weeks following the maternal infection.[53]

Patients presenting with fetal hydrops

These cases should be managed at a specialised fetal medicine unit where protocols for management of fetal hydrops exist. These will include serological maternal investigations for possible causes of hydrops, including parvovirus B19 antibodies. However, the results of these tests and other tests for causes of hydrops will not be available for a few days and delaying treatment might result in fetal loss. It is therefore advisable to initiate treatment without awaiting confirmation of the cause of hydrops. Fetal blood sampling should be performed with blood ready for intravascular fetal transfusion if anaemia is confirmed.

Several reports have described intravascular transfusion for treatment of parvovirus-related fetal anaemia with a fetal survival rate of more than 80%.[42,43,54-56] As in the case of anaemia due to rhesus alloimmunisation, more than one transfusion will usually be

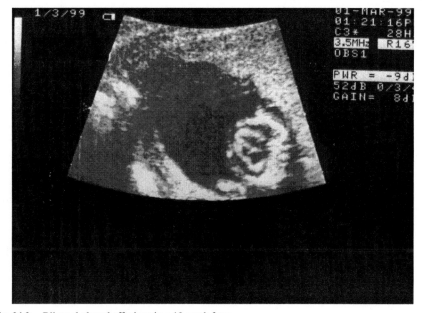

Fig. 24.2.   Bilateral pleural effusions in a 13-week fetus

required for the complete correction of fetal anaemia. If the reticulocyte count in the fetal blood is relatively normal, this might signify that the fetal erythropoiesis is in the recovery stage. In this case, further transfusions might not be necessary but careful monitoring for resolution of hydrops should still be undertaken.[53] One report noted a longer duration of bleeding from the puncture site in the umbilical cord following a transfusion in a case of parvovirus as compared with several transfusions in rhesus cases.[42] This might be explained by the associated thrombocytopenia and the authors recommended having platelets ready for transfusion, together with the blood, in these cases. However, this was reported in only one case and it has not been shown to be a significant problem in other reports. Platelet transfusion therefore does not need to be a part of the routine procedure.

Conservative management of fetal hydrops

There have been some reports of spontaneous resolution of fetal hydrops in cases of congenital parvovirus infection. The severity of hydrops varied from severe forms with ascites, pleural and pericardial effusions, bilateral hydroceles and abdominal wall oedema in some fetuses[57,58] to only moderate ascites in others.[59] This was also described in the first trimester in three cases.[60] Hydrops demonstrated spontaneous gradual improvement within days and resolved completely in all three cases within a few weeks of the original diagnosis. Such reports have led to a policy of conservative management of fetal hydrops in some cases. Advocates of this policy explain that the pathophysiology and natural history of congenital parvovirus infection are not fully understood and that the infection of the erythroid precursor cells is self-limiting with spontaneous recovery of fetal red cell production.[58,61] It was also speculated that fetuses treated by intravascular transfusions might have improved spontaneously if no intervention had been undertaken.

Interestingly, the haemoglobin level of all reported conservatively managed fetuses whose blood was sampled by cordocentesis was either normal or showed only mild anaemia. This is contrary to normal expectations in hydrops related to anaemia, when the haemoglobin is expected to be at least six standard deviations below the normal mean for gestational age.[47] It was speculated that at the time of diagnosis and cordocentesis the fetuses were already in the stage of recovering from a more severe but self-limiting anaemia.[57,58] Although this approach might be appealing, as it avoids intrauterine transfusion with its associated risks, it should be noted that there is no available reliable means to predict whether a hydropic fetus will improve or deteriorate. In 1995, Fairley et al.[62] reviewed reported cases of fetal hydrops due to parvovirus infection in England and Wales. Of 12 fetuses treated by intrauterine transfusions, three died (25%), while 13 of the 26 fetuses managed conservatively died (50%). After adjustment for the severity of hydrops and for gestational ages, the odds of fetal death after transfusion were significantly less than conservative management (OR 0.14; 95% CI 0.02–0.96).

Postmortem findings

The main feature in autopsies of fetal deaths due to congenital parvovirus infection is the presence of characteristic intranuclear inclusion bodies in the erythroid precursors. These have been shown to contain virus particles by electron microscopy, *in situ* hybridisation and PCR.[63] These viral inclusions are also commonly found in the fetal liver (as a major site of erythropoiesis in early fetal life), the placenta, heart and lungs and are also found in the thymus. In addition, inflammatory changes are noted in the myocardium, with evidence of subendocardial fibroelastosis, further supporting the role of cardiac infection by the virus in the development of fetal hydrops and as a contributory cause of fetal death.[27,28] Interestingly, one study demonstrated that viral inclusions were found in only two of five placentas, suggesting that histopathological examination of the placenta alone is probably an inappropriate method for ruling out parvovirus infection.[40]

Most of the studies defining pathological features of congenital parvovirus infection were undertaken by retrospectively reviewing cases of non-immune hydrops fetalis. One study, however, examined 66 autopsies of nonmalformed cases of intrauterine fetal deaths, including hydropic and nonhydropic fetuses.[64] The authors identified 11 cases of parvovirus infection at gestational ages ranging from 11 to 26 weeks. Of those, only three had hydrops. The remaining eight cases had no evidence of hydrops, either on antenatal ultrasound or on postmortem pathological examination. Maternal parvovirus B19 infection should be excluded in cases of intrauterine fetal death, even in the absence of hydrops.

Long-term effects

The current available evidence suggests that parvovirus infection in pregnancy is not associated with long-term adverse effects in the infant. The large study conducted by the Public Health Laboratory Service in the UK in 1990 followed 186 women with confirmed parvovirus infection during pregnancy.[23] They retrieved information on 114 infants up to the age of one year, and none had signs of neurodevelopmental or other serious health problems that could be attributed to parvovirus. Another study[25] gathered information from 129 infants to ages 7–10 years and confirmed the absence of late effects that may have been attributed to intrauterine exposure to parvovirus B19 infection. Five children had mild haematological conditions (three with iron deficiency anaemia, one with transient idiopathic thrombocytopenic purpura and one with transient eosinophilia). However, these findings would be expected in the general population.[65] Two percent of the children in this study had mild developmental delay, which again would be expected in any unselected group of children.[25]

Most infants treated by intrauterine transfusion because of parvovirus-related anaemia have been found to have normal neonatal outcomes. However, repeated intrauterine transfusions in rhesus-positive fetuses caused suppression of fetal erythropoiesis resulting in fetal dependence and the need for neonatal transfusions. Therefore, close follow-up of parvovirus-infected fetuses who have received several intrauterine transfusions is mandatory.[53] One report of three infants who required repeated intrauterine transfusions for parvovirus infections, described persistent red cell aplasia resulting in one death at nine months of age and transfusion dependency in the other two infants.[66]

Summary

About 50% of women at childbearing age are immune to parvovirus B19 infection and 50% are therefore susceptible to infection during pregnancy. The disease is mild in adults but the virus may be transmitted transplacentally and can cause severe destruction of erythroid progenitor cells in the fetus, with the risk of developing fetal anaemia, hydrops and intrauterine death. The virus may also affect the fetal heart, causing myocarditis and heart failure. The risk of fetal death is higher in cases of maternal infection before 20 weeks of gestation, although with present data we cannot be certain that fetal death will not occur at later gestational ages. In general, the risk of fetal loss is less than 9% and may be as low as 3–4%. Pregnant women with parvovirus B19 infection should be referred to specialised fetal medicine units for monitoring, advice and management of fetal infection.

Fetal hydrops can develop up to 12 weeks, and possibly 18 weeks, following the maternal infection. Therefore detailed ultrasound examination for signs of fetal hydrops should be undertaken for at least 12 weeks from the date of the original exposure or proven maternal infection. If hydrops develops, it should be treated by intravascular fetal blood transfusion. Parvovirus B19 infection should be considered in any case of fetal hydrops diagnosed on a routine scan, even with no history of maternal infection or contact with a parvovirus case. Fetal parvovirus B19 infection is not known to be associated with congenital malformations and fetuses surviving the initial hydropic effect have good long-term outcomes.

References

1. Levy R, Weissman A, Blomberg G, Hagay Z. Infection by Parvovirus B19 during pregnancy: A review. *Obstet Gynecol Surv* 1997;**52**:254–9.
2. Brown KE, Anderson SM, Young NS. Erythrocyte P antigen: Cellular response for B19 parvovirus. *Science* 1993;**262**:114–7.
3. Brown KE, Hibbs JR, Gallinella G, Anderson SM, Lehman ED, McCarthy P, *et al*. Resistance to parvovirus B19 infection due to lack of virus receptor (erythrocyte P antigen). *N Engl J Med* 1994;**330**:1192–6.
4. Cossart YE, Field AM, Cant B, Widdows D. Parvovirus-like particles in human sera. *Lancet* 1975;**i**:72–3.
5. Gillespie SM, Cartter ML, Asch S, Rokos JB, Gary GW, Tsou CJ, *et al*. Occupational risk of human parvovirus B19 infection for school and day-care personnel during an outbreak of erythema infectiosum. *JAMA* 1990;**263**:2061–5.
6. Anderson MJ. Parvoviruses as agents of human disease. *Prog Med Virol* 1987;**34**:55–69.
7. Török TJ. Parvovirus B19 and human disease. *Adv Intern Med* 1992;**37**:431–55.
8. Gratacós E, Torres PJ, Vidal J, Antolín E, Costa J, Jiménez de Anta MT, *et al*. The incidence of human parvovirus B19 infection during pregnancy and its impact on perinatal outcome. *J Infect Dis* 1995;**171**:1360–3.
9. Skjöldebrand-Sparre L, Fridell E, Nyman M, Wahren B. A prospective study of antibodies against parvovirus B19 in pregnancy. *Acta Obstet Gynecol Scand* 1996;**75**:336–9.
10. Yaegashi N, Niinuma T, Chisaka H, Uehara S, Okamura K, Shinkawa O, *et al*. Serologic study of human parvovirus B19 infection in pregnancy in Japan. *J Infect* 1999;**38**:30–5.
11. Jensen IP, Thorsen P, Jeune B, Møller BR, Vestergaard BF. An epidemic of parvovirus B19 in a population of 3596 pregnant women: a study of sociodemographic and medical risk factors. *BJOG* 2000;**107**:637–43.
12. Anderson LJ, Hurwitz ES. Human parvovirus B19 and pregnancy. *Clin Perinatol* 1988;**15**:273–86.
13. Thurn J. Human parvovirus B19: Historical and clinical review. *Rev Infect Dis* 1988;**10**:1005–11.

14. Pattison JR. Human parvovirus B19. *BMJ* 1994;**308**:918–19.
15. Blacklock H, Mortimer P. Aplastic crisis and other effects of the human parvovirus infection. *Clin Haematol* 1984;**13**:679–91.
16. Serjeant GR, Topley JM, Mason K, Serjeant BE, Pattison JR, Jones SE, *et al.* Outbreak of aplastic crises in sickle cell anaemia associated with parvovirus-like agent. *Lancet* 1981;**ii**:595–7.
17. Rao KRP, Patel AR, Anderson MJ, Hodgson J, Jones SE, Pattison JR. Infection with parvovirus-like virus and aplastic crisis in chronic hemolytic anemia. *Ann Intern Med* 1983;**98**:930–2.
18. Cohen B. Parvovirus B19: an expanding spectrum of disease. *BMJ* 1995;**311**:1549–52.
19. Koch WC, Massey G, Russell CE, Alder SP. Manifestations and treatment of human parvovirus B19 infection in immunocompromised patients. *J Pediatr* 1990;**116**:355–9.
20. Brown T, Anand A, Ritchie LD, Clewley JP, Reid TMS. Intrauterine parvovirus infection associated with hydrops fetalis. *Lancet* 1984;**ii**:1033–4.
21. Knott PD, Welply GAC, Anderson MJ. Serologically proved intrauterine infection with parvovirus. *BMJ* 1984;**289**:1660.
22. Mortimer PP, Cohen BJ, Buckley MM, Cradock-Watson JE, Ridehalgh MK, Burkhardt F, *et al.* Human parvovirus and the fetus [letter]. *Lancet* 1985;**ii**:1012.
23. Public Health Laboratory Service working party on fifth disease. Prospective study of human parvovirus (B19) infection in pregnancy. *BMJ* 1990;**300**:1166–70.
24. Rodis JF, Quinn DL, Gary GW, Anderson LJ, Rosengren S, Cartter ML, *et al.* Management and outcomes of pregnancies complicated by human B19 parvovirus infection: A prospective study. *Am J Obstet Gynecol* 1990;**163**:1168–71.
25. Miller E, Fairley CK, Cohen BJ, Seng C. Immediate and long term outcome of human parvovirus B19 infection in pregnancy. *Br J Obstet Gynaecol* 1998;**105**:174–8.
26. Skjöldebrand-Sparre L, Tolfvenstam T, Papadogiannakis N, Wahren B, Broliden K, Nyman M. Parvovirus B19 infection: association with third-trimester intrauterine fetal death. *BJOG* 2000;**107**:476–80.
27. Porter HJ, Quantril AM, Fleming KA. B19 parvovirus infection of myocardial cells. *Lancet* 1988;**i**:535–6.
28. Morey AL, Keeling JW, Porter HJ, Fleming KA. Clinical and histopathological features of parvovirus B19 infection in the human fetus. *Br J Obstet Gynaecol* 1992;**99**:566–74.
29. Smoleniec JS, Pillai M, Caul EO, Usher J. Subclinical transplacental parvovirus B19 infection: an increased fetal risk? [letter] *Lancet* 1994;**343**:1100–1.
30. Smulian JC, Egan JF, Rodis JF. Fetal hydrops in the first trimester associated with maternal parvovirus infection. *J Clin Ultrasound* 1998;**26**:314–16.
31. Sohan K, Carroll S, Byrne D, Ashworth M, Soothill P. Parvovirus as a differential diagnosis of hydrops fetalis in the first trimester. *Fetal Diagn Ther* 2000;**15**:234–6.
32. Weiland HT, Vermey-Keers C, Salimans MM, Fleuren GJ, Verwey RA, Anderson MJ. Parvovirus B19 associated with fetal abnormality. *Lancet* 1987;**i**:682–3.
33. Tiessen RG, van Elsacker-Niele AMW, Vermeij-Keers CHR, Oepeks D, van Roosmalen J, Gorsira MCB. A fetus with a parvovirus B19 infection and congenital anomalies. *Prenat Diagn* 1994;**14**:173–6.
34. Katz VL, McCoy C, Kuller JA, Hansen WF. An association between fetal parvovirus B19 infection and fetal anomalies: A report of two cases. *Am J Perinatol* 1996;**13**:43–5.
35. Zerbini M, Musiani M, Gentilomi G, Venturoli S, Gallinella G, Morandi R. Comparative evaluation of virological and serological methods in prenatal diagnosis of parvovirus B19 fetal hydrops. *J Clin Microbiol* 1996;**34**:603–8.
36. Dieke D, Schild RL, Hansmann M, Eis-Hubinger AM. Prenatal diagnosis of congenital parvovirus B19 infection: Value of serological and PCR techniques in maternal and fetal serum. *Prenat Diagn* 1999;**19**:1119–23.
37. Salimans MM, van de Rijke FM, Raap AK, van Elsacker-Niele AM. Detection of parvovirus B19 DNA in fetal tissues by *in situ* hybridisation and polymerase chain reaction. *J Clin Pathol* 1989;**42**:525–30.
38. Schwarz TF, Nerlich A, Hottentrager B, Jager G, Wiest I, Kantimm S, *et al.* Parvovirus B19 infection of the fetus: Histology and *in situ* hybridisation. *Am J Clin Pathol* 1991;**96**:121–6.
39. Mark Y, Rogers BB, Oyer C. Diagnosis and incidence of fetal parvovirus infection in an autopsy series, II: DNA amplification. *Pediatr Pathol* 1993;**13**:381–6.
40. Rogers BB, Mark Y, Oyer C. Diagnosis and incidence of fetal parvovirus infection in an autopsy series, I: Histology. *Pediatr Pathol* 1993;**13**:371–9.
41. Jordan JA. Identification of human parvovirus B 19 infection in idiopathic nonimmune hydrops fetalis. *Am J Obstet Gynecol* 1994;**174**:37–42.
42. Peters MT, Nicolaides KH. Cordocentesis for the diagnosis and treatment of human fetal parvovirus infection. *Obstet Gynecol* 1990;**75**:501–4.

43. Sahakian V, Weiner CP, Naides SJ, Williamson RA, Scharosch LL. Intrauterine transfusion treatment of nonimmune hydrops fetalis secondary to human parvovirus B19 infection. *Am J Obstet Gynecol* 1991;**164**:1090–1.

44. Carrington D, Gilmore DH, Whittle MJ, Aitken D, Gibson AA, Patrick WJ, *et al.* Maternal serum alphafetoprotein – a marker of fetal aplastic crisis during intrauterine human parvovirus infection. *Lancet* 1987;**i**:433–5.

45. Bernstein IM, Capeless EL. Elevated maternal serum alpha-fetoprotein and hydrops fetalis in association with fetal parvovirus B19 infection. *Obstet Gynecol* 1989;**74**:456–7.

46. Saller DN Jr, Rogers BB, Canick JA. Maternal serum biochemical markers in pregnancies with fetal parvovirus B19 infection. *Prenat Diagn* 1993;**13**:467–71.

47. Nicolaides KH, Soothill PW, Clewell WH, Rodeck CH, Mibashan RS, Campbell S. Fetal haemoglobin measurement in the assessment of red cell iso-immunisation. *Lancet* 1988;**i**:1073–75.

48. Welch R, Rampling MW, Anwar A, Talbert DG, Rodeck CH. Changes in hemorheology with fetal intravascular transfusion. *Am J Obstet Gynecol* 1994;**170**:726–32.

49. Vyas S, Nicolaides KH, Campbell S. Doppler examination of the middle cerebral artery in anemic fetuses. *Am J Obstet Gynecol* 1990;**162**:1066–8.

50. Mari G, Adrignolo A, Abuhamad AZ, Pirhonen J, Jones DC, Ludomirsky A, *et al.* Diagnosis of fetal anaemia with Doppler ultrasound in the pregnancy complicated by maternal blood group immunization. *Ultrasound Obstet Gynecol* 1995;**5**:400–5.

51. Mari G. For the collaborative group for Doppler assessment of the blood velocity in anaemic fetuses. Noninvasive diagnosis by Doppler ultrasonography of fetal anaemia due to maternal red-cell alloimmunization. *N Engl J Med* 2000;**342**:9–14.

52. Smoleniec J, James D. Predictive value of pleural effusions in fetal hydrops. *Fetal Diagn Ther* 1995;**10**:95–100.

53. Moise KJ Jr, Schumacher B. Anaemia. In: Fisk NM, Moise KJ Jr, editors. *Fetal Therapy, Invasive and Transplacental*. Cambridge: Cambridge University Press; 1997. p. 141–63.

54. Schwarz TF, Roggendorf M, Hottentrager B, Deinhardt F, Gloning KP. Schramm T, *et al.* Human parvovirus B19 in pregnancy. *Lancet* 1988;**ii**:566–7.

55. Soothill P. Intrauterine blood transfusion for nonimmune hydrops fetalis due to parvovirus B19 infection. *Lancet* 1990;**336**:121–2.

56. Smoleniec JS, Pillai M. Management of fetal hydrops associated with parvovirus B19 infection. *Br J Obstet Gynaecol* 1994;**101**:1079–81.

57. Humphrey W, Magoon M, O'Shaughnessy R. Severe nonimmune hydrops secondary to parvovirus B19 infection: Spontaneous reversal in utero and survival of a term infant. *Obstet Gynecol* 1991;**78**:900–2.

58. Sheikh AU, Ernest JM, O'Shea M. Long-term outcome in fetal hydrops from parvovirus B19 infection. *Am J Obstet Gynecol* 1992;**167**:337–41.

59. Pryde PG, Nugent CE, Pridjian G, Barr M Jr, Faix RG. Spontaneous resolution of nonimmune hydrops fetalis secondary to human parvovirus B19 infection. *Obstet Gynecol* 1992;**79**:859–61.

60. Petrikovsky BM, Baker D, Schneider E. Fetal hydrops secondary to human parvovirus infection in early pregnancy. *Prenat Diagn* 1996;**16**:242–4.

61. Morey AL, Nicolini U, Welch CR, Economides D, Chamberlain PF, Cohen BJ. Parvovirus B19 infection and transient fetal hydrops. *Lancet* 1991;**337**:496.

62. Fairley CK, Smoleniec JS, Caul OE, Miller E. Observational study of effect of intrauterine transfusions on outcome of fetal hydrops after parvovirus B19 infection. *Lancet* 1995;**346**:1335–7.

63. Berry PJ, Gray ES, Porter HJ, Burton PA. Parvovirus infection of the human fetus and newborn. *Semin Diagn Pathol* 1992;**9**:4–12.

64. Wright C, Hinchliffe SA, Taylor C. Fetal pathology in intrauterine death due to parvovirus B19 infection. *Br J Obstet Gynaecol* 1996;**103**:133–6.

65. Grant GA. Prevalence of iron deficiency anaemia in rural pre-school children in Northern Ireland. *Br J Gen Pract* 1990;**40**:112–13.

66. Brown KE, Green SW, Antunez de Mayolo J, Ballanti JA, Smith SD, Smith TJ, *et al.* Congenital anaemia after transplacental B19 parvovirus infection. *Lancet* 1994;**343**:895–6.

Chapter 25

Viruses and pregnancy II

Discussion

Discussion following Professor McIntyre's paper

Newell: Your last point concerned caesarean section and viral load. There has recently been a meta-analysis[1] looking at the rate of transmission in women with a viral load of less than 1000 copies/ml. In a multivariate analysis, caesarean section had an independent effect even in those women with a very low viral load. That is an important observation.

It is also important to realise that in Europe the rate of vertical transmission has now reduced to 1%, through a combination of the 076 zidovudine regimen, elective caesarean section and advising infected women not to breastfeed. The rates are similar to what you see in the WITS study,[2] with highly active anti-retroviral therapy and many fewer elective caesarean sections.

Discussion following Dr Simmonds' paper

Newell: I would like to urge caution in the interpretation of the Gibb paper[3] on vertical transmission of hepatitis C and the possible benefit of an elective caesarean section. In this study, although they had information on 400 or so women and children in the UK and Ireland, they did not have follow-up information on more than half of the children. They therefore employed a statistical imputation method, which was developed for HIV infection some years ago. On the basis of that, they did their multivariate analysis, but the assumptions underlying this method are questionable.

Indeed, in a large cohort of about 1500 European children born to hepatitis C-infected mothers, we saw such a large interaction between HIV co-infection and mode of delivery that we decided that we could only do a stratified analysis.[4] We found that an elective caesarean section was only beneficial in co-infected women, to reduce both HIV infection and hepatitis C infection transmission. The same was true for breastfeeding, but no effect of either caesarean section or breastfeeding was seen in women who were only hepatitis C infected.

We ought to be very careful about starting to recommend elective caesarean section for women infected with hepatitis C only.

Simmonds: Yes, there is no real disagreement about breastfeeding. Clearly, there is no evidence for an increased risk of transmission by that route.

Elective caesarean makes sense, given that hepatitis C is usually acquired perinatally.

Carrington: Dr Newell, are there any guidelines in existence to cover hepatitis C? I would be particularly interested to know, because clearly scalp electrodes, mechanical delivery and so on could increase risk. Could I ask the obstetricians whether these are in existence?

Newell: There are certainly no European guidelines on hepatitis C at the moment, because it has been very difficult to collect the data. It is premature to start making recommendations. Our analysis from the larger datasets in Europe would strengthen the argument for an elective caesarean section in women who are HIV infected, as well as for those with hepatitis C infection. It also strengthens the argument for screening women infected with HIV for hepatitis C. However, there are no formal guidelines.

[The discussion then moved on to considering hepatitis B in pregnancy.]

Brocklehurst: There has been a reported randomised controlled trial from Japan,[5] giving mothers, who are hepatitis B virus e-antigen-positive, hepatitis B-specific immunoglobulins during pregnancy. This showed a further reduction in mother-to-child transmission, compared with postnatal treatment alone. Is anyone else familiar with that?

Newell: All I remember, like you, is that there was the Japanese trial which used immunoglobulins during pregnancy and found a further reduction. The study was trying to address the remaining 5% transmission rate that still exists even with immunisation and vaccination.

MacLean: Could I ask about the availability of immunoglobulin? I seem to remember that there were recently some concerns for those mothers who were hepatitis B e-antigen-negative.

Miller: There was a shortage a few years ago, which meant that the recommendation that the infant of any carrier mother should have immunoglobulin as well as vaccine was amended. Only those who were at higher risk – the e-antigen-positive group – were prioritised. I am not aware of a systematic review of the literature but there is evidence that the addition of immunoglobulin to the mothers in the low-risk category may reduce that residual few percent a little further. Since there is no longer an issue about supply for all mothers carrying the virus, that is a question that could be revisited.

In relation to other ways of reducing the risk of vertical transmission, a simple way is to complete the immunisation course of the infant. The evidence is that only about two-thirds of the infants complete the course and receive all three doses. Concentrating on implementing the current policy, rather than necessarily doing fancy things as a result of clinical trials elsewhere, should be a major recommendation of this group. This is notwithstanding the fact that it is a paediatric rather than an obstetric action that is required.

Carrington: I am aware that the rules on the vaccination of infants have changed and that we should now be adopting the accelerated programme of doses at 0, 1, 2 and 12 months of age, rather than at 0, 1 and 6 months.

Brink: That is correct. It was amended a year or so ago to 0, 1, 2 and 12 months.

Discussion following Professor Soothill's paper

Jauniaux: It is interesting to realise that the same virus, in a similar population, has a different effect. The American paper[6] published in 1998, which followed up more than 600 women with symptoms of parvovirus and serologic evidence, showed no hydrops and no intrauterine fetal deaths.

Soothill: Could that be partly due to gestational age? Gestational age has not been adequately included in the assessment of maternal infection.

Jauniaux: There was quite a wide spectrum of gestational age. This was also a prospective study, which is rare. Most of the studies are retrospective.
  Doppler and more sophisticated investigations will not be available in most units. Even in fetal medicine units, most obstetricians are not performing sophisticated Doppler scans. How predictive are these techniques in the case of parvovirus? Are they really useful tools?

Soothill: I do not really know the answer to your question. What I do know is that you can have anaemic fetuses that can compensate for quite a long time – we know that from several other conditions. If we recognise hyperdynamic bloodflow – and we have to look at that prospectively in terms of prediction of hydrops – then that is an important sign.

Jauniaux: In rhesus disease, we know that you can have a perfectly normal-looking baby, with severe anaemia and abnormal bloodflows. In parvovirus, however, it seems that ascites and hydrops will be quite quick to develop, and it is likely that the middle cerebral artery studies will have little impact in predicting this sort of complication.

Soothill: I do not totally agree with that. If you have infection at, say, 15 weeks of pregnancy, then you would need to follow that fetus right through to 30 weeks. If you had a progressive rise in the peak velocity in the middle cerebral artery, that would be a useful warning, perhaps combined with a maternal serum alphafetoprotein test, that that baby is getting into trouble.
  I am using an analogy from another cause of anaemia, and we need to do that work. However, we know that you get hyperdynamic circulation in anaemic fetuses with parvovirus infection. How long that happens before they develop hydrops, I am not sure, but the haemoglobin level needs to be down at around 6 g/dl before you get hydrops. You are talking about quite severe anaemia and, from the American data,[7] the peak velocity is going up at lower levels of haemoglobin than that.

Jauniaux: In rhesus disease?

Soothill: The point I have been trying to make to this group is that we do not know a great deal about parvovirus. We need to do much more follow-up, which we are now doing. However, we do have extensive experience of the treatment of fetal anaemic hydrops. There is no evidence at all that it does not behave in the same way as other causes of anaemic hydrops.

Jauniaux: I was quite shocked by the reported data[8] of three dead in 12 fetal transfusions. This is very high, and perhaps they should have referred the patients to a unit that was capable of performing transfusions with lower mortality.

Soothill: I agree but I would also emphasise that, in my own series of parvovirus transfusions, we have higher rates of death than in rhesus disease. However, that is entirely because two of those cases were done at 17 and 18 weeks of gestation. Once again, the gestation factor is important.

Miller: I was a co-author of that paper. Some of the cases were transfused at a very late stage. They were seriously ill and severely hydropic when they were transfused. The cases were collected over a period of time and, with the state-of-the-art fetal transfusion available now, and with the current prospective follow-up and early detection of cases of fetal hydrops, that would not necessarily be the experience now. I cannot remember whether we analysed the data according to gestational age, but we still have it and I could go back to look at that. It would not reflect current experience, however.

Soothill: Thank you. As well as that you are absolutely right that, if we pick up early ascites, with a hyperdynamic circulation, the prognosis will be much better than if we wait until the baby has severe polyhydramnios, severe skin oedema, severe pleural effusion and severe ascites. You are right: picking it up before the baby becomes moribund is an important reason for monitoring recently infected cases intensively.

Miller: The question is how frequently? Would you need to do a scan every week? Or every two weeks?

Soothill: At the moment we are scanning every week. The interval between the first sign of hydrops and death can be quite short. The discussion of Dr Jauniaux's paper reflected that it is possible that the hypervelocity Doppler studies may allow us to spread that out a little, to two weeks, but we do not have the data to say that. I am therefore encouraging these patients to come every week.

References

1. Ioannidis JP, Abrams EJ, Ammann A, Bulterys M, Goedert JJ, Gray L, *et al.* Perinatal transmission of human immunodeficiency virus type 1 by pregnant women with RNA virus loads <1000 copies/ml. *J Infect Dis* 2001;**183**:539–45.
2. Blattner W. Antenatal ART and MTCT in WITS 1990–1999. Women and Infants Transmission Study. XIII International AIDS Conference, 9–14 July 2000, Durban, South Africa. Abstract LBCr4.
3. Gibb DM, Goodall RL, Dunn DT, Healy M, Neave P, Cafferkey M, *et al.* Mother-to-child transmission of hepatitis C virus: evidence for preventable peripartum transmission. *Lancet* 2000;**356**:904–7.
4. European Paediatric Hepatitis C Virus Network. Effects of mode of delivery and infant feeding on the

risk of mother-to-child transmission of hepatitis C virus. *BJOG* 2001;**108**:371–7.

5. Qirong Z, Xinhuan G, Huafang, Shucheng D. A preliminary study on interruption of HBV transmission in uterus. *Chin Med J* 1997;**110**:145–7.

6. Harger JH, Adler SP, Koch WC, Harger GF. Prospective evaluation of 618 pregnant women exposed to parvovirus B19: risks and symptoms. *Obstet Gynecol* 1998;**91**:413–20.

7. Mari G, Deter RL, Carpenter RL, Rahman F, Zimmerman R, Moise KJ Jr, *et al*. Noninvasive diagnosis by Doppler ultrasonography of fetal anemia due to maternal red-cell alloimmunization. Collaborative Group for Doppler Assessment of the Blood Velocity in Anemic Fetuses. *N Engl J Med* 2000;**342**:9–14.

8. Fairley CK, Smoleniec JS, Caul OE, Miller E. Observational study of effect of intrauterine transfusions on outcome of fetal hydrops after parvovirus B19 infection. *Lancet* 1995;**346**:1335–7.

SECTION 7

INFECTION I

Chapter 26

Infection and pregnancy loss

Lesley Regan and Shehnaaz Jivraj

Introduction

Maternal infections during pregnancy are common – at least one in twenty women will experience an infective illness when pregnant. In the vast majority of cases, they prove to be harmless. However, a minority of these infections have the potential to cause damage to the mother, her fetus or her newborn baby. There are many different possible outcomes for pregnancies that are complicated by an infection. They range from an early miscarriage occurring during the first trimester to late miscarriage at any gestational age between 13 and 24 weeks. Infections are also a recognised cause of complications in the third trimester of pregnancy such as preterm delivery, intrauterine death, stillbirth and the delivery of a baby with a congenital abnormality.

Although the most likely outcome of maternal infection in pregnancy is the birth of a completely normal baby, the emotional distress and healthcare resources expended on those pregnancies that are miscarried or develop serious complications at a later stage are highly significant. As we enter the 21st century, it is sobering to reflect on the fact that our ability to predict those pregnancies at risk of an adverse outcome is poor. In this chapter, the contribution of infection to pregnancies lost before 24 weeks is reviewed. The contribution that infections make to the problems of preterm delivery, neonatal morbidity and mortality are addressed by other authors in this book.

Miscarriage definitions

A miscarriage is the spontaneous loss of a pregnancy before the fetus has reached a viable gestational age. The World Health Organization defines miscarriage as the spontaneous loss of a fetus weighing 500 g or less. The term miscarriage therefore includes all pregnancy losses occurring between 5 and 24 weeks. As will be discussed below, pregnancies that are lost after this gestational age are fortunately rare.

There are two distinct types of miscarriage. Sporadic miscarriage – due to an isolated or random event (the most common of which is a fetal chromosomal abnormality) – is the most common complication of pregnancy. At least 25% and probably as many as 50% of all women experience at least one sporadic miscarriage during their reproductive life. However, these clinically recognised pregnancies that are known to end in miscarriage represent the tip of the iceberg of reproductive loss. Epidemiological data have demonstrated that the fate of a fertilised egg is not a happy one.[1] Among 100 conceptions, only 73 implantations can be expected and of these a significant number will be lost before achieving a positive pregnancy test. Around 57 will be recognised clinically by positive human chorionic gonadotrophin testing and subsequent ultrasound scan documentation of an intrauterine pregnancy sac. Only 51 of the original conceptions will progress to the fetal stage (heart beat visualised) and 50 will eventually result in a live birth. In summary, 50% of all conceptions are miscarried and 15% of all clinically recognised pregnancies end in sporadic miscarriage.[2]

In contrast, recurrent miscarriage, defined as three or more spontaneous pregnancy losses, affects 1% of couples. Many clinicians choose to include couples who have had two or more losses in their definition, in which case the scale of the problem increases from 1% of all couples to 5% of all couples trying to achieve a live take-home baby. It is important to appreciate that this has a dramatic impact on the resources needed to investigate and care for these patients.

By convention, the miscarriage is termed early if it occurs before the 13th week of pregnancy and late when the miscarriage involves the loss of a fetus between 13 and 24 weeks in size, confirmed on ultrasound or postmortem measurement. Importantly, 98% of sporadic miscarriages occur before 13 weeks, which means that women who suffer a sporadic miscarriage can be reassured that when their next pregnancy reaches the second trimester their chances of a successful live birth are high. However, it is known that 75% of women who suffer recurrent miscarriage lose their pregnancies in the first trimester and that 25% of these women will experience a late miscarriage as well as early losses.[3] The dilemma for the clinician is that it is often difficult to decide whether the woman has two different and recurring causes for her early and late miscarriages, or has a recurrent cause for the late losses and in addition has suffered an early loss due to fetal chromosomal abnormality, which is usually a sporadic pregnancy loss.[4]

The checklist of causes for both sporadic and recurrent miscarriage can be divided into broad categories: genetic, anatomical, infective, environmental, immune, endocrine and unexplained. Most recently, it has been recognised that prothrombotic abnormalities are also important – some of which have an autoimmune and others a genetic basis. The majority of sporadic miscarriages are usually attributed to fetal genetic abnormalities or maternal acute infective episodes, whereas the less random nature of recurrent miscarriage has led to the belief that endocrine and immune causes are the more likely aetiology. However, it is important to remember that the majority of couples who present with recurrent pregnancy loss will do so because they have experienced several episodes of bad luck. Many couples feel distressed that the investigations they undergo prove to be negative, but in fact the prognosis for couples with 'unexplained recurrent miscarriage' is invariably better than if they are found to have an underlying abnormality. A successful outcome in the next pregnancy can be expected for 75–80% of couples with unexplained recurrent loss if they are offered supportive care in a dedicated early-pregnancy clinic.[5,6]

Potential mechanisms of infective pregnancy loss

Infections have been cited as a potential cause of pregnancy loss for the last 50 years. However, the precise role of infection as a cause of early miscarriage is poorly and inconsistently reported. In a minority of cases, maternal infections are capable of causing congenital infections (*in utero*), infection during the intrapartum period or a postnatally acquired infection. Infections that occur during pregnancy are the cause of less than 3% of all congenital abnormalities. The majority of these infections are completely harmless.[6]

Different theories have been proposed to explain how an infectious agent can lead to miscarriage and a summary of the these, together with likely candidate organisms, is listed below:[7,8]

- direct effect on the ovum or the fertilisation process by infected spermatozoa (*Ureaplasma urealyticum,* chlamydia)
- unfavourable implantation due to endometrial infection or inflammation caused by ascending spread of organisms from the lower genital tract (mycoplasmas, herpesvirus, chlamydia, bacterial vaginosis)
- induction of an anatomically and genetically altered embryo or fetus by viral infection during early gestation (rubella, cytomegalovirus, parvovirus B19)
- placental and blood-borne agents (*Treponema pallidum, Toxoplasma gondii,* listeria, malaria)
- amniotic infection from ascending bacteria (group B streptococcus, bacterial vaginosis).

There are many maternal infections that could cause sporadic miscarriages. Organisms that have been associated with sporadic loss are:

- *Chlamydia trachomatis*
- cytomegalovirus (CMV)
- gonorrhoea
- group B streptococcus
- hepatitis B virus
- herpes simplex virus (HSV)
- HIV
- *Listeria monocytogenes*
- parvovirus B19
- rubella
- syphilis
- *T. gondii*
- varicella-zoster virus.

The mechanisms are poorly understood but have traditionally been assumed to be secondary to an acute maternal pyrexia, bacteraemia or viraemia. This viewpoint has been challenged in a cohort study published in 1996 suggesting that the contribution of maternal infections to the incidence of early sporadic miscarriage is less common than previously believed.[9]

There are many reports in the literature that have implicated a large number of infective agents in the aetiology of recurrent miscarriage. The theories put forward have included:

- the possibility that these infective organisms cause a chronic infection of low virulence leading to implantation problems
- the stimulation of a maternal inflammatory response, either systemically or in the decidual bed
- the development of repeated fetal or placental infections.

None of these anecdotal studies and their accompanying theories has been conclusive, since adequate control groups have never been included. As a result, those reports claiming benefit from empirical antibiotic drug regimens require cautious interpretation until well-designed placebo-controlled treatment studies have been conducted.

For an organism to be capable of causing recurrent pregnancy loss, it must be able to persist in the genital tract for a long period of time, produce minimal symptoms in the affected woman in order to avoid detection and also be resistant to treatment with the powerful antibiotic drugs available today. In reality, many infective organisms may cause miscarriage during the primary stages of infection but are an unlikely cause of recurrent miscarriage in an immunocompetent mother, who produces specific antibodies to protect subsequent pregnancies. Hence the routine use of infective screening for women with recurrent miscarriage is difficult to justify.[8,10]

The TORCH screen is, in my opinion, unhelpful and should be considered a burnt-out methodology. T stands for toxoplasmosis. O does not stand for any specific organism but could be interpreted as 'other organisms'. Nonetheless, it conveniently makes up the TORCH acronym. R stands for rubella and, as will be discussed below, it is highly unlikely that rubella is ever a cause of recurrent miscarriages. Historically, the C stood for CMV but should nowadays also include chlamydia. H stands for HSV and, more recently, HIV.

The problem with the TORCH screen is that it fails to identify recurrent causes of miscarriage, and offers the clinician no understanding or insight into the temporal relationship that a woman had with an infective organism when one of the antibody titres is reported as positive. In any case (with the exception of HIV), once a woman has been exposed to an infection, she is in most cases immune from future infections. Indeed, this is the principle underlying vaccination.

The data that have led to some of these organisms being considered causative in the aetiology of pregnancy loss are reviewed below. Space precludes this from being an exhaustive list. Hence, parvovirus B19, group B streptococcus, malaria, varicella-zoster virus, listeria and syphilis are discussed in other chapters.

Toxoplasmosis infection and miscarriage

The prevalence of primary toxoplasmosis infection in pregnant women in the UK is 2 per 1000. This is an important figure since fetal infections only occur when the mother acquires her primary infection during pregnancy – except in the unusual case of an immunocompromised woman, who occasionally may be susceptible to reinfection. There is no evidence that latent toxoplasmosis infection in healthy mothers causes congenital infection or miscarriage.

The primary maternal illness is often subclinical. However, the risk and severity of the fetal infection depends on the gestational age of the pregnancy. Overall, the fetus becomes infected in about 40% of primary maternal infections. The incidence of fetal infection is highest (90%) when a non-immune mother is infected during the third trimester or at the time of delivery, resulting in congenital disease or subclinical infection. Fetal infection follows in only 10% of cases when maternal infection occurs in the periconceptual period or in the first trimester, but severity of fetal injury is greatest at this stage and may result in miscarriage, later intrauterine death or a liveborn child with severe neurological lesions.[11] However, it is debatable whether maternal treatment with spiramycin improves outcome for the fetus infected during pregnancy.[12]

The prevalence of previous toxoplasmosis infection in pregnant women in the UK is more difficult to establish but is quoted as 10%. In France, the figure is much higher (about 55%).[13,14] Toxoplasmosis is acquired by ingestion of viable tissue cysts in meat or oocysts excreted by cats and left in soil.[15] In Western Europe, toxoplasmosis is mainly acquired by consuming undercooked meat. In a case–control study published in 2000 involving six European cities, the odds ratio and population-attributable fraction associated with food and environmental risk factors for acute toxoplasmosis in pregnancy was determined.[16] The risk factors most strongly predictive of acute infection in pregnant women were eating uncooked lamb, beef or game, contact with soil and travel outside Europe, the USA and Canada. Between 30% and 63% of infections in the six different centres were attributed to consumption of undercooked or cured meat products and between 6% and 17% to soil contact.

Although contact with cats is most commonly cited as a risk factor, this study concluded that this makes only a small contribution to the problem.[16] Cats excrete toxoplasma oocysts when they first acquire infection, but the oocysts become infective one to five days after excretion and can survive in soil for more than a year.[17] Thus, contact with contaminated soil and water, rather than direct contact with cats, is the more important risk factor. Pork and lamb carry a higher risk of infection with *T. gondii* than beef or poultry. The recent European decline in beef consumption has led to an increased consumption of pork and lamb products and ready prepared quick chill meals and burgers may have further increased exposure to *T. gondii*.[18] Although the consumption of unpasteurised milk or milk products from goats, sheep or cows was previously thought to be an unlikely cause of toxoplasmosis infection, there is evidence that suggests that the tachyzoites are not always destroyed by gastric juices.[19] Indeed, a case of acute toxoplasmosis in a breastfed infant has been reported.[20]

In summary, toxoplasmosis is an established cause of sporadic miscarriage and fetal injury but there are no data to support its role in recurrent pregnancy loss.

Rubella infection and miscarriage

Primary rubella infection causes a widespread erythematous macular papular rash, typically covering the face and neck initially and then rapidly spreading to the rest of the body. The rash is typically non-itchy. Approximately 50% of children infected with rubella are asymptomatic. With increasing age, the proportion of subclinical infection falls and by adulthood, asymptomatic rubella infection is relatively uncommon.

In the mid-18th century, German physicians identified rubella as a distinct illness and hence the term German measles was applied to the disease. In 1940, a major epidemic of rubella occurred in Australia. The following year, Sir Norman Gregg, an Australian ophthalmologist noted an unusually high prevalence of congenital cataracts in Sydney. Subsequently, congenital heart disease and intrauterine growth restriction were found to be associated with rubella in pregnancy.[21] The rubella virus was successfully cultured in 1961[22,23] and the first live attenuated vaccine was licensed in 1969.[24]

Since 1988, all children in the UK have been offered vaccination against rubella (together with measles and mumps – the MMR injection) during the second year of life and targeted again at the time of preschool entry at 4–5 years. This vaccination policy is aimed at eradicating rubella from the community rather than simply targeting young women who may become pregnant. The policy has been so successful that it has now been possible to abandon the routine vaccination for teenage girls at school and the *ad hoc* screening that used to occur in general practice, occupational health, family planning and well-women clinics. Nonetheless, screening of male and female healthcare workers and routine antenatal screening for all women continues in order to ensure that vaccination failures are identified and the potential pool of risk to pregnant women is kept to the absolute minimum in the UK.[25] Concerns about the risk of fetal infection if vaccination is performed immediately prior to or during pregnancy have been unfounded. To date, there have been no reports of congenital rubella syndrome following maternal immunisation and no increase in the rate of pregnancy loss.

Primary maternal infection with rubella causes congenital abnormalities and sporadic miscarriage. However, the primary infection or the live vaccine stimulates maternal antibody production, which protects against subsequent fetal infection. Hence, recurrent pregnancy loss due to rubella would not be expected and has never been reported.

Cytomegalovirus infection and miscarriage

CMV is the most common viral infection transmitted to the fetus. It can be transmitted from mother to baby transplacentally during pregnancy, at the time of delivery and via breast milk. Now that congenital rubella has been largely eliminated in the West, CMV infection has become the leading congenital viral infection. It is a significant public health problem because CMV infection is common and, in a significant proportion of cases, central nervous system impairment follows, primarily affecting the baby's psychomotor and perceptual functions. Features of congenital CMV infection include microcephaly, choroidoretinitis, sensorineural hearing loss, cognitive and motor disability.[26]

The risk of primary CMV infection in pregnancy has been variably reported and depends on the population studied. Serological studies of pregnant women indicate that 50–80% of pregnant women in industrialised countries have had a primary CMV infection prior to pregnancy, the incidence being highest in lower socio-economic groups.[27] Of the remaining susceptible women, approximately 2% will develop a primary CMV infection during pregnancy and 40% of these women will transmit the virus to their fetus.[28] The maternal infection is often asymptomatic, although some women may develop a mononucleosis-like syndrome. It has thus been difficult to determine whether the gestational age at the time of the primary maternal infection affects the risk of fetal infection.

Primary infection during pregnancy may lead to early miscarriage but the magnitude of the problem remains unclear. Stagno *et al.*[29] reviewed 3712 pregnant women screened for CMV and documented 21 cases of primary maternal CMV during pregnancy, among which 11 resulted in a neonatal infection. No cases of miscarriage were reported but, since CMV screening took place at antenatal clinic registration, the contribution that CMV infection may make to early pregnancy loss remains unknown.[6]

However, routine CMV screening for pregnant women cannot be recommended since there remain significant limitations in the serological diagnosis of primary maternal CMV infection. Even when good immunoglobulin M (IgM) antibody assays are employed, a positive screening test for IgM is just as likely to represent a false positive test for primary infection as real evidence of recent infection.[30]

As noted earlier, in continuing pregnancies complicated by CMV infection, approximately 40% of the infants will be culture-positive at birth, of whom 10% will have clinical manifestations such as hepatosplenomegaly, jaundice, thrombocytopenia, chorioretinitis, microcephaly and cognitive disability.[27] However, culture-positive infants with no overt stigmata of disease are still at risk of sequelae. In total, 5–15% of infants with congenital CMV infection will develop significant hearing loss by the age of two years, and others are at risk for later developmental delays and learning disabilities.

After the primary infection, CMV enters a latent stage and is recoverable from the urine and genital secretions of 5–15% of pregnant women. CMV is one of the few viruses that can produce a secondary viraemia, which occurs during the latent phase of infection and is usually asymptomatic. Although uncommon, recurrent *in utero* infections have been reported – it has been estimated that fetal infection may occur in 0.5–1% of secondary CMV infections. Recurrent maternal infections could be due to reactivation of endogenous latent CMV, re-infection with new strains or possibly primary infection that occurred in the recent past. Recurrent infections are only recognised when a baby with congenital CMV is born to a mother known to have been immune prior to conception. Hence it has not been possible to determine the gestational age at which viral transmission occurs, nor what type of secondary maternal event (reactivation, reinfection or preconception primary infection) leads to fetal infection.

Limiting exposure is the only method available for the prevention of maternal and congenital CMV infection. Contact with preschool children and sexual contact appear to be important risks for primary maternal infection. Avoidance of the former is impractical for most women who are employed in child care or have young children of their own. General hygiene precautions such as hand washing and avoiding direct contact with body fluids are effective in preventing CMV acquisition from young children.[31] Antiviral agents are commonly used to prevent or treat CMV infections in immunocompromised patients but none of these agents has been approved for use in pregnancy and none has been shown to be effective in the treatment of congenital CMV infection. At the present time, no CMV vaccine is available to prevent maternal or congenital infection but candidate vaccines are undergoing clinical trials.[30]

In summary, there have been many reports of CMV-associated sporadic miscarriage in otherwise-healthy women. CMV infection may be a cause of recurrent pregnancy loss secondary to reactivation of latent CMV or re-infection with new strains of the virus. Concerns remain that reactivation may occur in immunocompromised women, resulting in recurrent pregnancy loss.

Chlamydia and miscarriage

The role of *C. trachomatis* as a causative agent in sporadic human miscarriage has been poorly documented, although bovine pregnancy loss with *C. psittaci* is well recognised. *C. trachomatis* is frequently isolated from the cervix in women examined for sexually transmitted diseases and can be recovered from 3–30% of pregnant women. The prevalence is greatest among young single women.[32] The maternal infection is often asymptomatic and therefore remains undetected. Chlamydia can evade host immune defence mechanisms, persist for long periods of time and ascend to the uterus and upper genital tract without clinical symptoms, and is an important cause of subfertility secondary to endometrial and tubal damage.

Over the last 20 years, serological studies have reported chlamydia to be a cause of sporadic miscarriage, recurrent miscarriage and pregnancy loss following *in vitro* fertilisation (IVF). Quinn *et al.*[33] investigated 66 women with two previous miscarriages and found a significantly higher prevalence of chlamydial antibodies in women with recurrent miscarriage compared with normal pregnant women. Witkin and Ledger[34] studied 30 women with three or more miscarriages and found a higher prevalence of immunoglobulin G (IgG) antibodies to *C. trachomatis* in the group with recurrent miscarriage (at least three miscarriages) compared with those with no history of miscarriage or those with one or two miscarriages. Licciardi *et al.*[35] noted an increased prevalence of IgG antibodies to chlamydia in women who miscarried after IVF treatment when compared with those who went on to have a successful pregnancy and those who failed to conceive with IVF. In a further IVF study, high chlamydia antibody titres identified women at greater risk of subsequent miscarriage.[36] However, in all of these serology-based studies, none of the women gave a history of chlamydial infection and all had negative cervical cultures. Furthermore, IgM antibodies were not tested for, which suggests that the presence of active chlamydial infection was unlikely.

A subsequent serological study of women with a history of three or more miscarriages concluded that there is no association between previous chlamydial infection and recurrent miscarriage.[37] Importantly, this study was able to determine the species-specificity for those women with chlamydial antibodies – information that was not available in the previous studies. Fourteen of 26 women with recurrent miscarriage carried antibodies directed towards *C. pneumoniae* rather than *C. trachomatis*. The authors concluded that there is no association between previous chlamydial infection and future fetal loss in women with a history of recurrent miscarriage.

Furthermore, a Swedish serological study[38] reported in 1996 that no significant cross-reactivity between *C. pneumoniae* and *C. trachomatis* and that there is no association between previous chlamydial infection and either single (sporadic) or repeated miscarriage. Moreover, several prospective studies[39,40] of pregnant women in which *C. trachomatis* was identified using cervical culture techniques found no association with pregnancy loss.

If chlamydia does cause miscarriage, the mechanism by which it does this remains to be determined. It has been postulated that a low-grade infection may persist in the endometrium and that pregnancy-related changes in immune and hormonal function may reactivate this latent infection. Another hypothesis is that prolonged exposure to chlamydia, which is an intracellular pathogen, may result in damage to the endometrial epithelium and induce scar tissue formation, thereby preventing successful implantation.[7] It has been suggested that chlamydia may cause pregnancy complications by producing heat-shock proteins that induce a delayed hypersensitivity reaction in the endometrium, which may have an adverse effect on implantation and the subsequent weeks of early pregnancy.[41]

C. trachomatis infections are frequently asymptomatic and may lead to endometritis and salpingitis. However, concrete evidence to confirm that chlamydia is a cause of early or late miscarriage is currently lacking.

Herpes simplex virus and miscarriage

HSV infections are one of the most common viral infections affecting humans. HSV infection may cause cold sores, genital herpes, ophthalmic herpes or herpes simplex encephalitis but most individuals remain asymptomatic.[42] The majority of maternal HSV infections acquired either before or during pregnancy are also asymptomatic and neonatal herpes infections secondary to these maternal infections are most prevalent when the mother suffers her primary infection and has no protective antibodies. Of all perinatally acquired HSV infections, *in utero* transmission occurs in 5% of cases and at the time of delivery in 85% of cases. In 10% of cases, the infection is acquired postnatally.[43,44]

The first report to link genital herpes infection in early pregnancy with an increased rate of miscarriage appeared in the literature in 1971.[45] Subsequent studies suggested that primary herpes infections before 20 weeks of pregnancy diagnosed by cytological methods (Papanicolaou staining) led to sporadic and recurrent miscarriages.[46,47] Serological studies then advocated the use of immunoglobulin A antibodies to HSV as a tool to predict which women would suffer a miscarriage.[39,48] A follow-up study undertaken in Oslo of 29,000 pregnant women failed to demonstrate an increase in the rate of sporadic miscarriage even when the primary infection occurred in early pregnancy and further concluded that women with recurrent HSV infections share the same 1% risk of recurrent miscarriage as the general population.[49]

HIV and miscarriage

HIV is a potentially significant cause of sporadic and recurrent miscarriage since the infection has a major impact on the woman's systemic health and her HIV infectivity continues after she has mounted an antibody response. Currently, in the UK, routine screening for HIV in women is only conducted in inner-city antenatal clinics and for individuals considered to be at high risk of infection. Whether HIV infection is an important cause of early pregnancy loss is not known, since these limited screening programmes only include women whose pregnancies have reached a gestational age of 12 weeks or more. The true burden of miscarriage has occurred before this date and the majority of HIV-positive mothers and their babies only come to the attention of obstetricians following their antenatal booking visit and consequent blood tests.

One USA prospective study[50] has suggested an increased rate of early miscarriage. These workers isolated HIV in placental and fetal tissues obtained from 50% of the miscarriages that occurred in their population and reported that mothers who subsequently went on to develop full-blown AIDS suffered a high fetal wastage rate.

These data need cautious interpretation since it is not known whether it is the presence of the virus, the mother's general health or her immunocompromised status that is the cause of the reported increase in fetal loss rates.

Bacterial vaginosis and miscarriage

Bacterial vaginosis (BV) is defined as an alteration in vaginal flora associated with absent or reduced lactobacilli and a rise in vaginal pH to greater than 4.5. The presence of BV before pregnancy and during early pregnancy has been associated with a seven-fold increase in risk of premature rupture of membranes and a two-fold increase in risk of preterm labour.[51] At the Recurrent Miscarriage Clinic at St Mary's Hospital, London, 199 women who presented with a history of early miscarriage alone and a history at least one late miscarriage were screened. BV was diagnosed in 22% of the women with a history of at least one late miscarriage screened before pregnancy, compared with 9.7% of women with a history of early miscarriages only ($P = 0.02$).[52]

In a study[53] carried out in women undergoing IVF treatment, the presence of BV at the time of egg retrieval was shown to have no detrimental effect on conception rates. Furthermore, there was no difference in the miscarriage rate at 7 and 12 weeks between those patients with BV and those without. However, this study did report a two-fold increase in the risk of miscarriage at or before six weeks of gestation, suggesting that BV may contribute to the problem of fetal loss by reducing the number of subclinical or biochemical pregnancies.

If this is the case, the possibility should be considered that BV may induce a noninflammatory endometrial response in the host that, despite the absence of classical markers of inflammation or infection, is capable of disturbing the normal process of implantation. The concept of 'bacteria endometrialis' has been put forward by Viniker[54] and suggests that we should be investigating whether the presence of BV in the vagina is a marker of a subclinical and disordered host response in the higher genital tract underlying many common gynaecological and obstetric disorders such as subfertility, miscarriage, pelvic pain, premature delivery, placental insufficiency and pre-eclampsia.

For the clinician, confusion remains: should all pregnant women be screened and treated for BV? Many studies have shown an increased risk of late miscarriage and preterm labour in women with BV.[51,52,55,56] One randomised and controlled study[57] of antibiotic therapy conducted in Australia reported that the benefit of treatment with metronidazole in pregnancy for women with proven BV is confined to a subgroup of women with a history of previous preterm labour. It is tempting to speculate that this finding reflects the possibility that some women have an increased susceptibility (or alternatively a suboptimal immune response) to the presence of bacterial colonisation and that, in a different host mother, the same organisms do not lead to any clinical sequelae. However, a more recent dataset obtained from a large multicentre study conducted in the USA has demonstrated that the use of metronidazole and other antibiotics in women with BV does not reduce the late miscarriage or preterm delivery rate.[58]

Inherited immunodeficiency and miscarriage

To date, the search for infectious causes of miscarriage has been limited to the identification of organisms in maternal and fetal blood, the genital tract or placenta. However, as noted earlier in this chapter, the identification of individual organisms has proven to be a disappointing method for predicting miscarriage and other pregnancy complications. This suggests that the outcome of pregnancy is determined by the maternal or fetal host response to the infection, not merely the presence of an infective organism.

Reports of the importance of molecular mutations in the aetiology of severe neonatal and infant infections in babies with mannose-binding protein (MBP) deficiency has raised the exciting possibility that gene mutations inherited by the fetus are a cause of both sporadic and recurrent episodes of miscarriage, secondary to an increased fetal susceptibility to infection *in utero*. Of course, it is likely that there are a multitude of gene mutations involved, since the innate and acquired human immune systems are complex and have many components. Nonetheless, a brief summary of what is known concerning MBP mutations and their effect on immunodeficiency serves as a useful introduction to a potentially productive avenue of research for the future.

MBP is a calcium-dependent plasma lectin synthesised by the liver and secreted as an acute-phase protein in response to infection. MBP is an essential component of the innate immune system. MBP binds to sugars on the surface of microbes and activates complement. Deficient levels of MBP are the most common cause of inherited immunodeficiency worldwide.[59] In populations in the West, serum levels of MBP are determined by three common mutations of the MBP gene. Severe recurrent infections are seen in neonates and young children who are homozygous for these MBP gene mutations,[60–62] and preterm infants have a higher prevalence of homozygosity for this gene.[63]

The possibility that MBP gene mutations are a cause of fetal loss *in utero* is suggested firstly by the small number of homozygote liveborn fetuses who carry this mutation (significantly fewer than would be expected by Hardy–Weinberg calculations) and secondly because low serum levels of MBP have been reported in couples with recurrent miscarriage.[64,65] Whereas MBP polymorphisms are associated with susceptibility to infection, tumour necrosis factor (TNF) polymorphisms are associated with severity of infection. Elevated maternal and fetal levels of TNF-α have been found in cases of premature membrane rupture and preterm delivery[66] and may therefore be additionally associated with late miscarriage due to genital tract infection.

In a study[67] at St Mary's Hospital, London, we recruited 77 white couples with a history of three consecutive miscarriages who had undergone detailed investigation and been found to have no established abnormality to account for their pregnancy losses, according to our established clinical protocol. The control group ($n=71$) comprised couples who had at least one previous live birth at term and no history of miscarriage. State-of-the-art assays (hybridisation to immobilised sequence-specific oligonucleotides) were used to determine the MBP and TNF genotypes. In this carefully defined population, no association was found between recurrent miscarriage and variations of the MBP and TNF genes. However, a trend in association with late miscarriage and preterm labour was noticed.

Conclusion

In the 21st century, advances in medical science will be led by new discoveries and a better understanding of molecular genetics. Clinicians interested in the aetiology of infections in pregnancy that determine fetal loss, perinatal mortality and morbidity need to ask themselves an important question: has any progress been made in the last 20 years?

Sadly, the answer has to be very little. Medical research into the infective causes of miscarriage is still in the dark ages. Clinical scientists have found an infective aetiology for ageing, gastric ulcers, cardiovascular disease and several autoimmune conditions but infective causes for the most common complication of pregnancy – miscarriage – are still speculative. Future research efforts need to be focused in a different direction. Instead of looking for organisms, factors that predispose a mother and her baby to being more susceptible to infection during pregnancy should be investigated. In simple terms, we should stop looking for 'bugs' and start looking for genetic susceptibility.

References

1. Kline J, Stein Z, Susser M. Conception and reproductive loss: probabilities. In: Kline J, Stein Z, Susser M, editors. *Conception to Birth: Epidemiology of Prenatal Development*. New York: Oxford University Press; 1989. p. 43–68.
2. Regan L. Sporadic and recurrent miscarriage. In: Grudzinskas JG, O'Brien PMS, editors. *Problems in Early Pregnancy: Advances in Diagnosis and Management*. London: RCOG Press; 1997. p. 31–52.
3. Clifford K, Rai R, Watson H, Regan L. An informative protocol for the investigation of recurrent miscarriage: preliminary experience of 500 consecutive cases. *Hum Reprod* 1994;**9**:1328–32.
4. Regan L. Recurrent miscarriage. In: Kurjak A, Exalto N, editors. *Textbook of Perinatal Medicine*. Carnforth: Parthenon; 1998. p. 953–1027.
5. Clifford K, Rai R, Regan L. Future pregnancy outcome in unexplained recurrent first trimester miscarriage. *Hum Reprod* 1997;**12**:387–9.
6. Regan L. *Miscarriage – What Every Woman Needs to Know*. London: Orion Publications; 2001.
7. Stray-Pedersen B. Genital tract infections and recurrent miscarriage. *Infertility and Reproductive Medicine Clinics of North America* 1996;**7**:795–806.
8. Summers P. Microbiology relevant to recurrent miscarriage. *Clin Obstet Gynecol* 1994;**37**:722–9.
9. Simpson JL, Gray RH, Queenan JT, Barbato M, Perez A, Mena P, et al. Further evidence that infection is an infrequent cause of first trimester spontaneous abortion. *Hum Reprod* 1996;**11**:2058–60.
10. Regan L. Recurrent miscarriage [editorial]. *BMJ* 1991;**302**:543–4.
11. Desmonts G, Daffos F, Forestier F, Capella-Pavlovsky M, Thulliez P, Chartier M. Prenatal diagnosis of congenital toxoplasmosis. *Lancet* 1985;**i**:500–4.
12. Wallon, M, Liou C, Garner P, Peyron F. Congenital toxoplasmosis: systematic review of evidence of efficacy of treatment in pregnancy. *BMJ* 1999;**318**:1511–14.
13. Allain JP, Palmer CR, Pearson G. Epidemiological study of latent and recent infection by *Toxoplasma gondii* in pregnant women from a regional population in the UK. *J Infect* 1998;**36**:189–96.
14. Ancelle T, Goulet V, Tirard-Fleury V, Baril L, du Mazaubrun C, Thulliez P, et al. La toxoplasmose chez la femme enceinte en France en 1995. Resultats d'une enquête nationale perinatale. *Bulletin Epidemiologique Hebdomadaire* 1996;**51**:227–9.
15. Remington JS, McLeod R, Desmonts G. Toxoplasmosis. In: Remington JS, Klein JO, editors. *Infectious Diseases of the Fetus and Newborn*. 4th ed. Pennsylvania: WB Saunders, 1995. p. 140–267.
16. Cook AJC, Gilbert RE, Buffolano W, Zufferey J, Peterson E, Jenum PA, et al. Sources of toxoplasma infection in pregnant women: European multicentre case-control study. European Research Network on Congenital Toxoplasmosis. *BMJ* 2000;**321**:142–7.
17. Dubey JP. Toxoplasmosis in sheep, goats, pigs and cattle. In: Dubey J, Beattie C, editors. *Toxoplasmosis in Animals and Man*. Boca Raton (FL): CRC Press; 1988. p. 61–114.

18. Eurostat. *Eurostat Agricultural Yearbook.* Luxembourg: Statistical Office for the European Community; 1996.
19. Dubey JP. Re-examination of resistance of *Toxoplasma gondii* tachyzoites and bradyzoites to pepsin and trypsin digestion. *Parasitology* 1998;**116**:43–50.
20. Bonametti AM, Passos JN, Koga de Silva EM, Macedo ZS. Probable transmission of acute toxoplasmosis through breast feeding. *J Trop Ped* 1997;**43**:116.
21. Burgess MA. Gregg's rubella legacy 1941–1991. *Med J Aust* 1991;**155**:355–7.
22. Weller TH, Neva A. Propagation in tissue culture of cytopathic agents from patients with rubella-like illness. *Proc Soc Exp Biol Med* 1962;**111**:215–25.
23. Parkman PD, Buescher EL, Artenstein MS. Recovery of rubella virus from army recruits. *Proc Soc Exp Biol Med* 1962;**111**:225–30.
24. Plotkin JA, Farquhar JD, Katz M. Attenuation of RA 27/3 rubella virus in WI-38 human diploid cells. *Am J Dis Child* 1969;**118**:178–85.
25. Morgan-Capner P. Rubella. In: Jeffries DJ, Hudson CN, editors. *Viral Infections in Obstetrics and Gynaecology.* London: Arnold; 1999. p. 15–35.
26. Boppana SB, Fowler KB, Britt WJ, Stagno S, Pass RF. Congenital cytomegalovirus infection following first trimester maternal infection. *Pediatrics* 1999;**104**:55–60.
27. Stagno S. Pass RF, Cloud G, *et al.* Primary cytomegalovirus infection in pregnancy. *JAMA* 1986;**256**:1904–8.
28. Griffiths PD, Baboonian C. A prospective study of primary cytomegalovirus infection during pregnancy: final report. *Br J Obstet Gynaecol* 1984;**91**:307–15.
29. Stagno S, Pass RF, Dwosky ME, Henderson RE, Moore EG, Walton PD. Congenital cytomegalovirus infection: The relative importance of primary and recurrent maternal infection. *N Engl J Med* 1982;**306**:945–9.
30. Boppana S, Pass RF. Cytomegalovirus. In: Jeffries DJ, Hudson CN, editors. *Viral Infections in Obstetrics and Gynaecology.* London: Arnold; 1999. p. 35–6.
31. Kinney JS, Onorato IM, Stewart JA, *et al.* Cytomegaloviral infection and disease. *J Infect Dis* 1985;**151**:772–4.
32. Watts DH, Eschenbach DA. Reproductive tract infections as a cause of abortion and preterm birth. *Semin Reprod Endocrinol* 1988;**6**:203–15.
33. Quinn PA, Petric M, Barkin M, Butany J, Derzko C, Gysler M, *et al.* Prevalence of antibody to *Chlamydia trachomatis* in spontaneous abortion and infertility. *Am J Obstet Gynecol* 1987;**156**:291–6.
34. Witkin SS, Ledger WJ. Antibodies to *Chlamydia trachomatis* in sera of women with recurrent spontaneous abortions. *Am J Obstet Gynecol* 1992;**167**:135–9.
35. Licciardi F, Grifo JA, Rosenwaks Z, Witkin SS. Relation between antibodies to *Chlamydia trachomatis* and spontaneous abortion following *in vitro* fertilisation. *J Assist Reprod Genet* 1992;**9**:207–10.
36. Lunefeld E, Shapiro BS, Sarov B, Sarov I, Insler V, DeCherney A. The association between chlamydia specific IgG and IgA antibodies and pregnancy outcome in an *in vitro* fertilisation program. *J In Vitro Fert Embryo Transf* 1989;**6**:222–7.
37. Rae R, Smith JW, Liston WA, Kilpatrick DC. Chlamydia serologic studies and spontaneous abortion. *Am J Obstet Gynecol* 1994;**170**:782–5.
38. Osser S, Persson K. Chlamydial antibodies in women who suffer miscarriage. *Br J Obstet Gynaecol* 1996;**103**:137–41.
39. Gronroos M, Honkonen E, Terho P, Punnonen R. Cervical and serum IgA and serum IgG antibodies to *Chlamydia trachomatis* and herpes simplex virus in threatened abortion: A prospective study. *Br J Obstet Gynaecol* 1983;**90**:167–70.
40. Munday PE, Porter R, Falder PF, Carder JM, Holliman R, Lewis BV, *et al.* Spontaneous abortion – an infectious aetiology? *Br J Obstet Gynaecol* 1984;**91**:1177–80.
41. Witkin SS, Sultan KM, Neal GS, Jeremias J, Grifo JA, Rosenwaks Z. Unsuspected *Chlamydia trachomatis* infection and *in vitro* fertilisation outcome. *Am J Obstet Gynecol* 1994;**171**:1208–14.
42. Mindel A. Genital herpes – the forgotten epidemic. *Herpes* 1994;**1**:39–48.
43. Whitely R. Herpes simplex virus infection of women and their offspring: implications for a developed society. *Proc Natl Acad Sci U S A* 1994;**91**:2441–7.
44. Mindel A. Herpes simplex virus infections in pregnancy. In: Jeffries DJ, Hudson CN, editors. *Viral Infections in Obstetrics and Gynaecology.* London: Arnold; 1999. p. 115–34.
45. Nahmias AJ, Josey WE, Naib ZM, Freeman MG, Fernandez RJ, Wheeler JH. Perinatal risk associated with maternal genital herpes simplex virus infection. *Am J Obstet Gynecol* 1971;**110**:825–37.
46. Grossman JH, Wallen WC, Sever JL. Management of genital herpes simplex virus infection during pregnancy. *Obstet Gynecol* 1981;**58**:1–4.

47. Harger JH, Pazin GJ, Armstrong JA, Breinig MC, Ho M. Characteristics and management of pregnancy in women with genital herpes simplex virus infection. *Am J Obstet Gynecol* 1983;**145**:784–91.
48. Stray-Pedersen B, Stray-Pedersen S. Etiologic factors and subsequent reproductive performance in 195 couples with a prior history of habitual abortion. *Am J Obstet Gynecol* 1984;**148**:140–6.
49. Stray-Pedersen B. New aspects of perinatal infections. *Ann Med* 1993;**25**:295.
50. Langston C, Lewis DE, Hammill HA, Popek EJ, Kozinetz CA, Kline MW, *et al*. Excess intrauterine fetal demise associated with maternal human immunodeficiency virus infection. *J Infect Dis* 1995;**172**:1451–60.
51. Kurki T, Sivonen A, Renkonen O, Savia E, Ylikorkala O. Bacterial vaginosis in early pregnancy and pregnancy outcome. *Obstet Gynaecol* 1992;**80**:173–7.
52. Llahi-Camp JM, Rai R, Ison C, Regan L, Taylor-Robinson D. Association of bacterial vaginosis with a history of second trimester miscarriage. *Hum Reprod* 1996;**11**:1575–8.
53. Ralph SG, Rutherford AJ, Wilson JD. Influence of bacterial vaginosis on conception and miscarriage in the first trimester: cohort study. *BMJ* 1999;**319**:220–3.
54. Viniker DA. Hypothesis on the role of sub-clinical bacteria of the endometrium (bacteria endometrialis) in gynaecological and obstetric enigmas. *Hum Reprod Update* 1999;**5**:373–85.
55. Hay PE, Lamont RF, Taylor-Robinson D, Morgan DJ, Ison C, Pearson J. Abnormal bacterial colonisation of genital tract and subsequent preterm delivery and late miscarriage. *BMJ* 1994;**308**:295–8.
56. Hillier SL, Nugent RP, Eschenback DA, Krohn MA, Gibbs RS, Martin DH, *et al*. Association between bacterial vaginosis and preterm delivery of a low-birth-weight infant. *N Engl J Med* 1995;**333**:1737–42.
57. McDonald HM, O'Loughlin JA, Vigneswaran R, Jolley PT, Harvey JA, Bof A, *et al*. Impact of metronidazole therapy on preterm birth in women with bacterial vaginosis flora (*Gardnerella vaginalis*): a randomised, placebo controlled trial. *Br J Obstet Gynaecol* 1997;**104**:1391–7.
58. Carey JC, Klebanoff MA, Hauth JC, Hillier SL, Thom EA, Ernest JM, *et al*. Metronidazole to prevent preterm delivery in pregnant women with asymptomatic bacterial vaginosis. National Institute of Child Health and Human Development Network of Maternal-Fetal Medicine Units. *N Engl J Med* 2000;**342**:534–40.
59. Sumiya M, Summerfield JA. The role of collectins in host defense. *Semin Liver Dis* 1997;**17**:311–18.
60. Summerfield JA, Ryder S, Sumiya M, Thursz M, Gorchein A, Montei MA, *et al*. Mannose binding protein gene mutations associated with unusual and severe infections in adults. *Lancet* 1995;**345**:886–9.
61. Summerfield JA, Sumiya M, Levin M, Turner MW. Association of mutations in mannose binding protein gene with childhood infection in consecutive hospital series. *BMJ* 1997;**314**:1229–32.
62. Sumiya M, Super M, Tabona P, Levinsky RJ, Arai T, Turner ME, *et al*. Molecular basis of opsonic defect in immunodeficient children. *Lancet* 1991;**337**:1569–70.
63. Lau YL, Chan SY, Turner MW, Fong J, Karlberg J. Mannose-binding protein in preterm infants: developmental profile and clinical significance. *Clin Exp Immunol* 1995;**102**:649–54.
64. Kilpatrick DC, Bevan BH, Liston WA. Association between mannan binding protein deficiency and recurrent miscarriage. *Hum Reprod* 1995;**10**:2501–5.
65. Kilpatrick DC, Starrs L, Moore S, Souter V, Liston WA. Mannan binding lectin concentration and risk of miscarriage. *Hum Reprod* 1999;**9**:2379–80.
66. Roberts AK, Monson-Bordonoba F, Van Deerlin PG, Holder J, Macones GA, Morgan MA, *et al*. Association of polymorphism within the promoter of the tumor necrosis factor alpha gene with increased risk of preterm premature rupture of the fetal membranes. *Am J Obstet Gynecol* 1999;**180**:1297–302.
67. Baxter N, Sumiya M, Cheng S, Erlich H, Regan L, Simons A, *et al*. Recurrent miscarriage and variant alleles of mannose binding lectin and tumour necrosis factor genes. *Clin Exp Immunol* 2001. In press.

Chapter 27

Infection in preterm labour

Ronald F Lamont

Introduction

Preterm birth is the major cause of death and handicap in the neonate in the developed world. The aetiology of spontaneous preterm labour and birth is multifactorial but there is strong evidence to implicate infection as a possible cause. Our knowledge of the microbiology and biochemistry of normal and abnormal genital-tract flora in relation to spontaneous preterm labour is increasing. It is not enough to concentrate on the exposure of the mother and fetus to abnormal genital-tract flora – the potential adverse effects of the fetomaternal immune response and the susceptibility of the mother and fetus to such a reaction must be considered.

Importance of preterm birth

With the improvement in operators' skills and technological advances in obstetric ultrasound, preterm birth, i.e. birth before 37 completed weeks of gestation, has overtaken congenital malformations as the major cause of death and handicap in the developed world. Approximately 13 million preterm births occur annually worldwide. The incidence ranges from 5.6% in Oceania to 11% in North America. Europe, with an incidence of 5.8%, accounts for approximately 400 000 cases annually.[1] Despite the use of tocolytics to delay or prevent preterm birth,[2] the use of antepartum glucocorticoids to reduce the incidence and severity of idiopathic respiratory distress syndrome (IRDS)[3] and the improvements in neonatal intensive care facilities, the mortality and morbidity following preterm birth has remained relatively constant over the last 20 years. At 24 weeks of gestation, 80% of babies die and it is not until 30 weeks that 90% of babies survive. While most preterm births occur after 35 weeks of gestation, virtually all of the mortality and morbidity occurs in babies born before 34 weeks of gestation.[4] A recently reported Epicure study[5] examined the outcome of over 1100 babies born between 22 and 26 weeks of gestation in the UK and Ireland over a nine-month period from March to December in 1995. Approximately 65% of these babies died in the delivery suite or in the neonatal intensive care unit. Of those babies whom it was possible to follow up at 30 months, approximately half were found to be suffering from some form of disability and in 50% of these the disability was severe. The estimated weekly cost of neonatal intensive care in the USA is approximately $10,000 per week, with an annual total cost of approximately $5 billion.[6]

The heterogeneity of preterm birth

Spontaneous preterm labour is either a physiological process occurring too early in pregnancy or a pathological process as a result of an abnormal trigger such as infection. While the final endocrine and paracrine process of labour may be the same, the nearer to 37 weeks of gestation at which labour occurs, the more likely labour is to be physiological. Conversely, the earlier in gestation at which spontaneous preterm labour occurs, the more likely this is to be due to a pathological process such as infection. The heterogeneity of preterm birth dictates that the following are all considered as preterm births but they are clearly due to different aetiologies and require different approaches to management:

- spontaneous preterm labour and birth at 36 completed weeks of gestation
- iatrogenic elective preterm birth at 34 weeks of gestation, as a result of fulminating pre-eclampsia
- spontaneous preterm labour and birth at 30 weeks of gestation, following an antepartum haemorrhage due to placental abruption
- spontaneous preterm labour and birth at 26 weeks of gestation, following spontaneous preterm prelabour rupture of the membranes (PPROM).

Evidence implicating infection as a cause of spontaneous preterm labour and birth

The aetiology of preterm birth is multifactorial but there is strong evidence to implicate infection as a possible cause[7–10] in up to 40% of cases.[11] In the 1960s, urinary tract infection was found to be associated with preterm birth.[12] Some investigators claimed that asymptomatic bacteriuria was associated with preterm birth but others suggested that pyelonephritis had to be present. It is known that 3% of pregnant women develop asymptomatic bacteriuria and 30% of these develop a symptomatic urinary tract infection. In a meta-analysis,[13] women with asymptomatic bacteriuria who were untreated had a statistically significantly increased risk of giving birth prematurely to low-birthweight (LBW) babies. Retrospective data from the 1970s from more than 1000 consecutive neonatal postmortems showed that, of those babies who died because of congenital pneumonia, a significant proportion had been born in the presence of chorioamnionitis. Of those who were born in the presence of chorioamnionitis, a significant proportion had been born preterm. The conclusion, in retrospect, was that infection was a cause of spontaneous preterm labour and birth.[14] Sixteen percent of women with intact membranes in spontaneous preterm labour will have positive cultures of amniotic fluid obtained at amniocentesis. At least 30% of those with ruptured membranes will have positive cultures. Chorioamnionitis and all forms of neonatal sepsis (e.g. congenital pneumonia, septicaemia and meningitis) and maternal sepsis (e.g. postpartum endometritis) are much more common after preterm than after term birth.[15] A past medical history of pelvic inflammatory disease or even intrauterine contraceptive device usage without such disease is associated with a 2.4-fold increased risk in the incidence of spontaneous preterm labour and birth. C-reactive protein (CRP) is an acute-phase protein secreted by the liver in response to inflammation. Women admitted in spontaneous preterm labour have significantly increased mean levels of CRP compared with women of the same gestation who are not in labour.[16] Women with increased levels of CRP are refractory to the use of tocolytics.[17] PPROM is associated with infection but whether this is cause or effect is not known and it is likely to be due to a combination of the two.[18]

Biochemical mechanisms of spontaneous preterm labour and birth

Labour is a dual process involving a decrease in cervical resistance leading to progressive effacement and dilatation, accompanied by an increase in uterine contractility resulting in longer, stronger, more frequent and more synchronous contractions. Prostaglandins induce both of these processes. Prostaglandins are synthesised from arachidonic acid, which is the obligate precursor of prostaglandin synthesis. Arachidonic acid is released from glycerophospholipids in the cell membrane by specific phospholipase enzymes such as phospholipase A_2 (PLA_2). Microorganisms are known to produce PLA_2[19] and microorganisms added to amnion *in vitro* can be shown to produce an increase in prostaglandin production.[20-22] By producing other enzymes such as proteases or mucinases, microorganisms may penetrate the cervical mucus plug. Thereafter, by producing enzymes such as collagenases or elastases, they may cause membrane disruption, which either leads to PPROM or release of PLA_2 enzymes from intracellular organelles (lysosomes) resulting in an increased release of arachidonic acid with prostaglandin synthesis.[7,8,23] Finally, by producing endotoxins, microorganisms induce macrophages to produce cytokines, which also drive the arachidonic acid cascade towards production of prostaglandins.[7,24] Pro-inflammatory cytokines such as interleukin-1, interleukin-6, interleukin-8 and tumour necrosis factor alpha are found in significantly increased concentrations in the amniotic fluid of women in spontaneous preterm labour with infection compared with women without infection.[25] The presence of these cytokines in amniotic fluid and fetal blood has been shown to be associated with fetal and neonatal tissue damage to brain and lung resulting in bronchopulmonary dysplasia[26] and periventricular leukomalacia.[27] Those babies born preterm in the presence of increased concentrations of interleukin-6 or interleukin-8 in amniotic fluid, increased white blood cell concentrations or funisitis (inflammation of umbilical cord vessels) are statistically significantly more likely to develop cerebral palsy by the age of three years.[28]

Normal and abnormal genital-tract flora

The vaginal flora is normally dominated by lactobacillus species, which produce lactic acid that maintains vaginal pH below 4.5. At this acidic pH, the growth of other organisms is suppressed. As normal pregnancy progresses, the total number of organisms in the vagina, both aerobes and anaerobes, increases. Aerobic organisms dominate so that, by term, the vagina is colonised by organisms of low virulence, which pose no significant threat to the fetus passing through the birth canal. At this low pH, lactobacilli produce hydrogen peroxide (H_2O_2), which is toxic to bacteria, firstly by producing toxic hydroxyl radicals and secondly by combining with a large pool of chlorine ions in the vagina to produce chloradinium ions. Under circumstances of increased alkalinity, such as bleeding in pregnancy (blood pH = 7.4), or sexual intercourse (semen pH = 8) or vaginal douching, lactobacilli lose their ability to produce H_2O_2. As a result, the normal lactobacillus-dominated flora is replaced by a thousand-fold overgrowth of anaerobic organisms and other organisms such as *Gardnerella vaginalis*, *Mycoplasma hominis* and *Mobiluncus* spp. These organisms produce keto-acids such as succinate, which blunts the chemotactic response of polymorphonuclear leukocytes and also their killing ability. As a result, there is little leukocytic activity despite large numbers of potentially pathogenic organisms. As there is no cellular inflammatory process (there may be a chemical inflammatory process involving cytokines), the condition is known as bacterial vaginosis (BV) rather than vaginitis. The prevalence, aetiology, natural history, diagnosis, adverse sequelae and treatment of BV are discussed in Chapter 14.

Using Gram stain of vaginal secretions, vaginal flora can be classified as grade I: normal (predominantly lactobacillus morphotypes); grade II: intermediate (reduced lactobacillus morphotypes mixed with other bacterial morphotypes); or grade III: bacterial vaginosis (few or no lactobacillus morphotypes with greatly increased numbers of *G. vaginalis* and other morphotypes). By examining the detailed microbiology of these different grades of genital-tract flora on Gram stain, a different distribution of bacterial species can be observed. The ability to isolate some organisms, such as lactobacillus species, decreases linearly from 91% in grade I to 66% in grade II and 38% in grade III. Some, such as α-haemolytic streptococcus or corynebacterium, show a linear increase in colonisation species (9% to 36% to 56% and 36% to 56% to 84%, respectively). Some organisms, such as coagulase-negative staphylococcus species, were isolated from a similar number of grade I (58%), grade II (78%) and grade III (74%) smears. Some organisms, such as *G. vaginalis*, *M. hominis* and many anaerobes, were isolated rarely in grade I and grade II and were only fully manifest with high isolation rates in grade III Gram stain. In this way, it is possible, using a cheap and simple test such as Gram stain of vaginal secretions, to predict the likelihood of the presence of particular organisms (Table 27.1).[29].

Abnormal genital-tract flora and the prediction of spontaneous preterm labour and birth

Although there is strong evidence to implicate infection as a possible cause of spontaneous preterm labour and birth in up to 40% of cases, by the time a woman is

Table 27.1.   Isolation of different organisms from women with grade III flora (bacterial vaginosis) and grade I flora (normal) following Gram stain of vaginal secretions

Organism	Grade I flora (normal) (%)	Grade III flora (bacterial vaginosis) (%)
Pathogenic organisms		
Chlamydia trachomatis	0	12
Microaerophilic flora		
Lactobacillus spp.	91	38
Gardnerella vaginalis	5	72
Aerobic flora		
Corynebacterium spp.	36	84
Coagulase-negative staphylococcus	58	7
Staphylococcus aureus	9	14
Haemolytic streptococcus	9	56
β-haemolytic streptococcus	0	4
Gram-negative rods	0	12
Candida spp.	21	14
Ureaplasma/mycoplasma		
Mycoplasma hominis	6	58
Ureaplasma urealyticum	42	68
Anaerobes		
Gram-positive cocci (e.g. *Peptococcus* spp. and *Peptostreptococcus* spp.)	15	74
Gram-negative rods (e.g. *Bacteroides* spp., *Prevotella* spp. and *Fusobacterium* spp.)	9	66
Bifidobacterium spp.	12	94
Other Gram-positive rods (e.g. *Mobiluncus* spp. and *Propionibacterium* spp.)	15	48

Adapted from Rosenstein *et al.*[29]

admitted in labour, there may already be irreversible changes in the uterine cervix that render any attempts to inhibit or reverse the process unsuccessful. It would seem more logical to use the information that infection was a potential cause of spontaneous preterm labour and birth to identify a group of women at risk due to abnormal genital-tract flora in early pregnancy. Minkoff *et al.*[30] carried out detailed microbiology of 233 women between 14 and 18 weeks of gestation. Those women colonised by *Bacteroides* spp., *Trichomonas vaginalis* or *Ureaplasma* spp. were statistically significantly more likely to experience PPROM, spontaneous preterm labour and preterm birth. A screening test to identify abnormal genital-tract flora should be inexpensive, simple, safe and reproducible. Detailed microbiology is expensive and up to 26 different organisms may be detected in women in spontaneous preterm labour. Even in those women who are not in spontaneous preterm labour but require elective preterm delivery for maternal or fetal indications, up to 15 different organisms can be isolated.[31] A simple classification of abnormal genital flora is proposed in Table 27.2.

There are only three pathogens to consider, although *Haemophilus influenzae* often acts in a similar fashion to gonococcus (*Neisseria gonorrhoeae*), *T. vaginalis* and *Chlamydia trachomatis*. *Trichomonas vaginalis* infection is associated with a statistically significantly increased risk of LBW and preterm birth but not PPROM.[32] In

Table 27.2. Simple classification of abnormal genital tract colonisation in pregnancy

Class		Organism
I	Pathogens	*Chlamydia trachomatis*
		Neisseria gonorrhoea
		Trichomonas vaginalis
II	Group B haemolytic streptococcus	
III	Enteropharyngeal organisms	e.g. *Streptococcus faecalis*
		Escherichia coli
IV	Bacterial vaginosis-related organisms	*Mycoplasma hominis*
		Gardnerella vaginalis
		Anaerobes

women negative for both BV and *T. vaginalis*, 10.8% delivered preterm compared with 17.3% in those with both present. While *C. trachomatis* in pregnancy is associated with PPROM and LBW, there is no association with preterm birth.

Group B streptococcus (GBS) is worth considering in a class of its own because of the devastating effects this may have on LBW or preterm babies. Since a light colonisation with GBS is not associated with LBW or preterm birth,[33] GBS is currently only considered important with respect to the intrapartum chemoprophylaxis for the prevention of early-onset neonatal GBS infection.[34] However, a heavy growth of GBS is associated with an increased risk of LBW and preterm birth.[33]

The presence of enteropharyngeal organisms is relative. Up to 5% of asymptomatic women delivered preterm electively because of fetal or maternal indications may be colonised by *Escherichia coli* and if these are present in small numbers with no polymorphonuclear leukocytes in an otherwise asymptomatic woman, this should probably be considered as normal endogenous flora. However, if *E. coli* is detected in high numbers with polymorphonuclear leukocytes and another enteropharyngeal organism or BV-related organism in a symptomatic woman, then this should be considered abnormal.

Cohort studies from Europe, the USA and the Far East[33,35-42] and three case–control studies from the USA, Sweden and Australia[43-45] have used different methodologies to examine the association with BV or BV-related organisms and the adverse outcome of pregnancy. While all the studies have focused on preterm birth or gestational age as an outcome parameter, they used different diagnostic techniques at varying gestational ages of screening. The majority of these studies showed a statistically significant association between abnormal genital-tract flora and adverse pregnancy outcome, and the degree of risk of preterm birth was greater the earlier in pregnancy at which the abnormal colonisation was detected. A positive result from screening at around 26 weeks of gestation was associated with 1.4- to 1.9-fold increased risk of preterm birth.[33,35,39,42] In contrast, a positive result from screening in the second trimester was associated with a 2.0- to 6.9-fold increased risk of adverse outcome.[36,37,40,41] In a longitudinal study of women in Indonesia,[40] the risk was almost double for women with BV in early pregnancy (21%) compared with those women who developed the condition later in pregnancy (11%). Using multiple regression analysis, BV diagnosed before 16 weeks of pregnancy was found to be associated with a five-fold increased risk of preterm birth or late miscarriage, independent of recognised risk factors such as previous preterm birth, black race or smoking.[37]

The use of antibiotics for the prevention of spontaneous preterm labour and birth

There are a number of situations in which antibiotics might be employed in the prevention of morbidity and mortality associated with spontaneous preterm labour and birth:

- prophylactically for women at increased risk of spontaneous preterm labour and birth because of abnormal genital tract colonisation
- prophylactically for the prevention of PPROM, and therapeutically to delay delivery in women who present with PPROM
- prophylactically for the prevention of early-onset GBS neonatal infection
- therapeutically to delay the delivery of women who present in spontaneous preterm labour.

Prophylactic antibiotics for women at increased risk of spontaneous preterm labour and birth because of abnormal genital-tract flora

A number of studies have examined the use of antibiotics for the prevention of preterm birth in women identified as being at risk of spontaneous preterm labour and birth due to infection. Unfortunately, the studies have used different doses of different antibiotics by different routes of administration and regimens to women of varying risk, with varying outcomes.[46]

The route of administration is important. There is merit in treating with local intravaginal antibiotics since the 1000-fold increase in genital-tract flora associated with BV may require a heavy loading dose of antibiotics to the vagina. If, however, the imbalance of genital-tract flora has existed from early pregnancy, then systemic therapy may be necessary to eradicate those organisms that have already gained access to the decidua by ascending colonisation.

The gestational age at the time of treatment is also important. The study by McDonald *et al.*[47] showed no benefit if therapy was introduced at 24 weeks of gestation. In the Carey study,[48] which also showed no benefit of antibiotics, 50% of the patients were treated after 20 weeks of gestation and none before 16 weeks. There are two published studies of the use of clindamycin vaginal cream, both of which showed no benefit of antibiotics. In one study,[49] 100% of the women were treated after 20 weeks of gestation and, in the other,[50] 60% were treated after 20 weeks. In contrast, two UK studies, as yet unpublished, showed that oral clindamycin and clindamycin vaginal cream administered early in pregnancy produced a significant reduction in the incidence of spontaneous preterm labour and birth.

The degree of abnormality of the genital-tract flora is also potentially important. In a subgroup analysis of a tricentre, randomised, double-blind placebo-controlled trial, women with grade III flora were found to respond better to clindamycin vaginal cream than those with either grade II flora or grades II and III combined, resulting in a greater reduction in the incidence of spontaneous preterm labour and birth.[51]

Antibiotics used prophylactically for the prevention of PPROM and therapeutically after PPROM

The literature with respect to PPROM is voluminous but has been reviewed in two meta-analyses.[52,53] These concluded that the use of antibiotics following PPROM could prolong pregnancy but was not associated with a reduction in perinatal mortality and morbidity. Many of the studies reviewed were conducted at late gestational ages where the incidence of IRDS was low and perinatal death too rare for any benefit to be observed. Conversely, other studies were conducted at gestational ages as low as 20 to 23 weeks, which was too close to the limit of viability for a reduction in the incidence of IRDS to be evident. In a subsequent study where antibiotics were used at between 24 and 32 weeks of gestation following PPROM, a significant reduction in perinatal mortality and morbidity was found, together with a reduction in maternal infectious morbidity and an increase in latency and delay of delivery.[54] In women who are at risk of PPROM, prophylactic antibiotics have been shown to reduce the subsequent incidence of PPROM.[55]

Intrapartum chemoprophylaxis for the prevention of early-onset Group B streptococcal infection of the neonate

While a heavy growth of GBS is associated with LBW and preterm birth,[34] most of the literature with respect to GBS is concerned with the use of intrapartum chemoprophylaxis for the prevention of early-onset GBS infection. Data from the UK are sparse although there are efforts to gather data from multidisciplinary groups in the UK (see Chapter 9).

Up to 30% of pregnant and nonpregnant women can be found to be colonised by GBS. The Centers for Disease Control and Prevention (CDC) in Atlanta, USA, estimated that there were 7600 cases of GBS sepsis (1.8% per 1000 live births) in the USA in 1990, which resulted in 310 deaths. In 1997, the American Academy of Pediatricians, the American College of Obstetricians and Gynecologists and the CDC published revised guidelines for the use of intrapartum chemoprophylaxis for the prevention of early-onset GBS infection in the neonate. They recommended either screening, or treating on the basis of risk. If screening is to be used to achieve the best possible isolation rates (up to 27%), the combination of a low vaginal swab and rectal swab should be cultured in selective broth medium. A high vaginal swab will only detect 5% of GBS colonisation. Screening should only occur after 35 weeks of gestation since, before this time, swabs do not reflect the genital-tract flora at term. If swab results are not available or labour occurs before this time, then prophylaxis should be given on the basis of risk factors (pyrexia, duration of ruptured membranes, prematurity). Women with positive screening results, those with incidental findings of GBS colonisation or those with a history of previous invasive GBS disease should be given intrapartum chemoprophylaxis without further screening or treatment during the pregnancy. The only situation where antibiotics are recommended during pregnancy for GBS is following diagnosis of GBS urinary-tract infection.

Intrapartum chemoprophylaxis should be in the form of penicillin given intravenously four-hourly, rather than ampicillin, to reduce the risk of producing resistant strains. For those women allergic to penicillin, the combination of erythromycin and clindamycin is recommended.[34] In a study to assess the effectiveness and feasibility of the screening-based protocol, the prevalence of early-onset GBS sepsis was found to be 1.16 per 1000 live births prior to institution of the policy and 0.14 per 1000 after the policy was implemented ($P < 0.001$). This represented an 88% reduction in early-onset GBS sepsis.[56]

The use of antibiotics to delay delivery in women in spontaneous preterm labour

A number of studies have shown latency when antibiotics are used in women in spontaneous preterm labour,[57-65] whereas others have shown no latency.[66-70] Of those studies that did show latency, it may be relevant that four used antibiotics active against anaerobes,[60-62,65] compared with only one of those studies that showed no latency.[70] Two of the studies that showed no latency stopped antibiotic treatment when amniotic fluid cultures proved positive so it is not surprising that antibiotics showed no latency.[66,67] In another study that showed no latency, despite a power calculation requiring 2000 women to be recruited, only 277 took part and only 60% completed study medication.[69] No constant benefit has been found between antibiotic treatment and pregnancy prolongation or a decrease in perinatal mortality or morbidity rate. This may be because pregnancy prolongation *per se* in the presence of infection is undesirable and a relative risk for the mother and fetus, particularly at later preterm gestations. The lack of consistent benefit may also be explained by the different antibiotics used. Clindamycin and metronidazole, in contrast to erythromycin and ampicillin, are effective against anaerobes. While erythromycin may be partially active against BV-related organisms, it cannot be fully activated in vaginal fluid. The combination of erythromycin and co-amoxiclav may also be ineffective since this is a combination of a bactericidal and a bacteriostatic antibiotic whose actions may cancel out the effectiveness of the other.

Kenyon *et al.*[71,72] recently completed a multicentre study on the effect of antibiotics on adverse outcomes of pregnancy. Co-amoxiclav alone or in combination with erythromycin prolonged pregnancy, without significant benefit for the neonate. When the multicentre study was conceived, ureaplasmas were considered important in the neonatal mortality and morbidity associated with spontaneous preterm labour and preterm birth[73] and this probably influenced the choice of erythromycin, which is not advocated in BV and is ineffective against anaerobes and *M. hominis*. When the study started in 1994, the detrimental influence of BV on the outcome of pregnancy was apparent, but BV was not considered as part of the study. Co-amoxiclav is effective against some anaerobes but is not useful in BV. Clindamycin has a better spectrum of activity and was reportedly considered but the reason for its dismissal was not given.

In the multicentre study, the clinician's subjective assessment of the risk of preterm birth was used rather than any objective measure of risk due to infection since no screen for BV or other infections was performed. Kenyon *et al.* reported that 89.9% and 84.6% of women with spontaneous preterm labour and intact membranes remained undelivered after 48 hours and 7 days, respectively. Only 41.3% required β-agonist therapy. The median gestational age at delivery was more than 38 completed weeks. Since infection is thought to cause up to 40% of cases of spontaneous preterm labour, it would appear that most women were not in spontaneous preterm labour. Of those who were, probably less than half were in labour due to infection. Consequently, it is not surprising that antibiotics did not lead to improved outcome.

Once spontaneous preterm labour begins, there may be irreversible changes in the uterine cervix mediated in part by the inflammatory response to infection, which make attempts to reverse the process futile. Antibiotics alone at this stage are unlikely to help. The earlier an abnormal flora is detected in pregnancy, the greater the risk of subsequent adverse pregnancy outcomes. It is, therefore, logical that antibiotics used to prevent preterm birth should be given early in pregnancy.

In the Kenyon study, it is likely that the wrong antibiotics were used on the wrong women, too late in pregnancy. If antibiotics are to be helpful in reducing the morbidity and mortality associated with late miscarriage and preterm birth, they should be given early in pregnancy to women with abnormal genital-tract flora. The results suggest that ureaplasmas do not cause neonatal disease because erythromycin was of little benefit, although ureaplasmal infection was not assessed in the study. It would have been helpful to determine the extent to which BV was associated with neonatal diseases since this might then have influenced the antibiotic regimen.

Conclusion

Infection is an important cause of spontaneous preterm labour and preterm birth. Abnormal genital-tract flora in early pregnancy is a useful predictor of subsequent pregnancy loss in the form of late miscarriage or spontaneous preterm labour and birth. The earlier in pregnancy at which this abnormal colonisation is detected, the greater is the subsequent risk of spontaneous preterm labour and birth. Antibiotics have the potential to prevent spontaneous preterm labour and delay preterm birth but the evidence shows lack of consistent benefit. If antibiotics are to be successful, it is likely that these will have to be administered early in pregnancy, be active against those organisms associated with BV and be used in those women likely to mount a damaging immune response and those women with the greatest degree of abnormal genital tract colonisation.

References

1. Villar J, Ezcurra EJ, Gurtner de la Fuente V, Campodonica L. Preterm delivery syndrome: the unmet need. In: Kierse MJNC, editor. New Perspectives for the Effective Treatment of Preterm Labour – an International Consensus. *Research and Clinical Forums* 1994;**16**:9–38.
2. Greenfield P, Lamont RF. Tocolytics. In: *Current Obstetrics and Gynaecology*. London: Harcourt; 2001.
3. Crowley P, Chalmers I, Keirse MJNC. The effect of corticosteroid administration prior to preterm delivery: an overview from the evidence from controlled trials. *Br J Obstet Gynaecol* 1990;**97**:11–25.
4. Magowan BA, Bain M, Juszczak E, McInneny K. Neonatal mortality amongst Scottish preterm singleton births (1985–1994). *Br J Obstet Gynaecol* 1998;**105**:1005–10.
5. Wood NS, Marlow N, Costeloe K, Gibson AT, Wilkinson AR. Neurologic and developmental disability after extremely preterm birth. EPICure Study Group. *N Engl J Med* 2000;**343**:378–84.
6. Keirse MJNC. New perspectives for the effective treatment of preterm labor. *Am J Obstet Gynecol* 1995;**173**:618–28.
7. Lamont RF, Fisk N. The role of infection in the pathogenesis of preterm labour. In: Studd JWW, editor. *Progress in Obstetrics and Gynaecology 10*. Edinburgh: Churchill Livingstone; 1993. p. 135–58.
8. McGregor JA, French JI, Lawellin D, Todd JK. Preterm birth and infection: pathogenic possibilities. *Am J Reprod Immunol Microbiol* 1988;**16**:123–32.
9. Mazor M, Chaim W, Horowitz S, Romero R, Glezerman M. The biomolecular mechanisms of preterm labor in women with intrauterine infection. *Isr J Med Sci* 1994;**30**:317–22.

10. Gibbs RS, Romero R, Hillier SL, Eschenbach DA, Sweet RL. A review of premature birth and subclinical infection. *Am J Obstet Gynecol* 1992;**166**:1515–28.
11. Lettieri L, Vintzileos AM, Rodis JF, Albini SM, Salafia CM. Does 'idiopathic' preterm labor resulting in preterm birth exist? *Am J Obstet Gynecol* 1993;**168**:1480–5.
12. Kass EH. Pyelonephritis and bacteraemia: a major problem in preventive medicine. *Ann Intern Med* 1962;**56**:46–53.
13. Romero R, Oyarzun E, Mazor M, Sirtori M, Hobbins JC, Bracken M. Meta-analysis of the relationship between asymptomatic bacteriuria and preterm delivery/low birth weight. *Obstet Gynecol* 1989;**73**:576–82.
14. Naeye RL, Peters EC. Causes and consequences of premature rupture of fetal membranes. *Lancet* 1980;**i**:193–4.
15. Romero R, Mazor M. Infection and preterm labor. *Clin Obstet Gynecol* 1988;**31**:553–584.
16. Farb HF, Arnesen M, Geistler P, Knox GE. C-reactive protein with premature rupture of membranes and premature labor. *Obstet Gynecol* 1983;**62**:49–51.
17. Ismail MA, Zinaman MJ, Lowensohn RI, Moawad AH. The significance of C-reactive protein levels in women with premature rupture of the membranes. *Am J Obstet Gynecol* 1985;**151**:541–4.
18. Zaaijman J Du T, Wilkinson AR, Keeling JW, Mitchell RG, Turnbull AC. Spontaneous premature rupture of the membranes: bacteriology, histology and neonatal outcome. *J Obstet Gynaecol* 1982;**2**:155–60.
19. Bejar R, Curbelo V, Davis C, Gluck L. Premature labor II. Bacterial sources of phospholipase. *Obstet Gynecol* 1981;**57**:479–81.
20. Lamont RF, Rose M, Elder MG. Effect of bacterial products on prostaglandin E production by amnion cells. *Lancet* 1985;**ii**:1131–3.
21. Lamont RF, Anthony R, Myatt L, Booth L, Furr PM, Taylor-Robinson D. Production of prostaglandin E2 by human amnion *in vitro* in response to addition of media conditioned by microorganisms associated with chorioamnionitis and preterm labor. *Am J Obstet Gynecol* 1990;**162**:819–25.
22. Bennett PR, Elder MG, Myatt L. The effects of lipoxygenase metabolites of arachidonic acid on human myometrial contractility. *Prostaglandins* 1987;**33**:837–84.
23. McGregor JA, French JI, Lawellin D, Franco-Buff A, Smith BA, Todd JK. *In vitro* study of bacterial protease-induced reduction of chorioamniotic membrane strength and elasticity. *Obstet Gynecol* 1987;**69**:167–74.
24. Romero R, Kadar N, Hobbins JC, Duff GW. Infection and labor: the detection of endotoxin in amniotic fluid. *Am J Obstet Gynecol* 1987;**157**:815–19.
25. Romero R, Gomez R, Mazor M, Ghezzi F, Yoon BH. The preterm labour syndrome. In: Elder MG, Lamont RF, Romero R, editors. *Preterm Labour*, Vol. 2. New York: Churchill Livingstone; 1997. p. 29–49.
26. Yoon BH, Romero R, Yang SH, Jun JK, Kim IO, Choi JH, *et al*. Interleukin-6 concentrations in umbilical cord plasma are elevated in neonates with white matter lesions associated with periventricular leukomalacia. *Am J Obstet Gynecol* 1996;**174**:1433–40.
27. Yoon BH, Romero R, Jun JK, Park KH, Park JD, Ghezzi F, *et al*. Amniotic fluid cytokines (interleukin-6, tumor necrosis factor-alpha, interleukin-1 beta, and interleukin-8) and the risk for the development of bronchopulmonary dysplasia. *Am J Obstet Gynecol* 1997;**177**:825–30.
28. Yoon BH, Romero R, Park JS, Kim CJ, Kim SH, Choi JH, *et al*. Fetal exposure to an intra-amniotic inflammation and the development of cerebral palsy at the age of three years. *Am J Obstet Gynecol* 2000;**182**:675–81.
29. Rosenstein IJ, Morgan DJ, Sheehan M, Lamont RF, Taylor-Robinson D. Bacterial vaginosis in pregnancy – distribution of bacterial species in different Gram-stain categories of the vaginal flora. *J Med Microbiol* 1996;**45**:120–6.
30. Minkoff H, Grunebaum AN, Schwarz RH, Feldman J, Cummings M, Crombleholme W, *et al*. Risk factors for prematurity and premature rupture of membranes: a prospective study of the vaginal flora in pregnancy. *Am J Obstet Gynecol* 1984;**150**:965–72.
31. Lamont RF, Taylor-Robinson D, Newman M, Wigglesworth JS, Elder MG. Spontaneous early preterm labour associated with abnormal genital bacterial colonisation. *Br J Obstet Gynaecol* 1986;**93**:804–10.
32. Cotch MF, Pastorek JG 2nd, Nugent RP, Hillier SL, Gibbs RS, Martin DH, *et al*. Trichomonas vaginalis associated with low birthweight and preterm delivery. The Vaginal Infections and Prematurity Study Group. *Sex Transm Dis* 1997;**24**:353–60.
33. Hillier SL, Nugent RP, Eschenbach DA, Krohn MA, Gibbs RS, Martin DH, *et al*. Association between bacterial vaginosis and preterm delivery of a low-birth-weight infant. The Vaginal Infections and Prematurity Study Group. *N Engl J Med* 1995;**333**:1737–42.
34. American Academy of Pediatrics Committee on Infectious Diseases and Committee on Fetus and

Newborn. Revised guidelines for prevention of early-onset group B streptococcal (GBS) infection. *Pediatrics* 1997;**99**:489–96.

35. Meis PJ, Goldenberg RL, Mercer B, Moawad A, Das A, McNellis D, *et al*. The preterm prediction study: significance of vaginal infections. National Institute of Child Health and Human Development Maternal-Fetal Medicine Units Network. *Am J Obstet Gynecol* 1995;**173**:1231–5.

36. Kurki T, Sivonen A, Renkonen OV, Savia E, Ylkikorkala O. Bacterial vaginosis in early pregnancy and pregnancy outcome. *Obstet Gynecol* 1992;**80**:173–7.

37. Hay PE, Lamont RF, Taylor-Robinson D, Morgan DJ, Ison C, Pearson J. Abnormal bacterial colonisation of the genital tract as a marker for subsequent preterm delivery and late miscarriage. *BMJ* 1994;**308**:295–8.

38. Gratalos E, Figueras F, Barranco M, Vila J, Cararach V, Alonso PL, *et al*. Spontaneous recovery of bacterial vaginosis during pregnancy is not associated with an improved perinatal outcome. *Acta Obstet Gynecol Scand* 1998;**77**:37–40.

39. Gravett MG, Nelson HP, DeRouen T, Critchlow C, Eschenbach DA, Holmes KK. Independent association of BV and chlamydia trachomatis infection with adverse pregnancy outcome. *JAMA* 1986;**256**:1899–903.

40. Riduan JM, Hillier SL, Utomo B, Wiknjosastro G, Linnan M, Kandun N. BV and prematurity in Indonesia: association in late and early pregnancy. *Am J Obstet Gynecol* 1993;**169**:175–8.

41. McGregor JA, French JI, Jones W, Milligan K, McKinney PJ, Patterson E, *et al*. Bacterial vaginosis is associated with prematurity and vaginal fluid mucinase and sialidase: Results of a controlled trial of topical clindamycin cream. *Am J Obstet Gynecol* 1994;**170**:1048–60.

42. Wennerholm UB, Holm B, Mattsby-Baltzer I, Nielsen T, Plats-Christiansen J, Sundell G, *et al*. Fetal fibronectin, endotoxin, bacterial vaginosis and cervical length as predictors of preterm birth and neonatal morbidity in twin pregnancies. *Br J Obstet Gynaecol* 1997;**104**:1398–404.

43. Holst E, Goffeng AR, Anersch B. Bacterial vaginosis and vaginal microorganisms in idiopathic premature labor and association with pregnancy outcome. *J Clin Microbiol* 1994;**32**:176–86.

44. Eschenbach DA, Gravett MG, Chen KC, Hoyme UB, Holmes KK. Bacterial vaginosis during pregnancy. An association with prematurity and postpartum complications. *Scand J Urol Nephrol Suppl* 1984;**86**:213–22.

45. McDonald HM, O'Loughlin JA, Jolley P, Vigneswaran R, McDonald PJ. Prenatal microbiological with factors associated with preterm birth. *Br J Obstet Gynaecol* 1992;**99**:190–6.

46. Lamont RF. Antibiotics for the prevention of preterm birth. *N Engl J Med* 2000;**342**:581–3.

47. McDonald HM, O'Loughlin JA, Vigneswaran R, Jolley PT, Harvey JA, Bof A, *et al*. Impact of metronidazole therapy on preterm birth in women with bacterial vaginosis flora (*Gardnerella vaginalis*): a randomised, placebo controlled trial. *Br J Obstet Gynaecol* 1997;**104**:1391–7.

48. Carey JC, Klebanoff MA, Hauth JC, Hillier SL, Thom EA, Ernest JM, *et al*. Metronidazole to prevent preterm delivery in pregnant women with asymptomatic bacterial vaginosis. National Institute of Child Health and Human Development Network of Maternal-Fetal Medicine Units. *N Engl J Med* 2000;**342**:534–40.

49. McGregor JA, French JI, Jones W, Milligan K, McKinney PJ, Patterson E, *et al*. Bacterial vaginosis is associated with prematurity and vaginal fluid mucinase and sialidase: results of a controlled trial of topical clindamycin cream. *Am J Obstet Gynecol* 1994;**170**:1048–60.

50. Joesoef MR, Hillier SL, Wiknjosastro G, Sumampouw H, Linnan M, Norojono W, *et al*. Intravaginal clindamycin treatment for bacterial vaginosis: effects on preterm delivery and low birth weight. *Am J Obstet Gynecol* 1995;**173**:1527–31.

51. Rosenstein IJ, Morgan DJ, Lamont RF, Sheehan M, Dore CJ, Hay PE, *et al*. Effect of intravaginal clindamycin cream on pregnancy outcome and on abnormal vaginal microbial flora of pregnant women. *Infect Dis Obstet Gynecol* 2000;**8**:158–65.

52. Mercer BM, Arheart KL. Antimicrobial therapy in expectant management of preterm premature rupture of membranes. *Lancet* 1995;**346**:1271–9.

53. Egarter C, Leitich H, Karas H, Wieser F, Husslein P, Kaider A, *et al*. Antibiotic treatment in preterm premature rupture of membranes and neonatal morbidity: a meta-analysis. *Am J Obstet Gynecol* 1996;**174**:589–97.

54. Mercer BM, Miodovnik M, Thurnau GR, Goldenberg RL, Das AF, Ramsey RD, *et al*. Antibiotic therapy for reduction of infant morbidity after preterm premature rupture of the membranes. A randomized controlled trial. National Institute of Child Health and Human Development Maternal-Fetal Medicine Units Network. *JAMA* 1997;**278**:989–95.

55. McGregor JA, Schoonmaker JN, Lunt BD, Lawellin DW. Antibiotic inhibition of bacterially induced fetal membrane weakening. *Obstet Gynecol* 1990;**76**:124–8.

56. Brozanski BS, Jones JG, Krohn MA, Sweet RL. Effect of a screening-based prevention policy on

prevalence of early-onset group B streptococcal sepsis. *Obstet Gynecol* 2000;**95**:496–501.

57. McGregor JA, French JI, Reller LB, Todd JK, Makowski EL. Adjunctive erythromycin treatment for idiopathic preterm labor: results of a randomised, double-blind, placebo-controlled trial. *Am J Obstet Gynecol* 1986;**154**:98–103.

58. Morales WJ, Angel JD, O'Brien WF, Knuppel RA, Finazzo M. A randomised study of antibiotic therapy in idiopathic preterm labor. *Obstet Gynecol* 1988;**72**:829–33.

59. Winkler M, Baumann L, Ruckhaberle KE, Schiller EM. Erythromycin therapy for subclinical intrauterine infections in threatened preterm delivery – a preliminary report. *J Perinat Med* 1988;**16**:253–6.

60. McGregor JA, French JI, Seo K. Adjunctive clindamycin therapy for preterm labor: results of a double-blind, placebo-controlled trial. *Am J Obstet Gynecol* 1991;**165**:867–75.

61. Norman K, Pattinson RE, deSouza J, deJong P, Moller G, Kirsten G. Ampicillin and metronidazole treatment in preterm labour: a multicentre, randomised controlled trial. *Br J Obstet Gynaecol* 1994;**101**:404–8.

62. McGregor JA, French JI, Witkin S. Infection and prematurity: evidence-based approaches. *Curr Opin Obstet Gynecol* 1996;**8**:428–32.

63. Nadisaukiene R, Bergstrom S, Kilda A. Ampicillin in the treatment of preterm labor: a randomised, placebo-controlled study. *Gynecol Obstet Invest* 1996;**41**:89–92.

64. Nadisaukiene R, Bergstrom S. Impact of intrapartum intravenous ampicillin on pregnancy outcome in women with preterm labor: a randomised, placebo-controlled study. *Gynecol Obstet Invest* 1996;**41**:85–8.

65. Svare J, Langhoff-Roos J, Andersen LF, Kryger-Baggesen N, Borch-Christensen H, Heisterberg L, *et al*. Ampicillin-metronidazole treatment in idiopathic preterm labour: a randomised controlled multicentre trial. *Br J Obstet Gynaecol* 1997;**104**:892–7.

66. Newton ER, Dinsmoor MJ, Gibbs RS. A randomized, blinded, placebo-controlled trial of antibiotics in idiopathic preterm labor. *Obstet Gynecol* 1989;**74**:562–6.

67. Newton ER, Shields L, Ridgway LE, Berkus MD, Elliott BD. Combination antibiotics and indomethacin in idiopathic preterm labor: a randomized double-blind clinical trial. *Am J Obstet Gynecol* 1991;**165**:1753–9.

68. McCaul JF, Perry Jr KG, Moore Jr JL, Martin RW, Bucovaz ET, Morrison JC. Adjunctive antibiotic treatment of women with preterm rupture of membranes or preterm labor. *Int J Gynaecol Obstet* 1992;**38**:19–24.

69. Romero R, Sibai B, Caritis S, Paul R, Depp R, Rosen M, *et al*. Antibiotic treatment of preterm labor with intact membranes: a multicenter, randomized, double-blinded, placebo-controlled trial. *Am J Obstet Gynecol* 1993;**169**:764–74.

70. Cox SM, Bohman VR, Sherman ML, Leveno KJ. Randomized investigation of antimicrobials for the prevention of preterm birth. *Am J Obstet Gynecol* 1996;**174**:206–10.

71. Kenyon SL, Taylor DJ, Tarnow-Mordi W. Broad-spectrum antibiotics for preterm, prelabour rupture of fetal membranes: the ORACLE I randomised trial. ORACLE Collaborative Group. *Lancet* 2001;**357**:979–88.

72. Kenyon SL, Taylor DJ, Tarnow-Mordi W. Broad-spectrum antibiotics for spontaneous preterm labour: the ORACLE II randomised trial. ORACLE Collaborative Group. *Lancet* 2001;**357**:989–94.

73. Cassell GH, Waites KB, Crouse DT, Rudd PT, Canupp KC, Stagno S, *et al*. Association of *Ureaplasma urealyticum* infection of the lower respiratory tract with chronic lung disease and death in very-low-birth-weight infants. *Lancet* 1988;**2**:240–5.

Chapter 28

Infection, inflammation and brain injury in newborn infants

Nigel Kennea, Phil Duggan and David Edwards

Introduction

In spite of the optimistic view that cerebral palsy would diminish with the improvement in obstetric and neonatal care, there has been little change in its frequency in the last few decades. The causes of cerebral palsy are still not completely understood. In the past, the majority of cerebral injury in newborn infants was assumed to result from hypoxic-ischaemic insults but perinatal infection and inflammation have now been clearly linked to brain injury in preterm infants and strongly implicated in the aetiology of cerebral palsy in infants born at term.

Placental inflammation and brain injury in preterm infants

Premature birth is strongly associated with brain damage and later neurodevelopmental impairment and it is often assumed that damage is due to cerebral hypoxia-ischaemia secondary to the extreme stresses induced by prolonged intensive care. Indeed, this may have been true in the early days of neonatal intensive care, when haemorrhagic parenchymal infarction and cystic periventricular leukomalacia (PVL) were the predominant disabling lesions. There was then a clear link between respiratory disease (especially pneumothorax) and brain damage, which suggested that postnatal hypoxic events with haemodynamic instability were important in the evolution of cerebral injury. However, improvements in neonatal care have changed the pattern of disease and throughout the world large focal haemorrhagic lesions are becoming less common. Noncystic PVL and telencephalic leucoencephalopathy are now seen as the most important disease types. These are predominantly, but not exclusively, diffuse white-matter lesions.

The primary pathological role of hypoxia-ischaemia and, in particular, reduced cerebral bloodflow has been questioned by the findings of several studies demonstrating that normal cerebral bloodflow can be as low as 5–10 ml/100 g/min in infants who have normal neurological outcome.[1,2] Indeed, some commonly used drugs, particularly indomethacin but also aminophylline, cause significant falls in cerebral bloodflow but there is no clear evidence that they lead to cerebral injury.[3,4] There is also conflicting evidence concerning the relevance of physiological variables which might relate to cerebral bloodflow: some studies suggest that systemic circulatory compromise is related to cerebral injury while others do not. This lack of a clear pathological model that accounts for the high incidence of cerebral damage in preterm infants has led to great interest among neonatologists in the recent evidence that a considerable number of extremely preterm infants may suffer some element of cerebral damage *in utero*. Previous results using cerebral ultrasonography suggested that less than one in twenty infants were delivered with definable cerebral abnormality.[5] However, in a study published in 1999, in which a consecutive cohort of extremely preterm infants born before 30 weeks of gestation was studied using magnetic resonance imaging at a median age of two days, over half the infants showed longstanding abnormalities.[6] These results are worrying not only for the high incidence of cerebral abnormality but also because they suggest that cerebral ultrasonography is an inaccurate tool for defining brain damage in preterm infants and call into question studies that rely solely on ultrasound as a predictor of outcome.

Several factors have led researchers to consider the possible role of intrauterine infection or inflammation in cerebral damage in preterm infants.

1. Paediatricians are familiar with the frequent neurological sequelae of meningitis and septicaemia in infants and older children.[7,8]

2. Intrauterine inflammation has been shown to be associated with lung damage and chronic lung disease in preterm infants.[9,10]

3. There is a strong relationship between preterm delivery before 30 weeks of gestation and infection and this offers the possibility of a unifying hypothesis connecting both delivery and brain injury.

The evidence that preterm birth is strongly associated with intrauterine infection and inflammation is strong. However, it is becoming increasingly apparent that such infection may be particularly chronic and persistent. Bacterial vaginosis is a strong predictor of preterm delivery and it has been shown to be associated with chronic endometritis, suggesting that the clinical appearance of bacterial vaginosis may indicate a more fundamental state of uterine inflammation.[11] This may be manifest in a systemic maternal immune response: maternal plasma immunoglobulin M concentrations were found to be elevated in mid-pregnancy in women who went on to deliver preterm.[12] Certainly, local uterine inflammation has been demonstrated in association with preterm delivery, and both chorioamnionitis and high amniotic fluid concentrations of the pro-inflammatory cytokines are found among infants born before 30 weeks of gestation.[13] Indeed, amniotic fluid pro-inflammatory cytokines may be increased some weeks before preterm birth, possibly indicating a more longstanding inflammatory process.[14]

Although the effects of a chronically inflamed intrauterine environment on the human fetus are poorly understood, the developing brain seems to be particularly vulnerable to inflammatory injury. In immature rat pups, inflammatory stimuli (interleukin-1β) cause increased blood–brain barrier breakdown with enhanced phagocyte diapedesis mediated by CXC chemokines, leading to more severe brain injury than in mature rats.[15] Pathological studies of brain tissue of patients who had PVL have demonstrated the presence of lymphocytes as well as increased tumour necrosis factor-α and interleukin-6 in many PVL lesions.[16]

There are some data from studies in animals that suggest that inflammation and infection may directly cause damage in the developing brain. In a groundbreaking study in 1976, Gilles *et al.*[17] showed that injection of endotoxin into kittens produced white-matter lesions similar to the telencephalic leucoencephalopathy described in preterm infants. Experimental intrauterine infection with *Escherichia coli* caused lesions in the cerebral white matter in fetal rabbits.[18] Nevertheless, it remains to be shown definitively that this effect is not due to systemic hypotension and changes in cerebral perfusion. Investigators at University College London have shown, in a preliminary study, that injection of bacterial lipopolysaccharide into the bloodstream of chronically catheterised fetal sheep leads to cerebral white-matter damage without any change in systemic blood pressure or cerebral bloodflow.[19]

At present, the evidence to support a role for intrauterine infection in human cerebral damage is largely circumstantial and, to some degree, inconsistent. A large epidemiological study has demonstrated that intraventricular haemorrhage diagnosed by cerebral ultrasound is associated with chorioamnionitis and funisitis in infants born within one hour of membrane rupture, but not later.[20] More recently, the same researchers have found that echolucencies on cerebral ultrasound are not associated with placental membrane inflammation but rather with indicators of maternal infection and fetal vasculitis.[21] Clinical studies have related evidence of intrauterine inflammation to cerebral injury. Pro-inflammatory interleukin-6 was found in high concentrations in the amniotic fluid and cord blood of infants who went on to develop ultrasound evidence of cerebral damage or neurodevelopmental impairment.[18,22]

However, these data are problematic: the relationship between maternal and fetal production of cytokines during preterm labour is not precisely defined, and, indeed, interleukin-6 is neuroprotective in some models of brain injury.[23,24]

These studies also use ultrasonography or neurological examination as measures of brain injury. Ultrasonography has particular problems, being both a sensitive and a specific test for haemorrhage but an insensitive (although specific) test for hypoxic-ischaemic lesions.[25] Its value in detecting diffuse white-matter damage has not been adequately assessed but is generally believed to be poor. Neurological examination can only be applied weeks or months after delivery, thus making it impossible to distinguish intrauterine from postnatal cerebral damage.

To begin to overcome this problem, our group has approached the question by using magnetic resonance imaging to define cerebral damage. We have installed within our neonatal intensive care unit a dedicated 1.0 T magnetic resonance system with full intensive care facilities, so that we are now able to obtain images of the brains of even the smallest and sickest infants soon after delivery.[26] In a consecutive cohort of over 40 infants born in our hospital, we have found a strong association between chorioamnionitis and white-matter damage detected by magnetic resonance imaging in the first two days after delivery (unpublished data). Pro-inflammatory cytokines were higher in umbilical cord blood of infants with white-matter disease. Brain abnormalities were also associated with higher fractions of CD45RO positive T cells, which are memory cells signifying exposure to antigen at least 7–10 days earlier.[27]

Thus although the data are not conclusive, there are lines of evidence suggesting that placental inflammation offers a causative mechanism for intrauterine brain injury. This mechanism must be considered alongside a number of others that may also play a significant role in causing neurodevelopmental impairment in this population. There remains the possibility that haemodynamic disturbances lead to injury and one particular complexity in separating the role of hypoxia-ischaemia and inflammation in brain injury is the fact that the neural response to hypoxia-ischaemia often involves inflammatory pathways.[28] The interrelation between hypoxia-ischaemia and inflammation may be profound: for example, it has recently been shown that hypoxia-ischaemia induces expression of Fas (a classical receptor for lymphocyte-mediated killing) on neural cells and that crosslinking of the receptor with antibodies is sufficient to cause neural apoptosis.[29] The picture is complex and placental inflammation may be only one factor in a subtle mechanism of damage and repair within the developing brain.

Brain injury in term infants

Considerable doubt has also been cast on the belief that perinatal hypoxia-ischaemia is the central cause of cerebral palsy in term infants. A consistent finding in various studies is that children with cerebral palsy rarely have evidence of perinatal hypoxia-ischaemia. Researchers are re-evaluating the factors associated with the development of cerebral palsy, with increasing emphasis on events occurring before the perinatal period. Several associations have been strongly endorsed. For example, maternal thyroid disease seems to play a role in some individuals[30] although the precise mechanism is not known. The genetic background of the individual and, in particular, the role played by inherited thrombophilic disorders in term infants suffering focal brain lesions may be important.[31] The possibility that intrauterine inflammation might play a role in cerebral damage at term is a provocative hypothesis that is relevant not only to brain damage in preterm infants but also to the possible understanding of the aetiology of the majority of children who develop cerebral palsy in whom neither a perinatal nor a genetic cause can be found. There is increasing epidemiological evidence of a link between maternofetal infection and neonatal encephalopathy in term infants.[30] Maternal fever in labour increases the risk of cerebral palsy in the child even when there is no clinical evidence of impaired intrauterine gas exchange.[32] Once again, inflammation may be the cause or result of ischaemia, but markers of inflammation, with or without coexistent ischaemia, are strongly associated with neonatal and long-term neurological morbidity.[33]

Conclusion

Current data suggest a role for inflammatory processes in newborn brain injury. However, such injury is multifactorial and inflammation may be only one element in a complex aetiology. More precise studies are needed to define precise mechanisms of inflammatory injury in the developing brain.

References

1. Greisen G, Pryds O. Low CBF, discontinuous EEG activity, and periventricular brain injury in ill, preterm neonates. *Brain Dev* 1989;**11**:164–8.
2. Edwards AD, Wyatt JS, Richardson C, Delpy DT, Cope M, Reynolds EOR. Cotside measurement of cerebral blood flow in ill newborn infants by near infrared spectroscopy. *Lancet* 1988;**ii**:770–1.
3. Edwards AD, Wyatt JS, Richardson C, Potter A, Cope M, Delpy DT, Reynolds EOR. Effects of indomethacin on cerebral haemodynamics in very preterm infants. *Lancet* 1990;**335**:1491–5.
4. McDonnell M, Ives NK, Hope PL. Intravenous aminophylline and cerebral blood flow in preterm infants. *Arch Dis Child* 1992;**67**:416–18.
5. Sinha SK, D'Souza SW, Rivlin E, Chiswick ML. Ischaemic brain lesions diagnosed at birth in preterm infants: clinical events and developmental outcome. *Arch Dis Child* 1990;**65**:1017–20.
6. Maalouf E, Duggan PJ, Rutherford MA, Counsell S, Fletcher AM, Battin M, *et al*. Magnetic resonance imaging of the brain in a cohort of extremely preterm infants. *J Pediatr* 1999;**135**:351–7.
7. Klinger G, Chin CN, Beyene J, Perlman M. Predicting outcome of neonatal bacterial meningitis. *Pediatrics* 2000;**106**:477–82.
8. Bennet R, Bergdahl S, Eriksson M, Zetterstrom R. The outcome of neonatal septicaemia during fifteen years. *Acta Paediatr Scand* 1989;**78**:40–3.
9. Ghezzi F, Gomez R, Romero R, Yoon BH, Edwin SS, David C, *et al*. Elevated interleukin-8 concentrations in amniotic fluid of mothers whose neonates subsequently develop bronchopulmonary dysplasia. *Eur J Obstet Gynecol Reprod Biol* 1998;**78**:5–10.
10. Yoon BH, Romero R, Jun JK, Park KH, Park JD, Ghezzi F, *et al*. Amniotic fluid cytokines (interleukin-6, tumor necrosis factor-alpha, interleukin-1 beta, and interleukin-8) and the risk for the development of bronchopulmonary dysplasia. *Am J Obstet Gynecol* 1997;**177**:825–30.
11. Mercer BM, Goldenberg RL, Mercer B, Iams J, Meis P, Moawad A, *et al*. The Preterm Prediction Study: prediction of preterm premature rupture of membranes through clinical findings and ancillary testing. The National Health and Human Development Maternal-Fetal Medicine Units. *Am J Obstet Gynecol* 2000;**183**:662–8.
12. Holzman C, Jetton J, Fisher R, Mohan M, Paneth N. Association of maternal IgM concentrations above the median at 15–19 weeks of gestation and early preterm delivery. *Lancet* 1999;**345**:1095–6.
13. Berry SM, Romero R, Gomez R, Puder KS, Ghezzi F, Cotton DB, *et al*. Premature parturition is characterized by *in utero* activation of the fetal immune system. *Am J Obstet Gynecol* 1995;**173**:1315–20.
14. Wenstrom KD, Andrews WW, Hauth JC, Goldenberg RL, DuBard MB, Cliver SP. Elevated second-trimester amniotic fluid interleukin-6 levels predict preterm delivery. *Am J Obstet Gynecol* 1998;**178**:546–50.
15. Anthony D, Dempster R, Fearn S, Clements J, Wells G, Perry VH, *et al*. CXC cytokines generate age-related increases in neutrophil-mediated brain inflammation and blood–brain barrier breakdown. *Curr Biol* 1998;**8**:923–6.
16. Yoon BH, Romero R, Kim CJ, Koo JN, Choe G, Syn HC, *et al*. High expression of tumor necrosis factor-alpha and interleukin-6 in periventricular leukomalacia. *Am J Obstet Gynecol* 1997;**177**:406–11.
17. Gilles FH, Leviton A, Kerr CS. Endotoxin leucoencephalopathy in the telencephalon of the newborn kitten. *J Neurol Sci* 1976;**27**:183–91.
18. Yoon BH, Jun JK, Romero R, Park KH, Gomez R, Choi JH, *et al*. Amniotic fluid inflammatory cytokines (interleukin-6, interleukin-1beta, and tumor necrosis factor-alpha), neonatal brain white matter lesions, and cerebral palsy. *Am J Obstet Gynecol* 1997;**177**:19–26.
19. DM Peebles, personal communication.
20. Di Salvo D. The correlation between placenta pathology and intraventricular haemorrhage in the preterm infant. The Developmental Epidemiology Network Investigators. *Pediatr Res* 1998;**43**:570.
21. Leviton A, Paneth N, Reuss ML, Susser M, Allred EN, Dammann O, *et al*. Maternal infection, fetal inflammatory response and brain damage in very low birth weight infants. Developmental Epidemiology Network Investigators. *Pediatr Res* 1999;**46**:566–75.
22. Yoon BH, Romero R, Yang SH, Jun JK, Kim IO, Choi JH, *et al*. Interleukin-6 concentrations in umbilical cord plasma are elevated in neonates with white matter lesions associated with periventricular leukomalacia. *Am J Obstet Gynecol* 1996;**174**:1433–40.
23. Loddick SA, Turnbull AV, Rothwell NJ. Cerebral interleukin-6 is neuroprotective during permanent focal cerebral ischemia in the rat. *J Cereb Blood Flow Metab* 1998;**18**:176–9.
24. Carlson NG, Wieggel WA, Chen J, Bacchi A, Rogers SW, Gahring LC. Inflammatory cytokines IL-1 alpha, IL-1 beta, IL-6, and TNF alpha impart neuroprotection to an excitotoxin through distinct

pathways. *J Immunol* 1999;**163**:3963–8.

25. Hope PL, Gould SJ, Howard S, Hamilton PA, Costello AM, Reynolds EO. Precision of ultrasound diagnosis of pathologically verified lesions in the brains of very preterm infants. *Dev Med Child Neurol* 1988;**30**:457–71.

26. Battin M, Maalouf E, Counsell S, Herlihy AH, Edwards AD. Magnetic resonance imaging of the brain of premature infants within a neonatal intensive care unit. *Lancet* 1997;**349**:1741.

27. Duggan PJ, Maalouf E, Watts TL, Sullivan MHF, Edwards AD. Fetal T-cell activation and cytokinaemia is related to cerebral injury at birth detected by magnetic resonance imaging. *Pediatr Res* 1999;**45**:908.

28. Rothwell NJ, Strijbos PJ. Cytokines in neurodegeneration and repair. *Int J Dev Neurosci* 1995;**13**:179–85.

29. Felderhoff-Mueser U, Taylor DL, Greenwood K, Kozma M, Stibenz D, Joashi UC, et al. Fas/CD95/APO-1 can function as a death receptor for neuronal cells *in vitro* and *in vivo* and is upregulated following cerebral hypoxic-ischemic injury to the developing rat brain. *Brain Pathol* 2000;**10**:17–29.

30. Badawi N, Kurinczuk JJ, Keogh JM, Alessandri LM, O'Sullivan F, Burton PR, Pemberton PJ, et al. Intrapartum risk factors for newborn encephalopathy: the Western Australian case–control study. *BMJ* 1998;**317**:1554–8.

31. Mercuri E, Cowan FM, Gupte G, Manning R, Laffan M, Rutherford M, et al. Prothrombotic disorders and abnormal neurodevelopmental outcome in infants with neonatal cerebral infarction. *Pediatrics* 2001. In press.

32. Grether JK, Nelson KB. Maternal infection and cerebral palsy in infants of normal birth weight. *JAMA* 1997;**278**:207–11.

33. Nelson KB, Dambrosia JM, Grether JK, Phillips TM. Neonatal cytokines and coagulation factors in children with cerebral palsy. *Ann Neurol* 1998;**44**:665–75.

Chapter 29

Infection I

Discussion

Discussion following Professor Regan's paper

Griffiths: Professor Regan, I think your point is very well made that clinical studies should always have matched controls in order to ensure that any infectious agent identified is not just a coincidental finding. I wonder whether either Mr Lamont or Dr Hay can give us any news on the cause of bacterial vaginosis (BV) yet.

Lamont: I have the advantage of having made a recent visit to Sweden where the concept of susceptibility was discussed in great depth. There are some data coming out just now about phage viruses causing BV. This makes looking at treatment regimens interesting. We have discussed the use of metronidazole or clindamycin. Perhaps you should consider metronidazole because it preserves the lactobacilli, whereas clindamycin decimates the lactobacilli. That may be why there is recurrence or failed treatment: if you use metronidazole, you retain the lactobacilli with the phage viruses, whereas with clindamycin, if you eradicate all the lactobacilli, you are eradicating the phage viruses as well. There is some movement on aetiology but I think you are right – it is a marker and we should look at host defence and susceptibility.

Hay: The phage story is interesting, although I am not sure that it is the solution to the cause of BV, which is probably multifactorial. Most women probably have a threshold to develop BV, if their vaginal ecosystem is insulted enough. That threshold is probably different in different women, which brings us back to genetics and susceptibility.

Peckham: I am surprised that people still talk about the TORCH (toxoplasmosis, other agents, rubella, cytomegalovirus, herpes simplex virus) screen because I thought that had disappeared about five years ago, following a Public Health Laboratory Service (PHLS) working group. I would agree that it should be abolished but it has been mentioned several times during the course of this meeting.

Holliman: Could I qualify some of Professor Regan's comments on toxoplasmosis? I would agree that toxoplasmosis is an uncommon cause of sporadic abortion and that it is not a cause of recurrent late abortion. We have to be rather more cautious when we talk about toxoplasmosis in early abortion, however. There is no doubt that acute toxoplasmosis is not the cause of recurrent early abortion, but I am not aware of any convincing evidence, one way or the other, regarding long-standing toxoplasma infection and recurrent early abortion.

There are animal models that show that it is undoubtedly a cause in rodents, and it is a big step – probably an inappropriate step – to translate those data to humans. However, there are studies showing an association and studies showing no association. There are even intervention studies from the Middle East, claiming to cure patients of recurrent abortion when intervening specifically for toxoplasmosis. I would be more guarded because I do not think we understand the association between long-standing toxoplasmosis and recurrent early abortion.

Regan: Thank you for that comment. I bow to your judgement on toxoplasmosis in general, in response to your comment about the Middle East and the treatment studies. However, that was in the 1970s, when everyone treated women for mycoplasmas or ureaplasmas and chlamydia. They all showed an improvement but then that is always what happens with recurrent miscarriage sufferers if you do not include control groups. You can never assess whether your 'improvement' is a genuine improvement.

Holliman: Absolutely, but that gives a verdict of 'case unproven', rather than disproven.

Discussion following Mr Lamont's paper

Soothill: That was a very exciting overview. I would like to make two points about maternal resistance to infection. The difficulty with BV might be the aspect of ascending through the cervix. As you know, we have been interested in the mucinase aspects of that. It is definitely true that the amount of mucinase that women with BV have varies greatly: some have very high levels, while others do not. That is a possible confounding factor. The second point we need to emphasise is cervical length, which is another confounding factor. However, that does not undermine anything you say – it just introduces noise and makes the associations more striking.

Lamont: I would agree with that. There are some data from Sabina Cauci in Udine in Northern Italy showing that women with BV could be divided into a low-risk group and a high-risk group with respect to preterm birth. The high-risk group comprises women who have cleavage of secretory immunoglobulin A (IgA), who produce no response to *Gardnerella vaginalis* haemolysin and who have high sialidase and high prolidase in the vagina. On the other hand, those women who have a good response to *Gardnerella vaginalis* haemolysin – those who have no cleavage of secretory IgA and have low sialidase and low prolidase – are at low risk of preterm birth. I agree with what Professor Regan said – that it may not be what organism is in the vagina that matters, but the response to it.

Discussion following Professor Edwards' paper

MacLean: Could you elaborate on C-reactive protein? We know that in some of these patients who we follow, there is quite a steep, sudden rise in C-reactive protein. Is it the duration for which the mother has an elevated C-reactive protein, or the peak, that is critical? I presume it is the duration of the insult.

Edwards: We have no data on that. The dataset that we have cannot answer that question. We recorded the mother's C-reactive protein just before and within 24 hours of delivery. I only have one measurement. One of the problems in this area is whether acute infection is more important than chronic infection, as I have tried to point out. I do not know the answer to that, and we need further infectious disease work in this field to understand that.

Regan: You made a throwaway comment about steroids affecting term babies. Do you mean that if you give a term baby steroids its postnatal development is poorer?

Edwards: Yes. In the dataset, there was a series of fetuses whose mothers were given repeated courses of steroids. Some mothers had four, even seven, courses of two doses of steroids, and then did not deliver and so went to term. There are about six children in the dataset, matched with normal term controls. Their cortical folding, cerebral volume and cerebral surface area are lower than those of a normal term control. So it is not an effect of prematurity itself but, if you give a steroid antenatally, you have an effect on growth.

They do not start off at the same size and the same surface area when the steroids are given. It is only several weeks later that you actually see the reduced growth. When we analyse it, we may find that endotoxin and other inflammatory mediators have the same sort of effect.

Regan: There is nothing to suggest that giving a term baby a dose of steroids, even post delivery, will affect its postnatal brain development?

Edwards: No, we have no data to suggest that, but these are crude measures of subtle events.

Holliman: I do not know what your rods and hollow rods are but I can suggest a way you may be able to find out, which you may have considered already. Rather than using conserved regions, if you use primers around hypervariable regions, look at the product, sequence it and then compare it to databases. You should be able to tell what species they are. Have you tried that?

Edwards: We have tried that. The first run was contaminated and the second run is being done. I do not know what a hollow rod is – it is a strange phenomenon.

General discussion

Regan: Mr Lamont made a comment about 20 weeks being too late. Although I am a great believer in the fact that most things in pregnancy are dictated by events that occur very early on, which are the data that you would flag up to support that, with respect to the BV antibiotic treatment.

Lamont: It is possible to try to use abnormal colonisation in early pregnancy as a way of identifying those women at risk of preterm birth. The earlier you pick up the presence of abnormal colonisation, the greater the subsequent risk of adverse outcome. Thus, if you screen at between 26 and 32 weeks of gestation, then there is a relative risk of adverse outcome of between 1.4 and 2. However, if you screen before 16 weeks of gestation and find abnormal colonisation the relative risk goes up to 5.5 or 7.5.

Another point is that, while the treatment studies are a nightmare because you use different antibiotics and different regimens by different routes of administration to women of different risk with differing outcomes, it seems clear that, if you are to achieve success, it is with earlier treatment. The earlier you treat, the more likely you are to be successful. There are three unpublished studies, one of which is ours and another which Dr Hay has presented. These again show that early treatment with systemic antibiotics works.

Then there was a study[1] from Kekki in Finland, showing that treatment did not work – except in those women who became recolonised. Those were the ones who, despite treatment, delivered preterm and became recolonised. That is the evidence that shows that we have to do something about it earlier in pregnancy. I also mentioned the Carey study, in which 50% of the women were treated after 20 weeks of gestation and 100% were treated after 16 weeks of gestation. In our study, we showed that 100% were treated before 20 weeks of gestation, and 60% were treated before 16 weeks of gestation.

Regan: Does it not then follow on logically that, if you believe it is important to treat early, you should repeatedly treat?

Lamont: I do not know. It may be that one good treatment might be enough. You may have to add anti-inflammatories to that treatment. Some antibiotics are anti-inflammatory – such as azithromycin, erythromycin, and clindamycin – and they are also membrane stabilisers. It may be that if you improved your choice of therapy, one treatment might be enough.

Hay: I agree with Mr Lamont. The two studies that used clindamycin cream showed a possible trend for an increase in adverse outcome – again, treated later in pregnancy than in his study. The difference between his study and Kekki's study[2] is probably the re-treatment – the fact that the women who still had BV were treated again three weeks later. I suspect that this made a difference to the amount of benefit that was shown for the treatment.

MacLean: Mr Lamont, in your studies you looked at antenatal patients in general. If a patient comes with a history of preterm delivery, do you have any recommendations as to when they should be seen for booking? What amount of investigation, bacteriologically, should they have? And would you manage these patients empirically with clindamycin cream from, say, 12 weeks?

Lamont: The aetiology of preterm labour is multifactorial and so the approach to it also has to be multifactorial. I discussed heterogeneity of preterm birth. If a woman came to you having had a previous preterm birth, but she was a white woman who, in the previous pregnancy had suffered an antepartum haemorrhage at 30 weeks of gestation, and delivered, that is very different from a black woman whose membranes ruptured at 24 weeks and who then delivered preterm.

We have not discussed whether we should screen in pregnancy – I do not screen, although I might if we had the resources. I thus treat on the basis of risk. If a patient comes to me and I think they are at high risk of adverse sequelae in their current pregnancy, because of complications in a previous pregnancy, I would give them antibiotics. The antibiotics I use are a combination of erythromycin and clindamycin, rather than metronidazole or cephalosporins. I like the thought of azithromycin and clindamycin.

Soothill: In response to Professor MacLean's question, in our study in Bristol[3] we have spent a long time worrying about cervical length and whether it was reasonable to observe a very short cervix and do nothing. After much thought, we decided that was not reasonable. We in fact insert a cervical suture if the cervix is less than 15 mm and the mother has a history of preterm birth. In the study so far, it appears that this was the right decision. There are many data on very short cervix in that group.

Ridgway: I wanted to comment on the erythromycin/clindamycin combination, which worries me a little. I cannot see the advantage of adding the macrolide into the lincosamine, as both antibiotics are acting at the same site. Clindamycin covers all the organisms you are interested in, whereas the macrolide does not – we were saying yesterday that all *Mycoplasma hominis* are universally resistant to macrolides. I can understand clindamycin, but clindamycin plus macrolide I cannot understand.

Lamont: What about group B streptococcus?

Ridgway: It is covered by clindamycin.

Regan: Can you take clindamycin orally, as well as in cream form?

Lamont: Yes.

Regan: I was struck by the paper[2] suggesting that if you use vaginal creams you do not achieve as good a response as you do with an oral preparation. That possibly leads on to the fact that the BV that you are treating in the vagina is a marker of something that is occurring higher up in the genital tract.

Lamont: There is logic in treating vaginally because that is the site of the greatest load of bacteria. That is the logic of trying to give intravaginal therapy to knock out that load. However, that treatment will not get access to the organisms which have already reached the decidua, and for that you would want to give systemic therapy. Perhaps there should be a combination of the two.

What about azithromycin and clindamycin? Does that not add anything to it either?
Ridgway: Azithromycin is also a macrolide.

Lamont: So it will not add anything – even with its anti-inflammatory and other properties?

Ridgway: That is the only thing you would add but, as you said, clindamycin is also anti-inflammatory. If I remember rightly, clindamycin's anti-inflammatory activity is stronger than that of the macrolides.

Hay: Coming back to Professor MacLean's question, I have slightly modified my recommendations, which will come up later for discussion. At the moment, the recommendations[4] from the Centers for Disease Control and Prevention (CDC) in Atlanta, USA, which were made before the Carey paper was published (but they were well aware of the data that had been presented in abstract), are that obstetricians may wish to screen and treat women with a prior preterm birth, on the basis of benefit shown in some of the studies. However, particularly with the Carey data, it is difficult to say that this should be considered as standard of care.

I would therefore agree with Mr Lamont: if you have a woman with a history of prior idiopathic or infective preterm birth, I would want to screen her for BV and offer her treatment. However, the data are not there to say that this should be the standard of care throughout the country at the moment.

Scott: I would like to ask Mr Lamont and Dr Hay how many patients would need to be treated with this antibiotic. I am rather worried about using clindamycin widely, because it is now recommended, following concerns in the 1970s over its association with pseudomembranous colitis, only for use in serious infections. The consequences of a woman who is 15 weeks pregnant developing pseudomembranous colitis are severe.

Lamont: The first thing to say is that we used intravaginal clindamycin for our study.

Scott: Did any of the patients have diarrhoea?

Lamont: Only 4% of the clindamycin cream is absorbed systemically, so we are not worried about that. We have safety and efficacy data, both for mother and baby, showing no difference in adverse outcome between clindamycin and placebo, with the use of intravaginal cream.

With systemic clindamycin, we use a short course – one week – but some of the studies have only used three days. Perhaps if you can get away with three days, that might be better. Nevertheless, we warn patients that if their stools are slightly loose, they should stop the treatment, and if they get watery diarrhoea, they must stop it immediately.

You will probably accept the fact that, while clindamycin got a bad name because it was the first one to be associated with pseudomembranous colitis, some people would say that ampicillin causes as much pseudomembranous colitis as clindamycin did.

Scott: There are not many good studies that compare the rate. There is one study[5] that suggests that the rate with clindamycin is slightly higher than with the others. As you say, however, all the antibiotics we use – even metronidazole – have been described as being associated with pseudomembranous colitis. I just have a slight anxiety about giving clindamycin to a large number of people. The toxicity is associated with the first dose, and does not increase with time: the first, single dose can precipitate this most extraordinary effect.

Hay: There is one case[6] reported in the literature of pseudomembranous colitis associated with the use of clindamycin cream, so it has been recorded even with the cream – although, presumably, one would expect less of it than otherwise. I agree with you: I worry that if 15% of pregnant women were to be treated with clindamycin we might have some disasters.

Emily Koumans from the CDC Atlanta has a paper in press where she is looking at the number needed to treat. If you look at some of the studies of high-risk women with a prior preterm birth, we are getting down to something like 6–10 women needing to be treated to prevent one preterm birth. That is reasonable. If you then look at Helen McDonald's study[7] in low-risk women, with no history of preterm birth, you are talking about 100 women, which is perhaps not so reasonable.

Fox: Mr Lamont, you talked about susceptibility and exposure. Would you like to comment on the role of nutrition in susceptibility?

Lamont: I do not know very much about that, so I cannot comment. However, I have had that question before, so perhaps I should learn more about it. Could you tell us a little more?

Fox: Not really. Delving back into the past, there was at one time great enthusiasm for the role of zinc. That enthusiasm has clearly waned but that does not mean that the importance has necessarily waned. Or has this issue just been thrown in the dustbin of history?

Lamont: Like many things, it has been forgotten about, Professor Fox. We need people such as you to remind us of it. For example, we have heard that there are trials being conducted in Sweden looking to see whether we should use metronidazole prophylactically for women undergoing hysterectomy. In the USA, cephalosporins are being used for prophylaxis for hysterectomy. This is because most literature searches only go back about 15 years and we forget much of the research that was done in the past. There was certainly zinc, and the other one was, of course, iron – ferritin.

Ridgway: Could I go back to what we were discussing and qualify it slightly? I am rather concerned at the comments I heard about clindamycin being effective against chlamydia. It has been used, but it should be stressed that it is not reliable. The full clinical trials that were done, certainly back in the late 1970s and early 1980s, came to the conclusion that you should not use it. It will have some effect, but it is not reliable. I do not think there is an antibiotic combination that satisfies all requirements in this situation. The qualification I would make is that clindamycin should not be used to treat chlamydia.

Regan: Professor Fox, do you know of any nutritional data that suggest that there may be an impaired, or an enhanced, inflammatory response?

Fox: There are so many confounding factors in all the studies – it is very difficult to sort it out.

Regan: It occurs to me that, in another branch of pregnancy, there are some thrombophilic disorders. A large proportion of our population carry a gene mutation, the MTHFR gene, but because most of us in our Western society have a folate-replete diet we do not end up with these prothrombotic disorders in pregnancy.

Lamont: I did not go through the list of factors associated with preterm birth, but for the first group of problems there were sociobiological variables – age, height, parity, nutritional status and smoking. Clearly, these are all linked in that those women who are of a poor socio-economic group may be undernourished, underfed, underweight, under-educated, have more children at an earlier age, and so on. In that sense, nutrition is obviously involved.

Smith: In the past, BV has been thought to be associated with increased nitrosamines, which was supposedly linked with BV and cervical intraepithelial neoplasia (CIN). Dr Hay and I have unpublished data showing that there is no increased association of nitrosamines and BV in relation to CIN. I know that is slightly off the subject, but such an association has been suggested in many publications yet does not appear to be true.

Lamont: In some ways, I am trying to get away from BV and more towards abnormal colonisation. It just so happens that one of the easiest ways to identify abnormal colonisation is the diagnosis of BV on a Gram stain in early pregnancy. It is not just the nitrosamines, however – there are many other compounds produced by the bacteria that may be a problem. I refer again to the data that Sabina Cauci has produced – some data on sialidase, prolidase, cleavage of secretory IgA, and IgA response to the haemolysin associated with *Gardnerella vaginalis*, elastase levels, and also even the presence or absence of inflammatory cells on the Gram stain. There is a great deal there, and not just the nitrosamines to worry about as compounding factors.

Soothill: I have a question for Professor Edwards about C-reactive protein in the mother, and also cytokines in the fetus. Is there any chance that tissue damage, for example infarction in the placenta, could be causing those, rather than infection?

Edwards: Yes, there probably is. The source of infection, or inflammation as I would really prefer to call it, is unclear in this situation. The evidence is that there is an increase in the amount of pro-inflammatory cytokines and, of course, the regulatory counter-inflammatory cytokines in amniotic fluid and cord blood.

I do not know of anyone who has got *in situ* staining of placental cytokines to work yet – we have not made it work yet. It is not fully known where the cytokines are in the maternal blood, nor where the receptors are turned on – where it is going to work. It is a very unclear story and all we know is that there is at least a focus around the uterus.

My guess is that there is a spreading inflammatory response coming out from a certain point, but where that point is needs to be defined. I would guess that it is the fetal membranes but that is nothing more than a guess. From there, you have the various mediators moving in an endocrine fashion through the body, or through the two bodies, and turning on inflammatory responses throughout both mother and fetus – although that is not clear and it needs to be proven.

The analogy is that people who have lung injury in adult intensive care develop a spreading inflammatory condition, which causes multiple organ failure – liver failure, renal failure and so on. You can think in those analogous terms for preterm birth as well, with the uterus as being the central point. That is a hypothesis.

Soothill: There is obviously some exciting research being conducted on the hypothesis you were discussing. We should just bear in mind the possibility that it is not infection but perhaps, for example, small placental infarctions that could produce both reactions.

Edwards: I have no problems with that. I would much rather discuss inflammation and immune responses than infection *per se*. Nevertheless, I have to say that three-quarters of these children have bacteria on their membranes and their placentas – and that is a high proportion. The bacteria may be entirely innocent bystanders to the whole proceedings, but you would need to demonstrate that.

References

1. Kekki M, Kurki T, Pelkonen J, Kurkinen-Raty M, Cacciatore B, Paavonen J. Vaginal clindamycin in preventing preterm birth and peripartal infections in asymptomatic women with bacterial vaginosis: a randomized, controlled trial. *Obstet Gynecol* 2001;**97**:643–8.
2. Joesoef MR, Hillier SL, Wiknjosastro G, Sumampouw H, Linnan M, Norojono W, *et al*. Intravaginal clindamycin treatment for bacterial vaginosis: effects on preterm delivery and low birth weight. *Am J Obstet Gynecol* 1995;**173**:1527–31.
3. Sohan K, Carroll SG, Kyle PM, Soothill PW. Cervical ultrasound at the 20-week scan in the prediction of preterm birth in low- and high-risk pregnancies. *J Obstet Gynaecol* 2001;**21** Suppl 1:S18–19.
4. Centers for Disease Control and Prevention. 1998 guidelines for treatment of sexually transmitted diseases. *MMWR Morb Mortal Wkly Rep* 1998;**47**:1–111.
5. Gerding DN, Olson MM, Peterson LR, Teasley DG, Gebhard RL, Schwartz ML, *et al*. *Clostridium difficile*-associated diarrhea and colitis in adults. A prospective case-controlled epidemiologic study. *Arch Intern Med* 1986;**146**:95–100.
6. Meadowcroft AM, Diaz PR, Latham GS. *Clostridium difficile* toxin-induced colitis after use of clindamycin phosphate vaginal cream. *Ann Pharmacother* 1998;**32**:309–11.
7. McDonald HM, O'Loughlin JA, Vigneswaran R, Jolley PT, Harvey JA, Bof A, *et al*. Impact of metronidazole therapy on preterm birth in women with bacterial vaginosis flora (*Gardnerella vaginalis*): a randomised, placebo controlled trial. *Br J Obstet Gynaecol* 1997;**104**:1391–7.

SECTION 8

INFECTION II

Chapter 30

Bacterial infection and the neonate

Paul T Heath

Introduction

The major part of this chapter will focus on neonatal aspects of group B streptococcal (GBS) infection. Not only is GBS the most important cause of early-onset bacterial infection in the newborn but many aspects of its pathogenesis, clinical presentation and management are relevant to consideration of the other major neonatal bacterial pathogens. Furthermore, it is a condition that can be prevented by the actions of the midwife or obstetrician. Other bacterial pathogens that cause early-onset infection will be discussed briefly. Late-onset neonatal bacterial infection will not be discussed because its pathogenesis is usually not related to the pregnancy or the birth process.

Epidemiology of neonatal bacterial infection

The range of organisms causing early-onset neonatal infection has been described in papers from Australia and the USA.[1,2] In Australia between 1991 and 1993, 67% of early-onset sepsis (defined as onset before 48 hours of age) was due to GBS, followed by *Escherichia coli* (18%), and *Haemophilus influenzae*, *Streptococcus pneumoniae* and *Listeria monocytogenes* (1–2% each). Other streptococci accounted for about 4% and enterococci about 2%. By the period 1995–97, the proportion due to GBS had fallen to 52% and the proportion due to *E. coli* had risen to 23%. The incidence of disease due to GBS was 1.7/1000 live births in 1991–93, falling to 1.1/1000 and then to 0.5/1000 in 1995–97. The rates of disease due to organisms other than GBS also fell during this period: 1.3/1000 in 1991–93, 0.8 in 1993–95 and 0.4/1000 in 1995–97.[1] This was a period in which intrapartum antibiotics were being increasingly used in Australia. In the USA between 1995 and 1996, the dominant organisms responsible for early-onset sepsis (defined as onset before seven days of age) were similar: GBS (40%) and *E. coli* (17%). Other organisms included *Streptococcus viridans* (7%), *Staphylococcus aureus* (6%), enterococcus (6%), and klebsiella species, pseudomonas species, serratia, *S. pneumoniae*, *H. influenzae* and listeria (1–4% each). The overall incidence of early-onset sepsis in this USA study was 3.5/1000 live births (similar to overall rates in Australia), with rates of GBS of 1.4/1000 and *E. coli* of 0.6/1000.[2]

In all studies of neonatal infections, the incidence of bacterial infection in premature neonates is at least ten times higher than that in term infants.

Recent data from the UK are not available but the organisms and their relative frequency are likely to be similar to those of Australia and the USA. The incidence of GBS is currently being assessed through a national surveillance study and is likely to be between 0.5/1000 and 1.0/1000 live births. A separate national surveillance study has revealed the rate of early-onset neonatal *H. influenzae* disease to be approximately 0.02/1000 live births, with more than 70% of cases occurring in premature infants.[3]

It should be emphasised that many more neonates are evaluated for early-onset sepsis and treated with antibiotics than actually have proven sepsis. For example, at St George's Hospital, London, approximately 13% of infants (i.e. 130/1000 live births) have a septic screen performed in the first six days of life and then receive antibiotics for at least 48 hours (unpublished data). This highlights the absence of clear clinical and laboratory markers for diagnosing neonatal sepsis and the non-specific manner in which neonatal sepsis may present, as well as the fact that sepsis can be present despite negative blood and cerebrospinal fluid (CSF) cultures. This is well demonstrated by postmortem studies of babies who clearly died from sepsis but had negative antemortem cultures.[4] Various factors are known to decrease the yield of blood and CSF cultures in the presence of true infection. This is particularly so in the case of bacterial pneumonia where accompanying bacteraemia is infrequent.[5] Increasingly, antibiotics are being administered to mothers during labour and this practice may suppress the growth of GBS (and other bacteria) in neonatal cultures. Additionally, cultures may not be taken prior to the administration of antibiotics. It is also possible that the volume of blood obtained from some neonates may be insufficient to grow the relevant organism.[6]

Pathogenesis of neonatal bacterial infection

The development of infection depends on the virulence of the bacteria, the degree of the exposure (the size of the inoculum) and the susceptibility of the neonate. The most important determinant of neonatal susceptibility is gestational age. Acquisition of the organisms responsible for early-onset bacterial sepsis occurs via three routes. The most common mode of neonatal infection is inhalation or ingestion of bacteria from infected amniotic fluid, the bacteria having ascended from the genital tract through ruptured membranes. Infection may also occur after contact with the organism in the genital tract during the birth process. Finally, maternal bacteraemia may allow infection of the neonate via the placenta. GBS disease usually occurs as a result of the first and second of these mechanisms.

Obstetric complications are frequently found in cases of early-onset bacterial sepsis. In one study, one or more of the following factors was found in 49% of cases of GBS disease and 79% of other cases of bacterial sepsis:

- gestation of less than 37 weeks
- intrapartum temperature of 38° C or higher
- rupture of membranes 18 or more hours before delivery.[2]

Outcome of neonatal bacterial infection

Most of the outcome data are available for neonatal meningitis only. In England and Wales, cases of neonatal meningitis were ascertained in 1985–86 and the overall case fatality rate was found to be 19.8%, with that of Gram-negative meningitis (mainly *E. coli*) being 32% and that of GBS 22%. The overall mortality of early-onset neonatal *H. influenzae* disease (mostly sepsis) in the UK in the period 1996–98 was 17%.[3] A USA review published in 2000 documented a higher mortality for non-GBS bacterial sepsis (mainly *E. coli*) of 22% versus 7% for GBS sepsis.[2] Long-term sequelae following neonatal meningitis are thought to occur in about 20–30% of cases.

Group B streptococcus

History

Streptococcus agalactiae, or group B streptococcus, was first isolated in 1887 but not reported as a cause of human disease until 1935.[7] In that year, Lancefield and Hare[8] identified the organism in vaginal cultures and Congdon[9] described a case of fatal puerperal sepsis. In 1938, three cases of fatal puerperal sepsis were reported.[10] Sporadic case reports appeared thereafter and it was not until the 1970s that GBS emerged as the most frequent cause of infection in newborn infants.

Microbiology

GBS are facultative Gram-positive cocci that grow on a variety of bacteriological media. To enhance the detection of GBS from sites such as the genital and gastrointestinal tracts, a number of selective media are used. On blood agar, colonies are surrounded by a narrow zone of β haemolysis (hence the term β-haemolytic). Definitive identification relies on detection of the group B-specific carbohydrate cell wall antigen. This can be done by a variety of methods but most commonly by using latex agglutination. GBS may be further subdivided into serotypes based on type-specific capsular polysaccharides. Eight serotypes currently exist.

To date, isolates of GBS remain susceptible to penicillin G. They are also susceptible to other β-lactams, cephalosporins, vancomycin and imipenem. Susceptibility to macrolides (erythromycin, clindamycin, clarithromycin) is less reliable and GBS are resistant to gentamicin. However, when gentamicin is combined with penicillin or ampicillin, *in vitro* and *in vivo* synergistic killing can be demonstrated.

Epidemiology

It is clear that GBS is the most frequent cause of significant infection in newborn infants. A bimodal distribution of cases by age of onset of disease is apparent. Early-onset infection is defined as the development of infection during the first six days of life (definitions of two days[1] and five days[11] have also been used) and late-onset GBS disease has its onset between seven days and three months of age. This distribution reflects differences in pathogenesis, incidence, clinical presentation and outcome. It also has implications for prevention: intrapartum antibiotic prophylaxis will have an impact on early-onset disease but minimal impact on late-onset disease, whereas a GBS vaccine may impact on both.

Reported attack rates for GBS disease in newborns and infants in the USA range from 0.7/1000 to 5.7/1000 live births. A multistate active surveillance program in 1990, which encompassed a population of 10 million people, reported a rate of early-onset disease of 1.4/1000 live births and late-onset disease of 0.3/1000 live births.[12]

In the UK, the situation has been less clear. A laboratory surveillance study involving 25 centres in the period 1978–79 yielded an incidence of disease (for infants younger than two months of age) of 0.3/1000 live births.[13] This led to the belief that GBS was much less common in the UK than it was in the USA. However, a number of studies have been published in the late 1990s suggesting that the transatlantic difference may not be so great. The first of these was from Oxford,[14] where active surveillance for neonatal infection has been in place since 1985. The 12-year experience of 75000 births revealed an incidence of definite disease (i.e. positive cultures from normally sterile sites) of 0.5/1000 (95% CI 0.4–0.7) with no significant change over time. Subsequently, three papers[15–17] have been published (or presented in abstract form) that report higher rates of disease. Fey *et al.*[15] analysed reports made and isolates sent to the Communicable Disease Surveillance Centre and Central Public Health Laboratory respectively for England and Wales. The overall rates of early- and late-onset disease were 0.4/1000 and 0.2/1000 respectively but for one region (South West) in which all laboratories reported in 1997, the rates were significantly higher at 0.7/1000 and 0.3/1000. The authors concluded that considerable under-reporting exists using current reporting systems.

Bignardi[16] reported the experience over a three-year period (1995–97) from one hospital in Sunderland. A total of 15 cases of definite disease occurred among 10500 live births. Ten of these were early in onset. The incidence of early-onset disease was 0.95/1000 (95% CI 0.36–1.54) and of late-onset disease 0.47/1000. Finally, Beardsall *et al.*[17] identified 34 cases of definite GBS disease over a six-year period (1993–98) at a hospital in south Bedfordshire. The calculated early-onset incidence figure of 1.15/1000 live births (95% CI 0.64–1.66) was again higher than that of previous studies. A significant increase in disease incidence was noted over time.

Another approach to this question is provided by data from the northwest of England. A retrospective study of deaths due to GBS calculated a mortality of 0.08/1000 live births; assuming a death rate of 10–20%, an incidence of disease of approximately 1.2/1000 live births can be calculated (1.2 = average of 0.8–1.6).[18]

A major criticism of these published studies is that major urban and deprived areas are not included. London in particular is missing. To attempt to correct this the Public Health Laboratory Service (PHLS) Working Group established a retrospective laboratory-based study of invasive GBS disease from five major London hospitals. This covered the period 1990–99 and the preliminary incidence figures are 0.7/1000 (early-onset) and 0.11/1000 (late-onset).[19]

If the published disease surveillance studies detailed above are combined, an incidence of 0.72 (95% CI 0.60–0.85) is yielded, similar to that of the London study.[19]

It is, however, difficult to proceed further with policy development in the UK without data from a larger population. To that end, a national 12-month surveillance study was initiated in February 2000. This is being conducted through the British

Paediatric Surveillance Unit (BPSU) and involves independent reporting from paediatricians, microbiologists and other groups such as parents of affected children reporting through the charity Group B Strep Support.[20]

As described earlier, there is also recognition that blood and CSF cultures may be negative for GBS (and other pathogens) despite the presence of invasive GBS infection. The concept of probable sepsis is therefore used. In one study,[21] the incidence of probable GBS disease (defined as surface swab positive for GBS, together with clinical sepsis) was 2.3/1000 live births, which was much higher than the culture-proven rate of 0.8/1000 live births. In the Oxford surveillance study,[14] probable disease incidence was also assessed and shown to be the same as that of definite GBS disease (0.5/1000 live births), thus doubling the estimate of the total GBS disease burden.

Pathogenesis

Group B streptococcal infection and disease in the newborn results from a complex interaction between the pathogen, which has its own unique virulence factors, and the neonate, who has a variety of deficiencies in host defence mechanisms. Early-onset infection in the neonate results from exposure to the organism in the maternal genital tract. Late-onset disease may also result from genital-tract exposure but may also result from postnatal exposure to other colonised babies, infected breast milk and a variety of other sources.[22–24]

In almost all cases of maternal genital-tract exposure, the mother is asymptomatically infected (colonised). Reported colonisation rates vary widely and depend on racial and demographic factors, as well as the method of detection used.[25] Acquisition of the organism by neonates born to colonised mothers occurs in 30–70% of cases[26,27] and is thought to occur either via the ascending route through ruptured membranes or via contact with the organism in the genital tract during birth. The former is likely to be the most critical. The most important factor associated with vertical transmission and infant colonisation is the size of the inoculum. The heavier the colonisation, the more likely transmission is to occur.[28] Intrapartum antibiotic prophylaxis has been shown to diminish the inoculum and to decrease infant colonisation.[29]

Vertical transmission is a prerequisite for the development of early-onset invasive disease in the neonate. The size of the inoculum also influences the risk of GBS disease: babies born to heavily colonised mothers are more likely to develop disease and babies who are themselves more heavily colonised are more likely to develop disease.[30] When exposure to the organism is prolonged by rupture of membranes for longer than 18 hours, the risk of disease is increased and the increase is directly related to the duration of membrane rupture.[31] It should also be noted, however, that GBS appear able to invade through intact placental membranes, as fulminant disease can develop in infants delivered by caesarean section. Other maternal factors associated with neonatal disease include premature rupture of membranes, prematurity and intrapartum fever.[32] The significance of prematurity as a risk factor for disease is complex as there is evidence that GBS *per se*, particularly heavy colonisation or GBS urinary infection, may result in premature delivery.[33]

Ascending infection by GBS leads to chorioamnionitis and bacterial proliferation in the amniotic fluid; aspiration of infected amniotic fluid then allows access to the fetal lung. It is likely that this mechanism of transmission, rather than contact with GBS during birth, is the critical one and results in the most severe early-onset disease.

Pneumonia is characteristic of early-onset disease. GBS are capable of invading alveolar epithelial and pulmonary endothelial cells and thus may gain access to the bloodstream. The newborn infant, and particularly the premature infant, is an immunosuppressed host with quantitative and qualitative deficiencies of phagocytes (both alveolar and bloodstream), antibody and complement. Furthermore, GBS possesses a number of unique attributes that account for its virulence, such as the production of β haemolysin, as well as possessing a polysaccharide capsule, which can itself inhibit macrophage and neutrophil phagocytosis.[34]

The importance of GBS serotype-specific antibody in particular has been demonstrated in several studies. These demonstrate that those infants at greatest risk of invasive disease are those with low concentrations of maternal antibody to the capsular antigen.[35] Premature infants, particularly those born most prematurely, will have low antibody concentrations, as placental transfer of antibody is less efficient prior to 34 weeks of gestation. The relationship between GBS antibody concentrations and susceptibility to GBS disease is the basis for considering vaccination as a prevention strategy. Once bacteraemia has been established, components of GBS appear capable of triggering the host cytokine cascade with resultant features of septic shock and multi-organ failure.

To produce meningitis, GBS must penetrate the blood–brain barrier. This can be done by transcytosis of endothelial cells or via damage and disruption of these cells. It appears that serotype III strains can do this more efficiently than other strains, which would account for the predominance of this serotype as a cause of meningitis.[34]

Clinical features

As described earlier, the timing of clinical presentation of GBS disease is characterised by a bimodal distribution. Early-onset disease occurs in the first six days of life with the majority presenting on the first day. The most common presentation is with sepsis followed by pneumonia and meningitis. The signs are similar in each of these and range from shock and respiratory failure at delivery to asymptomatic infection detected during evaluation prompted by maternal risk factors. Case fatality has ranged from 4% to 15% in different series. The USA active surveillance programme in 1990 reported a mortality of 6%.[12] A paper in 2000 reported, for the period 1993–98, a rate of 4%, which differed by gestational age: 30% for less than 34 weeks, 10% for 34–36 weeks and 2% for infants born after 36 weeks of gestation.[36] A review published in 1999 of GBS in Australia reported a mortality rate of 10% for the period 1991–97.[1] Unfortunately, there are no population-based studies of GBS mortality from the UK for comparison. However, it is anticipated that the current BPSU study will rectify this. Of the smaller UK studies, the Oxford study[14] reported a mortality of 9% for cases in the 1990s, the Bedfordshire study[17] reported 14% (1993–98) and the Newcastle study[18] reported an incidence of GBS-related deaths of 0.08/1000 live births.

Early-onset disease tends to occur in the setting of maternal complications as detailed above. Of the published UK studies, three have detailed maternal risk factors present among cases. Beardsall et al.[17] found that 32% of their 28 early-onset cases in Bedfordshire were born preterm (less than 37 weeks of gestation), but that no mother had a previously infected child, positive screening cultures or documented bacteriuria with GBS. Prolonged rupture of membranes was present in 46% of cases and maternal fever in 18%. There were four deaths and all were preterm infants (less than 28 weeks of gestation). Thus 64% had one or more risk factors present during labour. In the retrospective review of deaths due to GBS in the Northern Region, Embleton et al.[18] found that 41 of the 51 neonatal deaths (80%) were in premature infants. Their median gestational age was 31 weeks (range 21–41 weeks) and median birthweight 1770 g (range 520–4740 g). Of ten babies born at term, four mothers had prolonged rupture of membranes (longer than 24 hours). Thus 88% of the neonatal deaths due to GBS had one or more risk factors. Finally, in the Oxford study,[14] 63% of babies had one or more risk factors present at the time of delivery, the most frequent being prematurity (40%) and prolonged rupture of membranes (longer than 18 hours) (40%). It is the recognition of the frequency of these clinically identifiable factors among cases of early-onset disease that allows the possibility of a risk factor-based approach to be used for targeting preventive measures such as antibiotics.

Late-onset disease primarily affects term infants with an unremarkable maternal and neonatal history. The peak age of onset is approximately 36 days. Meningitis is a more common mode of presentation than it is in early-onset disease, pneumonia and sepsis occur, and a variety of focal infections may be seen, including osteomyelitis, septic arthritis, cellulitis and lymphadenitis. The mortality of late-onset disease is reported to be lower than that of early-onset disease.[11]

Sequelae are said to occur in 15–50% of survivors of GBS meningitis. However, there are no data from the 1990s. There are no published data from the UK, but unpublished five-year follow-up of infants with GBS meningitis admitted to hospital in the period 1985–86 reveals severe to moderate disability in 19% of survivors.[37]

Management: antibiotic treatment

Empiric treatment for early-onset bacterial disease will cover the organisms listed previously and will usually include penicillin or ampicillin together with an aminoglycoside. Some UK units prefer to use a third-generation cephalosporin with or without penicillin or ampicillin. Penicillin remains the antibiotic of choice for treatment of systemic GBS disease and, once GBS has been isolated, treatment courses can be completed with penicillin. Relatively high doses are recommended as these are usually well tolerated by neonates and will ensure rapid bacterial killing. Ampicillin is also acceptable but its broader spectrum of antibacterial activity is unnecessary once GBS has been confirmed. The addition of an aminoglycoside to penicillin or ampicillin in the treatment of established GBS infection is based upon animal model and in vitro studies that show the combination to be of the same or greater efficacy than ampicillin or penicillin alone.[38,39] There have been no clinical trials. It is probably reasonable to commence treatment with combination therapy but then rationalise to the single agent as clinical improvement occurs. Similarly, there are no clinical trials comparing third-generation cephalosporin treatment with penicillin and aminoglycoside combinations. Many clinicians would prefer to use cefotaxime or ceftriaxone in the presence of meningitis because of their superior CSF penetration.

The duration of antibiotic therapy for GBS infection will vary according to the clinical and laboratory response but, in general, at least 10 days of antibiotics will be given for bacteraemia without a focus, 14 days for soft-tissue infections, 14–21 days for meningitis and 3–4 weeks for osteomyelitis.

Recurrence of GBS disease occurs rarely and may indicate a persistent focus, immune deficiency or persistent mucous membrane infection.

Management of the infant where the mother has received antibiotics

One of the most difficult aspects of GBS and its prevention is the assessment and management of the infant whose mother has received antibiotics. It must be recognised that intrapartum antibiotic prophylaxis (IAP) is not 100% effective and this recognition will affect the practice of the paediatrician in terms of sepsis assessment of the baby, antibiotic use and duration of observation in hospital.[40] One study of the cost-effectiveness of IAP in the USA predicted that although IAP would be a cost-effective strategy this would not be the case if it resulted in neonates staying in hospital for one extra day of observation.[41] The options for paediatricians in this situation may include:

- observation of the baby for signs of disease, without antibiotic treatment
- taking blood (and CSF) cultures and observation, or antibiotic treatment which is then stopped when cultures are shown to be negative
- taking cultures and administering antibiotic treatment for a modified treatment course, e.g. five days or seven days
- antibiotics for a full treatment course.

In practice, this decision will be based on clinical findings in the neonate, the gestational age, the reasons that the mother was given antibiotics, the number of doses administered (and the timing of their administration) and the appropriateness of the dose and of the antibiotic administered. Thus a baby who is asymptomatic, is greater than 35 weeks of gestation and whose mother received two or more doses of penicillin for GBS colonisation might be observed carefully for 48 hours. A baby born at less than 30 weeks of gestation may still need to be treated with antibiotics despite adequate antibiotic prophylaxis to the mother.

Finally, there is an increasing number of reports of antibiotic-resistant bacteria and the emergence of unusual bacteria following the use of intrapartum antibiotic prophylaxis.[42,43] Careful surveillance will be required in order to document the impact of widespread antibiotic use in this setting.

References

1. Isaacs D, Royle JA. Intrapartum antibiotics and early-onset neonatal sepsis caused by group B Streptococcus and by other organisms in Australia. Australasian Study Group for Neonatal Infections. *Pediatr Infect Dis J* 1999;**18**:524–8.
2. Schuchat A, Zywicki SS, Dinsmoor MJ, *et al*. Risk factors and opportunities for prevention of early-onset neonatal sepsis: a multicenter case-control study. *Pediatrics* 2000;**105**:21–6.
3. Heath PT, Booy R, Azzopardi HJ, *et al*. Non-type B *Haemophilus influenzae* disease: clinical and epidemiological characteristics in the post-hib vaccine era. *Pediatr Infect Dis J* 2001;**20**:300–5.
4. Squire E, Favara B, Todd J. Diagnosis of neonatal bacterial infection: hematological and pathological findings in fatal and nonfatal cases. *Pediatrics* 1979;**64**:60–4.
5. Webber S, Wilkinson AR, Lindsell D, Hope PL, Dobson SR, Isaacs D. Neonatal pneumonia. *Arch Dis Child* 1990;**65**:207–11.
6. Isaacman DJ, Karasic RB, Reynolds EA, Kost SI. Effect of number of blood cultures and volume of blood on detection of bacteremia in children. *J Pediatr* 1996;**128**:190–5.
7. Nocard M. Sur une mammite contagieuse des vâches laitières. *Ann Inst Pasteur* 1887;**1**:109–27.
8. Lancefield RC, Hare R. The serological differentiation of pathogenic and non-pathogenic strains of hemolytic streptococci from parturient women. *J Exp Med* 1935;**61**:335–49.
9. Congdon PM. Streptococcal infection in childbirth and septic abortion. *Lancet* 1935;**ii**:1287–8.
10. Fry RM. Fatal infections by hemolytic streptococcus group B. *Lancet* 1938;**i**:199–201.

11. Edwards MS, Baker CJ. *Streptococcus agalactiae* (group B streptococcus). In: Mandell GL, Bennett JE, Dolin R, editors. *Mandell, Douglas, and Bennett's Principles and Practice of Infectious Diseases.* Philadelphia: Churchill Livingstone; 2000. p. 2156–67.
12. Zangwill KM, Schuchat A, Wenger JD. Group B streptococcal disease in the United States, 1990: report from a multistate active surveillance system. *Mor Mortal Wkly Rep CDC Surveill Summ* 1992;**41**:25–32.
13. Mayon-White RT. The incidence of GBS disease in neonates in different countries. *Antibiot Chemother* 1985;**35**:17–27.
14. Moses LM, Heath PT, Wilkinson AR, Jeffery HE, Isaacs D. Early-onset group B streptococcal neonatal infection in Oxford 1985–96. *Arch Dis Child Fetal Neonatal Ed* 1998;**79**:F148–9.
15. Fey R, Stuart J, George R. Neonatal group B streptococcal disease in England and Wales 1981–1997. *Arch Dis Child* 1999;**80**:A70,G202.
16. Bignardi G. Surveillance of neonatal group B streptococcal infection in Sunderland. *Commun Dis Public Health* 1999;**2**:64–5.
17. Beardsall K, Thompson M, Mulla R. Neonatal group B streptococcal infection in South Bedfordshire, 1993–1998. *Arch Dis Child Fetal Neonatal Ed* 2000;**82**:F205–7.
18. Embleton N, Wariyar U, Hey E. Mortality from early onset group B streptococcal infection in the United Kingdom. *Arch Dis Child Fetal Neonatal Ed* 1999;**80**:F139–41.
19. A Mifsud, personal communication.
20. Enhanced surveillance of neonatal group B streptococcal disease. *Commun Dis Rep CDR Wkly* 2000;**10**:21.
21. Bedford Russell A, Breathnach A, Sender P. Confirmed group B streptococcus infection: the tip of the iceberg. *Arch Dis Child* 2001;**84**:F140.
22. Noya FJ, Rench MA, Metzger TG, Colman G, Naidoo J, Baker CJ. Unusual occurrence of an epidemic of type Ib/c group B streptococcal sepsis in a neonatal intensive care unit. *J Infect Dis* 1987;**155**:1135–44.
23. Olver WJ, Bond DW, Boswell TC, Watkin SL. Neonatal group B streptococcal disease associated with infected breast milk. *Arch Dis Child Fetal Neonatal Ed* 2000;**83**:F48–9.
24. Easmon CS, Hastings MJ, Clare AJ, *et al.* Nosocomial transmission of group B streptococci. *BMJ* 1981;**283**:459–61.
25. Hastings MJ, Easmon CS, Neill J, Bloxham B, Rivers RP. Group B streptococcal colonisation and the outcome of pregnancy. *J Infect* 1986;**12**:23–9.
26. Baker CJ, Barrett FF. Transmission of group B streptococci among parturient women and their neonates. *J Pediatr* 1973;**83**:919–25.
27. Anthony BF, Okada DM, Hobel CJ. Epidemiology of the group B streptococcus: maternal and nosocomial sources for infant acquisitions. *J Pediatr* 1979;**95**:431–6.
28. Ancona RJ, Ferrieri P, Williams PP. Maternal factors that enhance the acquisition of group-B streptococci by newborn infants. *J Med Microbiol* 1980;**13**:273–80.
29. Boyer KM, Gadzala CA, Kelly PD, Gotoff SP. Selective intrapartum chemoprophylaxis of neonatal group B streptococcal early-onset disease. III. Interruption of mother-to-infant transmission. *J Infect Dis* 1983;**148**:810–16.
30. Lim DV, Kanerak KS, Peterson ME. Magnitude of colonization and sepsis by group B streptococci in newborn infants. *Curr Microbiol* 1982;**7**:99–101.
31. Stewardson-Krieger PB, Gotoff SP. Risk factors in early-onset neonatal group B streptococcal infections. *Infection* 1978;**6**:50–3.
32. Prevention of perinatal group B streptococcal disease: a public health perspective. Centers for Disease Control and Prevention. *MMWR Morb Mortal Wkly Rep* 1996;**45**:1–24.
33. Schuchat A. Group B streptococcus. *Lancet* 1999;**353**:51–6.
34. Nizet V, Ferrieri P, Rubens CE. Molecular pathogenesis of group B streptococcal disease in newborns. In: Stevens DL, Kaplan EL, editors. *Streptococcal Infections.* New York: Oxford University Press; 2000. p. 180–221.
35. Baker CJ, Kasper DL. Correlation of maternal antibody deficiency with susceptibility to neonatal group B streptococcal infection. *N Engl J Med* 1976;**294**:753–6.
36. Schrag SJ, Zywicki S, Farley MM, Reingold AL, Harrison LH, Lefkowitz LB, *et al.* Group B streptococcal disease in the era of intrapartum antibiotic prophylaxis. *N Engl J Med* 2000;**342**:15–20.
37. H Bedford, personal communication.
38. Bingen E, Lambert-Zechovsky N, Guihaire E, Mancy C, Aujard Y, Mathieu H. [Optimum choice of antibiotic treatment in neonatal infections due to group B streptococci]. *Pathol Biol (Paris)* 1986;**34**:530–3. French.
39. Kim KS. Effect of antimicrobial therapy for experimental infections due to group B streptococcus on mortality and clearance of bacteria. *J Infect Dis* 1987;**155**:1233–41.

40. Peralta-Carcelen M, Fargason CA Jr, Cliver SP, Cutter GR, Gigante J, Goldenberg RL. Impact of maternal group B streptococcal screening on pediatric management in full-term newborns. *Arch Pediatr Adolesc Med* 1996;**150**:802–8.

41. Benitz WE, Gould JB, Druzin ML. Preventing early-onset group B streptococcal sepsis: strategy development using decision analysis. *Pediatrics* 1999;**103**:e76.

42. Levine EM, Ghai V, Barton JJ, Strom CM. Intrapartum antibiotic prophylaxis increases the incidence of Gram-negative neonatal sepsis. *Infect Dis Obstet Gynecol* 1999;**7**:210–13.

43. McDuffie RS Jr, McGregor JA, Gibbs RS. Adverse perinatal outcome and resistant Enterobacteriaceae after antibiotic usage for premature rupture of the membranes and group B streptococcus carriage. *Obstet Gynecol* 1993;**82**:487–9.

Chapter 31

Infection and caesarean section

Peter Brocklehurst

Summary

Caesarean section is one of the most common operations performed in developed countries and accounts for a substantial proportion of the costs of maternity care. Relatively minor infections following caesarean section are common and although they appear to have few long-term consequences they contribute to longer hospital stay. More severe infections are less common but may cause substantial short- and long-term morbidity, including death in a very small number of women. Preventing infection following caesarean section by giving prophylactic antibiotics at the time of surgery has been clearly shown to decrease the incidence of infection. The role of other prophylactic procedures such as changes in surgical technique and attention to aseptic technique has been relatively poorly researched.

Once infection is diagnosed, treatment with antibiotics forms the mainstay of management but, in more severe infections, surgical management may be necessary. The long-term consequences of wound infection and endometritis on women's subsequent health, particularly in relation to future pregnancies, have been poorly described.

Epidemiology

In the UK, 17% of women were delivered by caesarean section in the 1997/98 financial year.[1] In other developed countries, the proportion of women undergoing delivery by caesarean section is even higher. The immediate consequences for the mother of caesarean section have not been well described but there is some evidence suggesting substantial short-term morbidity.[2] Among a cohort of 256795 women in Washington State from 1987 to 1996, 54074 (21%) were delivered by caesarean section. Of these women, the adjusted relative risk for subsequent re-admission to hospital compared with women having a vaginal delivery was 1.8 (95% CI 1.6–1.9). The single largest contributor to this re-admission was uterine infection (endometritis), with an incidence of 5.2 per 1000 live births compared with 2.9 per 1000 live births following vaginal delivery.[3]

There appears to be no agreed standard definition of infection following caesarean section. The usual conditions described are 'febrile morbidity', wound infection, endometritis, urinary tract infection and 'severe infectious morbidity'. Febrile morbidity describes women who develop fever after caesarean section which is either particularly high (i.e. 39° C or over) or which is persistent (38° C on two of the first ten days postpartum).[4] The proportion of women who develop febrile morbidity varies by study. In the 66 randomised controlled trials of prophylactic antibiotics associated with caesarean section included in the Cochrane database,[5] 34 reported 'fever' as an outcome. The median incidence of fever in the 'no prophylaxis' group was 35% (interquartile range 25–45%).

The diagnosis of wound infections or endometritis following caesarean section is also complicated by the lack of an agreed definition. For example, endometritis is variously diagnosed on the basis of the presence of fever, uterine tenderness, the presence of an offensive lochia and elevated white-cell counts.[5] However, definitions may depend on the duration and magnitude of fever, the subjective nature of assessing uterine tenderness and the difficulty of interpreting lochia which is not frankly offensive. The situation is even more difficult with wound infections, where slight erythema of the skin around the wound which resolves in the absence of antibiotic therapy may be taken by some clinicians as being evidence of wound infection whereas other clinicians may require evidence of discharge of pus from the wound before reaching the same diagnosis.

There does appear to be consensus, however, that a positive microbiological culture is not necessary for the diagnosis of wound infection, endometritis or other infectious complications following caesarean section before antibiotic therapy is initiated.

Wound infection

The proportion of women who develop a wound infection following their caesarean section is approximately 7%,[6] although estimates vary widely depending on the definitions used and the population being studied.[7] In the UK, a prospective study[8] estimated the incidence of wound infection using a standard definition in five maternity units over a three-month period. The incidence varied from 2.5% to 17.1% and this variation was greater than that expected by chance alone. Another important factor in assessing the incidence of wound infection appears to be the method of ascertainment. As postoperative hospital stay becomes shorter, more infections are being diagnosed after the mother is discharged home and thus studies that rely on estimating the number of infections in hospital may substantially underestimate the true incidence.[9] For example, in a study from New Zealand, 36% of all wound infections were diagnosed after the mother had been discharged home.[10]

Endometritis

The proportion of women who develop endometritis following delivery by caesarean section is approximately 5%[5] although, as with wound infections, the method of case ascertainment will influence the estimated incidence.[11] Unlike wound infections, where the majority of infections (although not all) are diagnosed in hospital, the majority of cases of endometritis are diagnosed after the woman has been discharged from hospital.

Urinary tract infection

Urinary tract infections appear to be common following urethral catheterisation. In the Cochrane review of antibiotic prophylaxis for caesarean section, 47 trials reported urinary tract infection as an outcome.[5] The median incidence of urinary tract infection was 7% (interquartile range 4–12%) in the 'no prophylaxis' arms of these trials. The diagnosis and management of urinary tract infections will not be considered further in this chapter.

Serious infectious morbidity

The definition of serious infectious morbidity varies. In the Cochrane review,[5] all episodes of bacteraemia were included in the definition of serious infectious morbidity, which also included pelvic thrombophlebitis and peritonitis.

Once again, the incidence of serious infectious morbidity varies depending on the definition used. Events such as bacteraemia will depend on how frequently blood cultures are performed for women with fever following caesarean section. Pelvic thrombophlebitis is uncommon and other serious complications such as pelvic abscesses are also relatively rare. In the Cochrane review, the median incidence of serious infectious morbidity in 28 trials that reported this outcome was 2% (interquartile range 0–4%) in the 'no prophylaxis' arms of these trials.[5]

Most infections after caesarean section are relatively mild. However, some infections will be severe and, even in the UK, postpartum sepsis following caesarean section still caused two maternal deaths in the period 1994–96.[12]

Costs associated with infectious morbidity

The cost to the health service of a caesarean section is not precisely known.[13] It is, however, widely accepted that the major contributor to the cost of this form of delivery is postnatal stay. The additional cost of treating wound infections and endometritis following a caesarean section is therefore likely to represent a considerable financial burden to the maternity care services. As caesarean sections are performed so frequently, any intervention that reduces the incidence of these infections, even slightly, is likely to have a substantial impact on the cost of maternity care provision nationally.

Risk factors for post-caesarean infection

Some of the major risk factors that have been associated with the development of an infection following a caesarean section are listed below:

- intrapartum caesarean section[14,15]
- prolonged labour[14,16,17]

- prolonged rupture of membranes[16]
- increasing number of vaginal examinations[8,16,17]
- maternal obesity[10,17,18]
- multiple pregnancy[19,20]
- preterm delivery[21,22]
- duration of internal fetal monitoring[16]
- bacterial vaginosis.[23]

The single most important risk factor appears to be whether the caesarean section was performed after the onset of labour. Other important risk factors include longer duration of labour and membrane rupture, an increasing number of vaginal examinations, maternal obesity, some of the surgical techniques used, increasing duration of the operation and increasing maternal age. Wound infections also appear to be more common with twin pregnancies. Many of these risk factors, however, may be interrelated. For example, increasing duration of labour is associated with an increased number of vaginal examinations.

Microbiology

Wound infection

The proportion of wound infections with positive microbiology will depend, in part, on the definition of wound infection used. Fever with some wound tenderness but no wound discharge will be less likely to yield a positive growth of bacteria than a wound where pus is present. The organisms commonly isolated from infected wounds are listed in Table 31.1.

Table 31.1.   Organisms commonly isolated from women with caesarean-section wound infections[6,28]

Group	Organism
Aerobic Gram-negative	*Escherichia coli* *Proteus* spp.
Anaerobic Gram-negative	*Bacteroides* spp.
Aerobic Gram-positive	*Staphylococcus aureus* *Staphylococcus epidermidis* *Staphylococcus faecalis* *Staphylococcus* spp. (other)
Anaerobic Gram-positive	*Peptostreptococcus* spp. *Clostridium* spp.
Other	*Mycoplasma* spp. *Ureaplasma urealyticum*

Table 31.2.   Organisms commonly isolated from women with endometritis[42,43]

Group	Organism
Aerobic Gram-negative	*Escherichia coli*
	Klebsiella pneumoniae
	Proteus spp.
	Enterobacter aerogenes
Anaerobic Gram-negative	*Bacteroides bivius*
	Bacteroides fragilis
	Bacteroides spp. (other)
	Fusobacterium spp.
Aerobic Gram-positive	*Streptococcus agalactiae*
	Streptococcus viridans
	Streptococcus faecalis
	Streptococcus spp. (other)
Anaerobic Gram-positive	*Peptococcus* spp.
	Peptostreptococcus spp.
Other	*Mycoplasma hominis*
	Ureaplasma urealyticum

Endometritis

Unless bacteriological specimens can be obtained from the upper genital tract without any evidence of contamination from the vagina, positive microbiology is often not found with endometritis. Bacteraemia may be present in up to 20% of cases with endometritis and blood cultures may therefore be useful when deciding on antibiotic treatment. The organisms most often isolated from women with endometritis are listed in Table 31.2.

Clinical manifestations and management

Wound infection

Wound infections can present early, within 48 hours, or late, four to seven days after the procedure. Early infections can present as early as 12 hours after surgery and the usual manifestations are either discolouration or cellulitis around the wound margins and fever. The immediate treatment of early wound infection consists of antibiotics although other agents such as honey have been used for mild infections with some success.[24,25] Incision and drainage of the wound or even debridement may be necessary if there is evidence of tissue necrosis. Infections that present later often present with discharge from the wound and fever is a variable feature. The immediate management of a late wound infection is incision and drainage of the wound and debridement as necessary. Antibiotics are indicated if the fever fails to settle shortly after incision and drainage.

In cases of severe wound infection where there is extensive necrosis the wound should be opened and debrided back to the level of healthy tissue. Current consensus appears to favour secondary closure after the open wound has started granulating, usually at least four days after debridement.[26,27]

Rarely, wound infections can become life threatening. Specific infections include necrotising fasciitis and clostridial gangrene.[28] Such serious wound infections are extremely uncommon and treatment includes extensive surgery to remove the affected tissue, appropriate antibiotic therapy and resuscitation if septic shock develops.

Endometritis

The antibiotic treatment of endometritis following any form of delivery has been systematically reviewed by the Cochrane Collaboration.[29] A total of 41 randomised controlled trials have been included and, although studies were generally methodologically poor, there is clear evidence that an antibiotic regimen containing gentamicin and clindamycin given intravenously is superior to any other antibiotic regimen tested in randomised controlled trials to date (summary relative risk for treatment failure for any antibiotic regimen versus clindamycin and gentamicin 1.37; 95% CI 1.10–1.70). In particular, those antibiotic regimens with poor activity against penicillin-resistant anaerobic bacteria were more likely to fail when compared with gentamicin and clindamycin. There is no evidence from this review that any particular antibiotic regimen has more adverse effects than any other regimen. Many of these trials had been performed before the widespread use of prophylactic antibiotics prior to caesarean section and the implications this has on the choice of subsequent therapy for endometritis are uncertain.

In studies that compared continued oral antibiotic therapy after intravenous therapy with intravenous therapy alone, no difference was found in recurrent endometritis or other infection-related outcomes. In this review, the authors concluded that the combination of gentamicin and clindamycin is the most effective treatment for endometritis. In addition, they concluded that 'once uncomplicated endometritis has clinically improved with intravenous therapy, oral therapy is not needed'. In the UK, the use of gentamicin for the treatment of endometritis appears to be uncommon. Only two randomised controlled trials in the Cochrane review included metronidazole. One compared metronidazole in combination with gentamicin with ampicillin and sulbactam (a β-lactamase inhibitor similar to clavulanate) in 70 women. The other compared metronidazole and ampicillin with amoxicillin and clavulanate in 73 women with 'mild' disease. In view of the small numbers of women included in these trials, the relative effectiveness of an antibiotic regimen containing metronidazole is not known.

Prevention

Antibiotic prophylaxis

The use of antibiotic prophylaxis for caesarean section has been reviewed by the Cochrane Collaboration. A total of 66 trials were included in this review[5] and the use of prophylactic antibiotics consistently and substantially reduced the incidence of fever (summary RR 0.46; 95% CI 0.41–0.50), endometritis (summary RR 0.37; 95% CI 0.33–0.42), wound infection (summary RR 0.40; 95% CI 0.33–0.47), urinary tract infection (summary RR 0.55; 95% CI 0.47–0.66) and serious infection following caesarean sections (summary RR 0.44; 95% CI 0.29–0.68). The size of the relative risk decrease was similar for elective and intrapartum caesarean sections. For example, the summary relative risk for endometritis was 0.25 (95% CI 0.11–0.55) for elective procedures and 0.39 (95% CI 0.33–0.46) for non-elective procedures. This substantial decrease in infectious complications, which is seen for all infectious sequelae of the procedure, 'justifies a policy of administering prophylactic antibiotics to women undergoing elective or non-elective caesarean section'.

In a related systematic review,[30] also published in the Cochrane database, the authors explored which antibiotic regimen was the most effective. This review included 51 randomised controlled trials that compared two or more different antibiotic regimens for the prevention of infectious complications following caesarean section. The review's conclusion was that both ampicillin and first-generation cephalosporins have similar effects in reducing the incidence of postoperative endometritis when compared with other antibiotic regimens. In addition there were no apparent benefits in using antibiotics with a broader spectrum of activity and the use of multiple doses of prophylactic antibiotics showed no advantage over a single-dose regimen (summary RR 0.94; 95% CI 0.74–1.18 comparing any single-dose regimen with any multiple-dose regimen). This review suggested that the only remaining questions to be addressed with respect to prophylactic antibiotics at caesarean section relate to determining the optimal timing of administration, in particular whether antibiotics should be given pre-operatively or after the umbilical cord has been clamped.[31,32]

It has been suggested that the incidence of infectious morbidity following caesarean section in these trials is very high and this does not reflect current experience, particularly for women undergoing elective caesarean section. Therefore, antibiotic prophylaxis may not be justified for women where the expected incidence of infection is low. This argument is not supported by current evidence and the relative risk decrease seen in existing trials is likely to be stable even if the baseline incidence of infection is low. In addition, it is important to remember that the incidence of postoperative infection will be artificially low if only infections diagnosed while a women is in hospital are included.[10] Clearly, if the true incidence is low the number needed to treat to prevent one infection will be relatively high. However, the use of a single dose of a narrow-spectrum antibiotic is unlikely to be associated with major adverse effects. The evidence therefore seems overwhelming that women undergoing caesarean section, whether after the onset of labour or electively, should receive prophylactic antibiotics.

The concern that widespread use of prophylactic antibiotics may lead to the development of antibiotic-resistant infections for both the mother and the neonate has some support. Prophylaxis alters the bacteriological flora of the uterus but whether it alters the natural history of any subsequent endometritis is less clear.[33,34] As the incidence of delivery by caesarean section is rising throughout the world it is likely that more antibiotics will be used in this context and the observation that broad-spectrum antibiotics offer no advantage over antibiotics with a narrower spectrum of activity[30] has important implications for practice if antibiotic resistance is to be minimised.

Other approaches to prevention

Although much attention has focused on the use of prophylactic antibiotics for decreasing the incidence of infectious complications following caesarean section, other factors may be amenable to intervention. Some of the risk factors known to be associated with infectious morbidity following caesarean section were listed earlier, and it is likely that interventions that decrease the incidence of intrapartum caesarean section and the duration of labour and membrane rupture will decrease subsequent morbidity. Although not confined to women who had a caesarean section, the large TERMPROM trial[35] suggested that immediate augmentation with oxytocin of women at term with ruptured membranes decreased the overall duration of membrane rupture and decreased the incidence of maternal postpartum infection.

Other risk factors that may also be amenable to intervention include the surgical techniques used at the time of caesarean section, other elements of infection control policies such as the environment in which the surgery is performed, the use of surgical masks, the use of antiseptic skin preparation agents and the use of antiseptic agents during vaginal examination for women in labour.[36] There are undoubtedly other components of the pre- and intra-operative process that could be modified which may also have an impact on the incidence of post-caesarean section morbidity.

Surgical techniques

Despite the fact that caesarean section is one of the most common operations performed in developed countries, there are wide variations in the surgical techniques used by obstetricians in the UK.[37] It is likely that some of these have an impact on the risk of infectious morbidity following the procedure. Randomised controlled trials have been performed comparing different elements of the operation and some of these have suggested that the incidence of infectious morbidity can be altered with different surgical techniques. All of these trials have been relatively small and have concentrated on 'febrile morbidity' as their major outcome. The impact of these various techniques on the incidence of clearly defined endometritis or wound infections is poorly reported.

This evidence has been reviewed[38] and the following techniques have been found to be associated with a lower incidence of infectious complications:

- spontaneous separation or controlled cord traction to remove the placenta is preferable to manual removal[39,40]
- peritoneal non-closure appears to result in less postoperative fever but with no impact on the incidence of endometritis
- the Joel Cohen approach to abdominal entry may result in a lower incidence of febrile morbidity when compared with the Pfannenstiel approach.

In general, however, none of these conclusions are particularly robust because of the small size of the trials included and the generally poor methodology.

Infection control measures

Feedback to clinicians about infectious complications and potential risk factors following caesarean section has resulted in a decrease in postoperative infectious morbidity.[41] No randomised controlled trials of this approach have been reported and there may be other reasons why infectious morbidity decreases after the introduction of these specific feedback mechanisms. However, it does raise the possibility that when greater attention is paid to the prevention of infectious complications of surgery, an impact can be made on the incidence of symptomatic disease.

Prognosis

The impact that wound infections, endometritis and other infectious morbidity have on women's subsequent health, particularly their subsequent reproductive health, has not been well reported. It would appear feasible that endometritis following caesarean section may result in a weaker uterine scar that is more likely to rupture during a subsequent labour. Similarly, infectious morbidity, whether wound infection or endometritis, may affect the incidence of subsequent subfertility, pelvic pain, wound dehiscence in labour and complications during future abdominal or pelvic surgery. These long-term consequences of post-caesarean morbidity need to be addressed in appropriate follow-up studies of subsequent randomised controlled trials of interventions aimed at preventing or treating infection following caesarean section.

References

1. Health Committee. *Public Expenditure on Health and Personal Social Services*. London: The Stationery Office; 1999.
2. Glazener C, Abdalla M, Stroud P, Naji S, Templeton A, Russell I. Postnatal maternal morbidity: extent, causes, prevention and treatment. *Br J Obstet Gynaecol* 1995;**102**:282–7.
3. Lyndon-Rochelle M, Holt, VL, Martin DP, Easterling TR. Association between method of delivery and maternal rehospitalization. *JAMA* 2000;**283**:2411–16.
4. Enkin M, Enkin E, Chalmers I, Hemminki E. Prophylactic antibiotics associated with caesarean section. In: Chalmers I, Enkin M, Keirse MJND, editors. *Effective Care in Pregnancy and Childbirth*. Oxford: Oxford University Press;1989. p. 1246–69.
5. Smaill F, Hofmeyr GJ. Antibiotic prophylaxis for cesarean section. *Cochrane Database Syst Rev* 2000;(2):CD000933.
6. Roberts S, Maccato M, Faro S, Pinell P. The microbiology of post-cesarean wound morbidity. *Obstet Gynecol* 1993;**81**:383–6.
7. Henderson J, Love EJ. Incidence of hospital-acquired infections associated with caesarean section. *J Hosp Infect* 1995;**29**:245–55.
8. Nice, C, Feeney A, Godwin P, Mohanraj M, Edwards A, Baldwin A, *et al*. A prospective audit of wound infection rates after caesarean section in five West Yorkshire hospitals. *J Hosp Infect* 1996;**33**:55–61.
9. Hulton LJ, Olmsted RN, Treston-Aurand J, Craig CP. Effect of postdischarge surveillance on rates of infectious complications after cesarean section. *Am J Infect Control* 1992;**20**:198–201.
10. Beattie PG, Rings TR, Hunter MF, Lake Y. Risk factors for wound infection following caesarean section. *Aust N Z J Obstet Gynaecol* 1994;**34**:398–402.
11. Baker C, Luce J, Chenoweth C, Friedman C. Comparison of case-finding methodologies for endometritis after cesarean section. *Am J Infect Control* 1995;**23**:27–33.
12. Drife J, Lewis G, editors. *Why Mothers Die. Report on Confidential Enquiries into Maternal Deaths in the United Kingdom 1994–1996*. London, The Stationery Office; 1998.
13. Henderson J, McCandlish R, Kumiega L, Petrou S. Systematic review of economic aspects of alternative modes of delivery. *BJOG* 2001;**108**:149–57.
14. Martens MG, Kolrud BL, Faro S, Maccato, Hammill H. Development of wound infection or separation after cesarean delivery. Prospective evaluation of 2,431 cases. *J Reprod Med* 1995;**40**:171–5.
15. Litta P, Vita P, Konishi de Toffoli, Onnis GL. Risk factors for complicating infections after cesarean section. *Clin Exp Obstet Gynecol* 1995;**22**:71–5.
16. Gibbs RS, Blanco JD, St Clair PJ. A case–control study of wound abscess after cesarean delivery. *Obstet Gynecol* 1983;**62**:498–501.
17. Moir-Bussy BR, Hutton RM, Thompson JR. Wound infection after cesarean section. *J Hosp Infect* 1984;**5**:359–70.
18. Tran TS, Jamulitrat S, Chongsuvivatwong V, Geater A. Risk factors for postcesarean surgical site infection. *Obstet Gynecol* 2000;**95**:367–71.
19. Suonio S, Huttunen S. Puerperal endometritis after abdominal twin delivery. *Acta Obstet Gynecol Scand* 1994;**73**:313–15.

20. Conde-Agudelo A, Beleizan JM, Lindmark G. Maternal morbidity and mortality associated with multiple gestations. *Obstet Gynecol* 2000;**95**:899–904.
21. Evans LC, Combs CA. Increased maternal morbidity after cesarean delivery before 28 weeks of gestation. *Int J Gynaecol Obstet* 1993;**40**:227–33.
22. Chaim W, Bashiri A, Bar DJ, Shoham-Vardi I, Mazor M. Prevalence and clinical significance of postpartum endometritis and wound infection. *Infect Dis Obstet Gynecol* 2000;**8**:77–82.
23. Newton ER, Prihoda TJ, Gibbs RS. A clinical and microbiologic analysis of risk factors for puerperal endometritis. *Obstet Gynecol* 1990;**75**:402–6.
24. Al-Waili NS, Saloom KY. Effects of topical honey on post-operative wound infections due to gram positive and gram negative bacteria following caesarean sections and hysterectomies. *Eur J Med Res* 1999;**4**:126–30.
25. Phuapradit W, Saropala N. Topical application of honey in treatment of abdominal wound disruption. *Aust N Z J Obstet Gynaecol* 1992;**32**:381–4.
26. Walters MD, Dombroski RA, Davidson SA, Mandel PC, Gibbs RS. Reclosure of disrupted abdominal incisions. *Obstet Gynecol* 1990;**76**:597–602.
27. Dodson MK, Magann EF, Sullivan DL, Meeks GR. Extrafascial wound dehiscence: deep en bloc closure versus superficial skin closure. *Obstet Gynecol* 1994;**83**:142–5.
28. Sweet R, Gibbs R. Wound and episiotomy infections. In: Sweet R, Gibbs R. *Gynecologic and Obstetric Infections*. Baltimore: Williams & Wilkins; 1995. p. 601–16.
29. French LM, Smaill FM. Antibiotic regimens for endometritis after delivery. *Cochrane Database Syst Rev* 2000;(2):CD001067.
30. Hopkins L, Smaill F. Antibiotic prophylaxis regimens and drugs for cesarean section. *Cochrane Database Syst Rev* 2000;(2):CD001136.
31. Wax JR, Hersey K, Phiput C, Wright MS, Nicols KV, Eggleston MK, *et al.* Single dose cefazolin prophylaxis for postcesarean infections: before vs. after cord clamping. *J Matern Fetal Med* 1997;**6**:61–5.
32. Cunningham FG, Leveno K, DePalma RT, Roark M, Rosenfeld CR. Perioperative antimicrobials for cesarean delivery: before or after cord clamping? *Obstet Gynecol* 1983;**62**:151–4.
33. Newton ER, Wallace PA. Effects of prophylactic antibiotics on endometrial flora in women with postcesarean endometritis. *Obstet Gynecol* 1998;**92**:262–8.
34. Gibbs RS, Blanco JD, St Clair PJ, Castaneda YS. Vaginal colonization with resistant aerobic bacteria after antibiotic therapy for endometritis. *Am J Obstet Gynecol* 1982;**142**:130–4.
35. Hannah M, Ohlsson A, Farine D, Hewson S, Hodnett E, Myhr T, Wang E, *et al.* Induction of labor compared with expectant management for prelabor rupture of the membranes at term. *N Engl J Med* 1996;**334**:1005–10.
36. Reid GC, Hartmann KE, McMahon MJ. Can postpartum infectious morbidity be decreased by vaginal preparation with povidone iodine prior to cesarean delivery? *Am J Obstet Gynecol* 2000;**182**:S96.
37. L Tully, personal communication.
38. Gates S, McKenzie-McHarg K, Hurley P. Effects of surgical techniques of caesarean section on maternal health. *Fet Mat Med Rev* 2001;**12**:105–37.
39. Lasley DS, Eblen A, Yancey MK, Duff P. The effect of placental removal method on the incidence of postcesarean infections. *Am J Obstet Gynecol* 1997;**176**:1250–4.
40. Magann EF, Washburne JF, Harris RL, Bass DJ, Duff PW, Morrison JC. Infectious morbidity, operative blood loss, and length of the operative procedure after cesarean delivery by method of placental removal and site of uterine repair. *J Am Coll Surg* 1995;**181**:517–20.
41. Evaldson GR, Frederici H, Jullig C, Mannerquist K, Nystrom B. Hospital-associated infections in obstetrics and gynecology. *Acta Obstet Gynecol Scand* 1992;**71**:54–8.
42. Casey, BM, Cox, SM. Chorioamnionitis and endometritis. *Infect Dis Clin North Am* 1997;**11**:203–22.
43. Duff P. Pathophysiology and management of postcaesarean endomyometritis. *Obstet Gynecol* 1986;**67**:269–76.

Chapter 32

Infection and maternal mortality

James Drife

Introduction

During the year 2001, about 600 000 women will die from causes directly related to pregnancy. This is equivalent to one death every minute of every day. About 99% of these tragedies will occur in developing countries. More than one-quarter of the deaths will be caused by infection, mainly in the form of either puerperal sepsis or septic abortion.[1]

Maternal mortality is defined as the death of a woman during pregnancy or up to six weeks after delivery due directly to the pregnancy or a condition exacerbated by pregnancy. In the UK, puerperal sepsis was the leading cause of maternal mortality throughout the 19th century and during the first third of the 20th century. After 1935, however, when antibiotics were introduced into clinical practice, the incidence of puerperal sepsis fell rapidly and by 1985 this disease had disappeared completely from the UK.[2]

In the 1960s, as other causes fell, infection again became the leading cause of maternal mortality in England and Wales, this time in the form of septic abortion. After the 1967 Abortion Act the incidence of this condition steadily decreased and by the 1980s criminal abortion had been eliminated as a cause of maternal death in the UK.[2]

During the 1990s, it became clear that the disappearance of puerperal sepsis from this country had been only temporary. Over that decade it again accounted for the deaths of a small number of women in the UK every year. Although the number of deaths is low – around five per year – it is important to remember that even today in a developed country a recently delivered woman can die quickly from overwhelming infection.[3]

History

The history of puerperal fever, in Britain and across the world, is discussed in several chapters of Irvine Loudon's masterly book, *Death in Childbirth: an International Study of Maternal Care and Maternal Mortality 1800–1950*. Most of what follows in this section is summarised from Dr Loudon's meticulous research.[4]

Between 1847 and 1903, the number of deaths from puerperal fever recorded in England and Wales was 93 342. Compulsory notification was introduced only in 1899, however, and this total was almost certainly an underestimate. At the start of the 20th century it was stated that the mortality from this cause was between 3000 and 5000 cases per annum in England and Wales. Despite notification, the number of nonfatal cases of puerperal sepsis remained difficult to define. In 1920, it was calculated that there may have been as many as 80 000 cases with about 2000 deaths, giving a fatality rate of about 2.5%.

In the 18th century and the first half of the 19th century, lying-in hospitals were susceptible to waves of puerperal infection. This was true everywhere, even in the leading hospitals of the day, whose standards of nursing were regarded as high. In such institutions the maternal mortality rate was often between 100 and 200 per 10 000 deliveries (i.e., 1–2%). In 1849, the maternal mortality rate at Queen Charlotte's Hospital in London rose to a peak of 932 per 10 000 deliveries and in 1861 at the Rotunda Hospital in Dublin the figure was 519. The rate was not linked to the frequency of obstetric operations and the great majority of cases occurred after non-instrumental deliveries; nor were the rates connected to the admission of especially complicated cases or to the social class of the women delivered.

In 1862, Florence Nightingale established a lying-in ward in King's College Hospital, London, where young women could be instructed in midwifery. From the start the ward was dogged by puerperal fever and she closed it in 1867. In the 1860s, obstetricians clearly recognised that the safest place for a woman to be delivered was in her own home, with skilled attendants available.

Nevertheless, puerperal sepsis was by no means confined to hospitals. On the contrary, in 19th century Britain the great majority of deliveries took place at home and, across the country, 97% of the deaths from puerperal sepsis occurred after home delivery. This explains why the introduction of antiseptic techniques into hospital practice in the second half of the nineteenth19th century had little effect on the national rate of maternal mortality (Figure 32.1).

During the 18th and 19th centuries a great deal of research was carried out on puerperal fever. It was known that the disease occurred in epidemics, during which the fatality rate of the condition could be extremely high – apparently reaching 100% at times. The first epidemic in Aberdeen occurred between 1789 and 1792 and was the subject of a treatise, published in 1795 by a local graduate, Alexander Gordon. He recognised that the disease appeared to be confined to the practice of a minority of midwives and that he himself had carried it from one patient to another. This was the first documentation of the contagious nature of puerperal fever. Unfortunately, Gordon believed that the disease could be cured by early and heavy bleeding and purging. For this reason, and because he himself had carried the disease, the women of Aberdeen turned against him.

Gordon's epidemiological observations were confirmed by others. For example, in 1815 William Hey described an epidemic in Leeds in which cases were confined to the patients of one practitioner but not of others. In the USA in 1843, Oliver Wendell Holmes read a paper on puerperal fever to the Boston Society for Medical Improvement. He concluded, from a study of the literature, that the disease 'is so far contagious as to be frequently carried from patient to patient by physicians and nurses'. This conclusion had already been reached by some other American doctors: one had

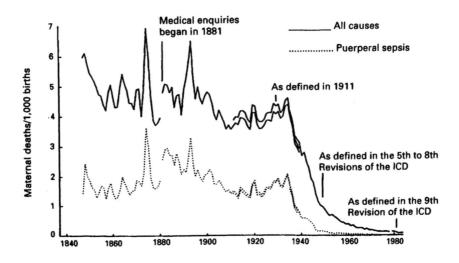

Fig. 32.1. Maternal mortality, England and Wales, 1847–1984; ICD, International Classification of Diseases (Source: OPCS mortality statistics)

retired after trying everything, including changes of clothing and equipment, to rid himself of the contagion, and another had managed to do so by washing his hands routinely in a solution of chloride of lime after every midwifery case. Nevertheless, the cause of the disease remained a mystery.

In 1846, Ignaz Semmelweis, then 28 years old, was appointed assistant in the Vienna Maternity Hospital, at that time one of the largest such hospitals in the world. It was divided into two clinics, one of which (the 'first') taught medical students, the other midwives. Patients were admitted to the two clinics on alternate days. The mortality rate from puerperal fever was known to be higher in the first clinic, although the reason was unknown. Medical students attended postmortem examinations on women who had died from puerperal fever. They then went on to the wards, where they carried out vaginal examinations. In 1847, Semmelweis introduced the practice of hand washing in disinfectant, after which the maternal mortality in the first clinic fell close to that in the midwives' clinic.

Semmelweis's innovation has become a medical legend but at the time it was not immediately followed by a widespread change of practice elsewhere. This was not because of poor communication – a paper about Semmelweis's results was read in London in 1849. One reason was that Semmelweis himself was slow to publish and was not a persuasive advocate of his own ideas; another was that the unifying cause of the disease still remained unknown.

Nevertheless, by this time analogies were being drawn between puerperal sepsis and surgical infection. In particular, it was realised that epidemics of puerperal fever coincided with epidemics of erysipelas, a wound infection, on surgical wards. In 1864, Rokitanski first observed organisms in the vaginal discharge of women with puerperal sepsis and these were identified as streptococci in 1865. In 1867, Joseph Lister, then working in Glasgow, published the first results of his introduction of antisepsis into surgical practice, showing how it markedly reduced the fatality rate after surgery.

In the 1870s, antiseptic techniques were introduced into maternity hospitals and maternal mortality rates in these institutions fell from levels well above the national average to the same or even lower levels. Antisepsis put an end to the dramatic epidemics of puerperal fever that had recurred through the previous decades. In Liège maternity hospital in Belgium, for example, maternal mortality fell from around 4% in 1860–70 to a tenth of that level after 1885. Nevertheless, as mentioned above, in Britain the national rate of puerperal sepsis remained unchanged.

By 1880, it was known that streptococcus was the main pathogen in most cases of puerperal sepsis. Early in the 20th century, *Streptococcus pyogenes* was shown to be the organism responsible for death in the great majority of cases. Elucidation of the cause, however, did not lead immediately to effective therapy. It was only with the introduction of effective treatment, in the form of sulphonamides, that the continuing death rate from puerperal fever was at last reduced.

In 1935, Domagk in Germany discovered that a single injection of a red dye, prontosil, could prevent the death of mice infected with streptococci. Leonard Colebrook, director of the Medical Research Council isolation block at Queen Charlotte's Hospital, London, managed to obtain some prontosil and, despite his misgivings about its safety, used it on a patient who seemed certain to die of puerperal septicaemia. Irvine Loudon described its effect: 'Prontosil was given to this patient late that day, and the staff watched her anxiously all night. Next morning her temperature was normal, and she made a full recovery'.

Some older obstetricians still remember hearing this story from those working in the hospital at the time. The drug must have seemed miraculous. Soon after the introduction of prontosil, the mortality rate of patients with puerperal fever at Queen Charlotte's Hospital was 4.7%, compared with a previous average of 25%.

Shortly afterwards, it was realised that the active metabolite of prontosil was sulphanilamide, which became widely available by 1937. The best-known proprietary brand, 'M&B' (for 'May and Baker'), appeared in 1938. The introduction of the sulphonamides appears to have coincided with a natural fall in the virulence of the streptococcus, from a high peak in 1934, but this was a minor factor in the decline of maternal mortality from sepsis compared with the part played by the introduction of antibiotics, first sulphonamides and then, in 1945, penicillin.

The dramatic fall in mortality from puerperal fever began the process of reducing or eliminating other causes of maternal mortality in Britain.[5] The history of puerperal fever is fascinating in its own right and is the subject of an award-winning book by Irvine Loudon.[6] It is sobering to consider how many women died in the past because insufficient attention was paid to accurate observations made by researchers over many years, and because controversy about the underlying cause led people to overlook the simple measures that could have saved lives.

The Confidential Enquiries into Maternal Deaths

The present system of Confidential Enquiries into Maternal Deaths (CEMD) was designed after the end of the Second World War and was implemented in England and Wales in the early 1950s. The first report,[7] published in 1957, covered the triennium

Table 32.1.   Number of maternal deaths[3,7]

Causes	1952–54[a]	1994–96[b]
Hypertensive disease	246	20
Haemorrhage	188	12
Abortion	153	1
Thromboembolism	138	48
Anaesthesia	49	1
Sepsis	42	14

[a] England and Wales; [b] UK

1952–54. That report included separate chapters on 'toxaemia of pregnancy', haemorrhage, pulmonary embolism and abortion, but – surprisingly, perhaps, in view of the pre-eminence of puerperal sepsis as a cause of death before 1945 – there was no chapter on infection. Sepsis, by far the leading cause of maternal mortality in England and Wales in the previous decade, now lagged far behind hypertensive disease and haemorrhage.

Over the next 40 years there was a further reduction in deaths from sepsis (Table 32.1), but the dramatic fall in mortality from sepsis had predated the CEMD.

Abortion

Table 32.1 also shows the high number of deaths from septic abortion in 1952–54. Although deaths from this cause had fallen because of the introduction of antibiotics, abortion continued to account for about 30 deaths a year in England and Wales throughout the 1950s and 1960s. The first CEMD report recorded the social status of those who died of abortion (Table 32.2).

Although its phraseology seems quaint to us nowadays, Table 32.2 shows that most of the women who died after criminal abortion were married and 'comfortable'.

By 1967, septic abortion had become the leading cause of maternal mortality in England and Wales, causing 19% of maternal deaths. The Abortion Act of 1967 was not, however, followed by an immediate fall in the number of deaths from this cause. It took 15 years before death from criminal abortion was finally eliminated from England and Wales, and during that time there was a period when deaths from legal abortion were as numerous as those from illegal abortion (Figure 32.2).

Table 32.2.   Social circumstances of women who died from abortion[7]

Circumstances	Single	Married
Well to do	1	1
Comfortable	12	42
Poor	3	20
Destitute	–	1
Not noted	6	21

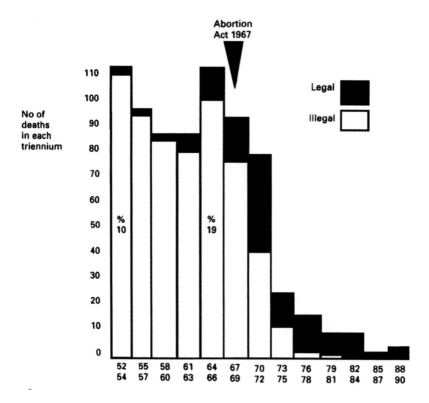

Fig. 32.2. Deaths from abortion, England and Wales, 1952–1994; percentages within columns indicate that, of all direct maternal deaths in that triennium, 10% and 19% were caused by abortion

The 1980s

Deaths from classic puerperal sepsis, already infrequent in the 1952–54 triennium, became steadily less common until, in the mid-1980s, this cause of maternal mortality seemed to have been eliminated completely. The *Report on Confidential Enquiries into Maternal Deaths in England and Wales 1982–84*[2] included the short, remarkable sentence 'No deaths could be directly attributed to puerperal sepsis'. In that triennium, only two deaths from sepsis were recorded. One was caused by haemolytic streptococcus after caesarean section. The other was of a woman who concealed her pregnancy and labour and who then died in the second stage of labour, which appeared to have lasted for days.

After 1982–84, however, the number of deaths from sepsis started to increase again: in each of the three triennia between 1988 and 1996, 15–17 women died from genital tract sepsis. This steady number masks a rise in puerperal sepsis in the most recent triennium (Table 32.3).

Table 32.3. Maternal deaths from genital tract sepsis including abortion and ectopic pregnancy: UK 1985–96

Triennium	Sepsis after abortion	Sepsis after ectopic pregnancy	Puerperal sepsis	Sepsis after surgical procedures	Sepsis before or during labour	Total	Rate per million maternities
1985–87	2	1	2	2	2	9	4.0
1988–90	7	1	4	5	0	17	7.2
1991–93	4	0	4	5	2	15	6.5
1994–96	2	0	10	3	1	16	7.3

The current report: 1994–96

The most recent CEMD report[3] covers the triennium 1994–96 and includes ten deaths from puerperal sepsis. In at least six of these cases, the causative organism was haemolytic streptococcus, and *Escherichia coli* and clostridium accounted for one case each. Haemolytic streptococcus also accounted for one death before delivery and three deaths after caesarean section.

The 1994–96 report collected data on the ethnic group of the women who died, and showed that, overall, the estimated rate of mortality per 100 000 maternities was higher among black women (31/100 000) than among white women (11/100 000), Indian/Bangladeshi/Pakistani women (8/100 000) or other women (4/100 000). When the 14 deaths from sepsis (excluding abortion) were examined, however, 12 of the women were white, one black and one unclassified – a distribution reflecting the national population.

In some of the cases, the diagnosis of infection was promptly made and treatment was given without delay but the case still had a fatal outcome. In other cases, apparently mild symptoms had given false reassurance but rapid deterioration then occurred. In a few cases, however, there was substandard care, when an obviously severe infection was not recognised as such and treatment with antibiotics was not promptly initiated.

Among the cases of puerperal infection, the interval between delivery and the onset of infection varied from 12 hours to two weeks. Risk factors such as prolonged rupture of the membranes or intrauterine death were present in some cases, but in others (including one home delivery and another in a GP unit) labour and delivery had been entirely straightforward. Continuing vigilance is important and the 'key recommendations' of this chapter of the report are reproduced here.

Genital sepsis: key recommendations from the CEMD[3]

- Puerperal sepsis is not a disease of the past, and GPs and midwives must be aware of the signs and be prepared to institute immediate treatment and referral of any recently delivered woman with a fever and/or offensive vaginal discharge.
- There is clear evidence from controlled trials showing the benefit of prophylactic antibiotics for caesarean section.
- When infection develops and the patient is systemically ill, urgent and repeated bacteriological specimens, including blood cultures, must be obtained. The advice

of a microbiologist must be sought at an early stage to assist with the use of appropriate antibiotic therapy. In serious cases, doctors should be prepared to give parenteral antibiotics before the diagnosis can be confirmed.

The global picture

'Every minute of every day, somewhere in the world, a woman dies as a result of complications arising during pregnancy and childbirth. The majority of these deaths are avoidable.'

This quotation, from a Joint Statement[1] published in 1999 by the World Health Organization (WHO), the World Bank and other United Nations organisations, reflects the WHO estimate that about 600 000 maternal deaths occur every year across the globe. Not only is each death an individual tragedy, but this total also reflects a much larger number of women affected by long-term morbidity. Maternal death has implications for the survival of the children: worldwide there are 3.4 million neonatal deaths (during the first week of life) every year.

Maternal mortality is an important indicator of women's health and of the status of women in society. Maternal health is important economically. In terms of 'disability adjusted life years' lost, poor maternal health far outstrips in importance other factors including HIV/AIDS, tuberculosis, war or alcoholism.[8]

The pattern of causes of maternal death will of course vary from area to area, but the broad picture globally is as shown in Table 32.4. It can be seen from this table that sepsis and unsafe abortion together account for 28% of deaths. In addition, the category 'indirect causes' includes malaria, hepatitis and, increasingly in some settings, HIV/AIDS.

A study[9] of maternal deaths in Anantapur District, Andhra Pradesh, India in 1988 concluded that about 36% of all deaths among females aged 15–49 years in the reference period were caused by complications of childbirth and these maternal deaths represented a maternal mortality ratio of 800 per 100 000 live births. In this study, infection accounted for a larger proportion than the 15% in other similar studies elsewhere. Of the total number of cases, 50% died at home or in transit to a healthcare facility and the other 50% died at a healthcare facility or hospital. In another study[10] in India, of 140 women moribund on admission to hospital, 97 arrived by bus, some came by bullock cart and only 12 arrived by ambulance.

Table 32.4. Proportion of maternal deaths worldwide due to specific causes

Cause	Proportion (%)
Haemorrhage	25
Indirect causes	20
Sepsis	15
Unsafe abortion	13
Eclampsia	12
Obstructed labour	8
Other direct causes	8

HIV/AIDS

In some countries, particularly in southern Africa, HIV/AIDS is now a leading cause of maternal mortality. Due to age asymmetry in sexual partnerships, HIV seroprevalence among women is highest in the 15–25 years age group, whereas men are typically ten years older when infected.[11]

Prevention and treatment

The joint WHO/UNFPA/UNICEF/World Bank statement includes the following observations on sepsis. 'Sepsis ... is often a consequence of poor hygiene during delivery or of untreated sexually transmitted diseases (STDs). ... Such infections can be effectively prevented by careful attention to clean delivery and by detection and management of STDs during pregnancy. Systematic postpartum care will ensure rapid detection of infection and its management by appropriate antibiotics.'

Better transport of women to hospital is important in many areas, but studies in India have concluded that often the woman is not recognised to be seriously ill by her immediate family members. When Indian states are compared with one another, some states such as Kerala have achieved relatively low levels of maternal mortality, and the same states have relatively high levels of contraceptive use and, perhaps most significantly, of female literacy.[9] This correlation supports the conclusion that reducing maternal mortality, from all direct causes including sepsis, involves attention to the social status of women as well as the provision of appropriate medical care.

Prevention and treatment of septic abortion

Prevention and management of unwanted pregnancies is a high priority among essential services for women's health.[11] Local initiatives to reduce the death rate from septic abortion include a project in West Bengal in which the UK Department for International Development is helping to strengthen local capacity to treat septic and incomplete abortion, including training in the use of manual vacuum aspiration.[12]

Prevention and treatment of HIV/AIDS

Efforts to reduce the risk of HIV/AIDS need to focus on women before pregnancy rather than during pregnancy. Such interventions can be effective, and include education, marketing of condoms, systematic treatment of other sexually transmitted infections, and voluntary testing and counselling.[11]

Conclusion

The underlying reason for the high rates of death from sepsis and infection in pregnancy is the unequal power distribution between men and women in many countries of the world. 'Women's low socio-economic status and reproductive role expose them to risks of poor health and premature death, yet many women's health problems can be prevented or mitigated through highly cost-effective interventions.'[11] Many international agencies are now involved in promoting the importance of strategies to improve health interventions for women. The last century saw huge improvements in women's health in developed countries such as the UK, and it is to be hoped that the 21st century will see similar progress worldwide.

References

1. World Health Organization. *Reduction of Maternal Mortality: a Joint WHO/UNFPA/UNICEF/World Bank Statement*. Geneva: WHO; 1999.
2. Turnbull A, Tindall VR, Beard RW, Robson G, Dawson IMP, Cloake EP, *et al. Report on Confidential Enquiries into Maternal Deaths in England and Wales 1982–84*. London: HMSO; 1989. Department of Health Report on Health and Social Subjects **34**.
3. Drife J, Lewis G, editors. *Why Mothers Die. Report on Confidential Enquiries into Maternal Deaths in the United Kingdom 1994–96*. London: The Stationery Office; 1998.
4. Loudon I. *Death in Childbirth: an International Study of Maternal Care and Maternal Mortality 1800–1950*. Oxford: Clarendon Press; 1992.
5. Drife J. Lessons to be learned from maternal mortality reports. *Curr Obstet Gynaecol* 1997;**7**:218–23.
6. Loudon I. *The Tragedy of Childbed Fever*. Oxford: Oxford University Press; 2000.
7. Walker AL, Wrigley AJ, Marston AD, Hirst KM, Martin WJ. *Report on Confidential Enquiries into Maternal Deaths in England and Wales 1952–1954*. London: HMSO, 1957. Ministry of Health Reports on Public Health and Medical Subjects No. 97.
8. Pittrof R. The sorry state of reproductive health of women – a global overview. *Contemp Rev Obstet Gynaecol* 1996;**8**:93–7.
9. World Bank. *Improving Women's Health in India*. Washington DC: World Bank; 1996.
10. Drife JO. We know why they die. *BMJ* 1996;**312**:1044.
11. Tinker A, Finn K, Epp J. *Improving Women's Health: Issues and Interventions*. Washington, DC: World Bank; 2000.
12. Department for International Development. *Time for Action: Reducing the Dangers of Pregnancy in Poor Societies*. London: Department for International Development, Health and Population Division; 1997.

Chapter 33

Infection II

Discussion

Discussion following Dr Heath's paper

Ridgway: I have two comments. The first is that, as this is a review, I am slightly surprised that you have not made any comment about ureaplasmas as a cause of neonatal infection. The second is that I would have thought that, provided our obstetric colleagues reduced the antibiotics to single intrapartum injections, we need not worry too much about the effect on the neonate, as far as the antibiotics that you should be using in the neonatal situation are concerned.

Heath: Thank you for those comments. In response to the first, I am speaking primarily of early-onset neonatal bacterial infection and ureaplasma is not really implicated in early-onset infection. With regard to the second, we know that, in the USA, much of the concern about the effect on the emergence of antibiotic resistance and other pathogens has been with using ampicillin. There was a phase recently in the USA where penicillin was not available and ampicillin was being used. If penicillin is being used for intrapartum antibiotic prophylaxis for group B streptococcus then, at least in theory, the effect on neonatal practice should be minimised.

Edwards: Could you comment on the evidence that treating a baby in the perinatal period affects the incidence of late-onset disease?

Heath: Do you mean intrapartum antibiotic prophylaxis, or treating the baby?

Edwards: Either intrapartum or strategies which give the baby antibiotics after birth.

Heath: A recently published paper[1] from the USA showed the impact in the USA from selected areas of intrapartum antibiotic prophylaxis on early-onset disease, with a significant reduction, and no impact on late-onset disease.

We still need to learn a great deal about late-onset group B streptococcal disease. Of the two, it is the one that has been the least well studied – epidemiologically, what are the risk factors? A figure of 50% has been given for vertical transmission and therefore the other 50% results from whatever happens in the nursery. However, that has not been well studied. You would think, however, that if that were the case then there should be an impact on late-onset disease, but that has not been seen in practice. So I am in fact not answering that, but raising some more questions.

Edwards: I am still not clear quite why you think there is a difference. It is rather strange that there should be a difference between those two things.

Heath: There is a difference probably because the pathogenesis of late-onset disease is different from that of early-onset disease. It is probably more different than we realise at the moment. I suspect that more late-onset disease is due to other factors not related to vertical transmission.

Discussion following Dr Brocklehurst's paper

MacLean: The recommendation that we should use a single dose of a narrow-spectrum agent perhaps flies in the face of what people are currently doing. In the study we conducted involving the Royal Free and University College Hospitals, the protocols encouraged the use of a single shot of Augmentin® (Glaxo Wellcome, Uxbridge). A good deal of metronidazole was used – metronidazole and a long-acting third-generation cephalosporin. That is perhaps inconsistent with what you are saying.

I know it is difficult to name brand names, but would you agree that it should be 'first-generation cephalosporin', or does Augmentin®, for instance, fall into this definition? There are some inconsistencies and I would welcome people's comments before we agree on a recommendation.

Brocklehurst: There are some inconsistencies. The use of a single dose is supported by the randomised trials.[2] The recommendation to use an antibiotic regimen with a narrow spectrum of activity is not based on randomised trials, because we have not been able to assess the possibility of antibiotic resistance in these trials. That would seem to be best practice but I would be interested in Dr Ridgway's view about whether that would constitute best practice in this situation.

Ridgway: I would suggest that a better choice of words is a 'relevant spectrum of activity', rather than a narrow spectrum of activity.

Regan: Following on from that point, perhaps I am out of touch, but what would our microbiological colleagues think about giving everybody who is going to have a caesarean section aminoglycoside? Would that have a major impact on other infectious problems?

Scott: That is not what is proposed.

Brocklehurst: No, I was not suggesting an aminoglycoside.

Scott: That is for the treatment of endometritis after delivery.

Regan: I beg your pardon, but you did say clindamycin –

Brocklehurst: Clindamycin and a gentamicin for established endometritis, not as prophylaxis.

Ridgway: I firmly believe that, if you have severe obstetric sepsis, clindamycin/gentamicin is the best possible combination. I would support that wholeheartedly.

Soothill: Could I just ask a question of fact about that? In the Cochrane review[3] on treating endometritis, did 'all other regimens' include not giving antibiotics? Or were they all treatment arms?

Brocklehurst: They were all treatment trials. There was a wide variety of antibiotic regimens but, to my knowledge, there have been no placebo-controlled trials of treatment for endometritis.

Soothill: Putting the same question in another way, did it include some arms that were illogical – in other words, that were not likely to be effective? Could that be the reason why that particular combination, and that particular analysis, appears to be the best? Did they include all the other possible cross-comparisons?

Brocklehurst: No, they did not include all the other possibilities. In particular, they did not include what many of us in the UK are currently using – many of which have not been subjected to randomised controlled trials. There may be arguments about how appropriate the antibiotic regimens were but all of them were considered to be appropriate treatments for endometritis and the trials were aiming to determine which was superior. If we looked at every one, I am sure there would be some discussion about that, but the aim was to treat endometritis.

Fox: How was the diagnosis of endometritis made in most of these studies?

Brocklehurst: That varies. Definitions were all a combination of uterine tenderness, offensive lochia and fever, in one combination or other. The definitions of fever, what constituted an offensive lochia and how severe uterine tenderness was, varied. However, whatever definition was used, it was standard in each trial. Therefore, within each randomised arm there was a decrease that was consistent across all the trials. This is, of course, a difficult diagnosis to be completely sure of.

Holliman: You mentioned that one-third of wound infections were picked up after the patient had left hospital, and commented that modern practice may elevate that figure. I think one-third is an underestimate now. I remember seeing a Department of Health study[4] from the mid-1990s that indicated that two-thirds of nosocomial infections were picked up after the patient had left hospital.

Hay: You have not said anything about outpatient treatment with oral antibiotics. The only patients I see regularly are the HIV-positive women, perhaps one or two weeks after caesarean section. My impression is that many of them are developing endometritis and I am generally treating them with oral co-amoxiclav. What do Mr

Smith and Professor McIntyre have to say about that, too? Do you have any data on it?

Brocklehurst: No, there are no randomised trials. All of those randomised trials for the treatment of endometritis were in hospital, with intravenous therapy, at least initially. I have seen no data about outpatient treatment. All of these were quite severe infections, because they came back to hospital.

Smith: Professor McIntyre and I have used the same thing in HIV-positive women as in HIV-negative women. Our standard protocol is just to use a shot of intravenous co-amoxiclav, intra-operatively. I have not seen much postpartum endometritis in that group – perhaps they have gone somewhere else, such as the HIV department.

Hay: I do not know whether our patients are receiving any intra-operative prophylaxis. I will have to check that.

Brocklehurst: Or, because you are giving prophylaxis, you are not seeing endometritis.

McIntyre: Our standard policy is to give one dose as prophylaxis for everybody, and we do the same with HIV. Our rates in HIV-positive women have not been high over the last couple of years, in sharp contrast to Pretoria and some of the other hospitals around us. I am not certain whether there is not some form of minimal antibiotic effect from zidovudine, for example. Many of our women have been on anti-retroviral therapy, whereas they are not in other African centres. I am not sure whether, in an African setting, we might need more than one dose, or whether it varies according to what other treatment is used.

Discussion following Professor Drife's paper

Ridgway: I would like to add a caveat to the recommendation where you say that early treatment with antibiotics still seems to be the best way to prevent death. As a bacteriologist, can I stress the importance of working with the surgeon to make sure that early hysterectomy is considered? Often, this is the only life-saving action you can take, after you have established the antibiotics. Antibiotics may hold it, but they will not always cure it, and you have to be prepared to go in.

Drife: Thank you very much for that point. The idea that early antibiotic treatment is the only way is not the case, for example, if the problem is necrotising fasciitis.

General discussion

Regan: Professor Drife, your comment about indirect deaths was interesting. You mentioned that women who had undergone transplant surgery had no increased risk of sepsis and were not counted as indirect deaths. Are there any other data from the most recent Confidential Enquiry into Maternal Deaths to suggest that the indirect death rate goes up because there are more women receiving sophisticated medical care for other problems, who then are considered able to become pregnant?

Drife: Yes, very much so. The most striking example of that is in the cardiac chapter, where it is no longer rheumatic heart disease but congenital heart disease being reported. The tragic cases we see are the people who have been determined to become pregnant, against medical advice in some cases.

It is evident to me, when I read the anonymised data I receive, that the cardiologists who see these women have never witnessed a maternal death. If you see somebody die before your eyes, as clinicians used to do, it gives you a certain emotional kick to try to prevent that. I do not think that the medical advice given to cardiac patients is particularly strong: it is more likely to be couched in terms of 'there is a risk' than 'do not get pregnant or you may die.' Furthermore, these women have been used to taking risks all their lives because they have lived with their cardiac condition.

It is very sad that some of these pregnancies have almost been connived at, to allow them to become pregnant. That may be putting it a little strongly but with the renal patients they will say 'this is a challenge to us as physicians but we will help you through it.' In cardiac cases, people die, but I do not think that comes across to the cardiologists quite as strongly as it should.

References

1. Schrag SJ, Zywicki S, Farley MM, Reingold AL, Harrison LH, Lefkowitz LB, *et al.* Group B streptococcal disease in the era of intrapartum antibiotic prophylaxis. *N Engl J Med* 2000;**342**:15–20.
2. Hopkins L, Smaill F. Antibiotic prophylaxis regimens and drugs for cesarean section. *Cochrane Database Syst Rev* 2000;(2):CD001136.
3. French LM, Smaill FM. Antibiotic regimens for endometritis after delivery. *Cochrane Database Syst Rev* 2000;(2):CD001067.
4. Plowman R, Graves N, Griffin M, Roberts JA, Swan AV, Cookson B, Taylor L. *The Socio-economic Burden of Hospital-acquired Infection*. Public Health Laboratory Service; 1999.

SECTION 9

RECOMMENDATIONS

Chapter 34

Recommendations arising from the 40th Study Group: Infection and Pregnancy

Recommendations fall into three categories:

1. Recommendations for **clinical practice** (principally aimed at Fellows and Members of the Royal College of Obstetricians and Gynaecologists) based upon research evidence (where available) and the consensus view of the Group. The clinical practice recommendations have been graded from 'A' to 'C' according to the strength of evidence on which each is based (Table 34.1). The scheme for the grading of recommendations is based on the system adopted by both the NHS Executive and the Scottish Intercollegiate Guidelines Network.

2. Recommendations for **future research** in those clinical areas where the Group identified a need for further evidence on which to base practice.

3. Recommendations relating to **health education** and **health policy**.

Recommendations for clinical practice

General

1. Sporadic miscarriage is so common that detailed infective screening cannot be justified economically. (Grade C)

Table 34.1. Grading of recommendations

Grade	Recommendation
A	Requires at least one randomised controlled trial as part of the body of literature of overall good quality and consistency addressing the specific recommendation.
B	Requires availability of well-conducted clinical studies but no randomised clinical trials on the topic of recommendation.
C	Requires evidence from expert committee reports or opinions and/or clinical experience of respected authorities. Indicates absence of directly applicable studies of good quality.

2. TORCH screening is unhelpful and should be abandoned in the investigation of recurrent miscarriage. (Grade C)

3. To prevent preterm labour and mid-trimester loss, any screening for abnormal genital tract colonisation should be done in early pregnancy. (Grade C)

4. Pregnancies complicated by congenital infection should preferably be referred to regional fetomaternal medicine centres. (Grade C)

5. Maternal investigations for possible infection causes in cases of fetal hydrops, fetal brain lesions, unexplained severe growth restriction or *in utero* demise are recommended. (Grade C)

6. Infants with the suspicion of congenital infection and those born preterm, where infection may have played a role, need neurological follow-up by a competent paediatrician. (Grade C)

Viral infections

7. All pregnant women presenting with a non-vesicular rash compatible with a systemic viral infection should be investigated for rubella and parvovirus B19 infection, irrespective of a prior history of rubella vaccination or previous positive rubella antibody tests. (Grade C)

8. All pregnant women with significant contact (defined as being in the same room for over 15 minutes or face-to-face contact) with a non-vesicular illness should be investigated for parvovirus B19 and rubella infection, irrespective of whether they develop a rash or not, unless there is satisfactory evidence of past rubella infection (two documented vaccinations, or one documented vaccination and one prior positive rubella antibody test, or two positive antibody tests). (Grade C)

9. All requests for laboratory investigation must give the following information in addition to the usual demographic details:
   - gestation of pregnancy (date of last menstrual period)
   - date of onset of rash, clinical features, type and distribution of rash
   - past history of rubella antibody tests or rubella vaccination
   - any known contact with rash illness and dates of contact. (Grade C)

10. Women found to be susceptible to rubella during prenatal screening or booking should receive appropriate vaccination before postnatal discharge. (Grade C)

11. When serology shows potential for early infection with parvovirus B19, the patient should be referred to a fetal medicine unit capable of fetal blood sampling and intravascular transfusion. (Grade C)

12. Amniocentesis is the method of choice for fetal sampling in the case of possible congenital infection but should be delayed until six weeks after maternal cytomegalovirus (CMV) seroconversion. (Grade A)

13. Neonates with congenital CMV infection and central nervous system signs at birth should be treated with ganciclovir according to the recent protocol from the Collaborative Antiviral Study Group. (Grade A)

14. Women without a previous history of varicella should be screened for varicella-

zoster virus antibodies, by a sensitive method, at booking or rapidly after contact or exposure, i.e. within 48 hours, so that patients qualifying can receive VZIG (varicella-zoster immunoglobulin) within the designated window period for efficacy. (Grade C)

15. After a significant varicella or zoster contact, a susceptible pregnant women (regardless of gestational age) should be given VZIG (up to 10 days after contact). (Grade B)

16. VZIG should be given to newborns, born to mothers who develop varicella seven days before and up to seven days after delivery, and they should be followed up for any subsequent infection. (Grade B)

17. Mothers developing chickenpox should be counselled concerning the risks of fetal varicella syndrome (approximately 2% risk in the first 20 weeks) and a risk assessment undertaken for severe maternal varicella. (Grade C)

18. Oral aciclovir should be recommended to women over 20 weeks of gestation on the first day of the rash. Oral aciclovir should be offered to women at less than 20 weeks of gestation. Full informed consent should be obtained because, although the safety profile is reassuring, approval for use in pregnancy does not yet exist. (Grade C)

19. Hospital assessment and, where appropriate with an infectious diseases physician, intravenous aciclovir should be given to those patients with varicella pneumonitis and in those over 36 weeks of gestation or with clinical deterioration after day six of appearance of rash, to avoid the consequences of varicella pneumonitis and other serious sequelae. Varicella of the newborn should be treated with intravenous aciclovir, regardless of the previous administration of VZIG. (Grade C)

20. If a patient presents with a primary episode of herpes simplex virus (HSV) and is in labour, caesarean section is advised. (Grade B)

21. If a patient presents with a primary episode of HSV after 34 weeks, and before the onset of labour, she should be commenced on aciclovir and continued until delivery. If the interval between initiating therapy and delivery is more than four weeks, vaginal delivery is appropriate. (Grade C)

22. If a patient presents with a primary episode of HSV before 34 weeks, e.g. first or second trimester, she should be treated with aciclovir from 36 weeks until delivery, and vaginal delivery would not be contraindicated. (Grade C)

23. There is no evidence to support routine antenatal screening for HSV 1 and 2 antibodies, or for virus detection in the cervix from patients with a history or recurrent HSV. (Grade B)

24. There is no agreement on the use of caesarean section or aciclovir in the management of patients with a history of recurrent HSV. If a patient presents in early labour with a visible herpetic lesion, caesarean section is recommended. If a patient has frequent symptomatic recurrences during pregnancy, the use of aciclovir from 36 weeks is recommended, and vaginal delivery would not be contraindicated. (Grade C)

25. Voluntary testing for HIV should be an integral part of antenatal care, offered and recommended to all pregnant women. (Grade C)

26. HIV-positive women should be offered a package of care that includes: safe obstetric practices; anti-retroviral treatment to reduce the risk of mother-to-child transmission of HIV, to the fullest extent that is available; information on infant feeding risks and benefits; and supportive counselling. (Grade C)

27. The care of HIV-positive women should include appropriate postpartum care with access to contraception and follow-up medical care for the woman and her child. (Grade C)

28. Hepatitis B and C viral infections are not contraindications to breastfeeding. (Grade C)

29. Hepatitis B immunoglobulin should be given to babies of mothers of high infectivity, e.g. those who are hepatitis Be antigen-positive. (Grade C)

Bacterial and other infections

30. Clinical trials of screening for and treatment of bacterial vaginosis have yielded conflicting results but treatment may reduce the risk of preterm birth in women with a previous preterm delivery. (Grade C)

31. There is no evidence to support the antenatal treatment of asymptomatic women colonised with the group B streptococcus (GBS). (Grade C)

32. Current recommendations are that all women with a history of having delivered an infant with GBS infection or of preterm rupture of the membranes, and all women found incidentally to have GBS in the urine or vagina during the current pregnancy should be offered intrapartum chemoprophylaxis. (Grade C)

33. Obstetricians must work with tuberculosis physicians to confirm and manage the disease. (Grade C)

34. Women with genital chlamydial infection need adequate chemotherapy and counselling, and a test of cure not less than three weeks after end of therapy. (Grade C)

35. Women with genital chlamydial infection must have contact tracing and appropriate management of their partners in a genitourinary medicine clinic. (Grade C)

36. Non-immune pregnant women should be advised against travel to a malarious area. If travel is unavoidable, advice should be given about personal protection and chemoprophylaxis. This advice also applies to previously immune women from malaria-endemic areas who have lived in the UK for more than two years and who will therefore have lost much of their pre-existing immunity. (Grade C)

37. Non-immune pregnant women with malaria need to be admitted to hospital, monitored closely (with particular attention to blood sugar and haemoglobin) and treated with an effective antimalarial such as quinine. (Grade C)

38. Recent immigrants from malaria-endemic areas are at risk of having placental malaria infection irrespective of whether they have a fever or peripheral parasitaemia. Malaria should be suspected and treated if women are anaemic or if there is evidence of intrauterine growth restriction. Unsuspected congenital

malaria may occur in their infants with onset between birth and several weeks of age. (Grade C)

39. There is no evidence currently to support routine screening for toxoplasmosis during pregnancy in the UK. (Grade C)

40. Data from the Cochrane Library support the use of prophylactic antibiotics for emergency and elective caesarean sections, unless there are clear reasons why they should not be given. (Grade A)

41. The antibiotic used for prophylaxis before caesarean section should be limited to one dose to reduce the possibility of antibiotic resistance. (Grade A)

42. The only surgical technique which can be unequivocally recommended at caesarean section is the avoidance of manual removal of the placenta. (Grade A)

43. When infection develops and the patient is systemically ill, urgent and repeated bacteriological specimens, including blood cultures, must be obtained. The advice of a microbiologist must be sought at an early stage to assist with the use of appropriate antibiotic therapy. In serious cases, doctors should be prepared to give parenteral antibiotics before the diagnosis can be confirmed. (Grade C)

44. Until further evidence becomes available, the optimum treatment for postpartum endometritis is clindamycin and an aminoglycoside. (Grade A)

Recommendations for future research

1. Research is needed to identify those factors that predispose a mother and her fetus to be susceptible to common infections during pregnancy.

2. Research must continue into understanding the risks of mother-to-fetus transmission, timing of acquisition and impact on subsequent morbidity and mortality.

3. Further research is required into the mechanisms and relationship between infection and brain damage in preterm and term infants.

4. Research is needed to define the precise role of molecular techniques in the diagnosis of fetal infections.

5. Future research on infection in preterm labour should include a measure of host defence response to identify those women with abnormal genital tract colonisation who by nature of the inflammatory response they evoke are at greater risk of adverse fetomaternal outcome.

6. There is good evidence that antibiotic treatment of women with preterm, prelabour rupture of the membranes prolongs pregnancy, although it has not been shown to improve neonatal outcome. Consideration should therefore be given to antimicrobial therapy in this group.

7. Interventions, including the use of antibiotics active against bacterial vaginosis-related organisms, should be conducted as early as possible in the second trimester and should use the reduction of fetomaternal infection as an outcome parameter rather than preterm birth.

8. Future studies should focus on identifying additional co-factors to bacterial vaginosis for adverse pregnancy outcome, the optimal gestational age for screening and for intervention and the optimal choice of treatment (systemic or intravaginal clindamycin, or metronidazole with or without macrolide).

9. A large study is required to determine whether screening for asymptomatic bacteriuria continues to be relevant in improving pregnancy outcome.

10. If screening for asymptomatic bacteriuria does remain relevant, inexpensive but effective techniques are required.

11. Consideration should be given to screening all antenatal women before delivery, i.e. in the third trimester, for genital chlamydial infection, preferably using a nucleic acid amplification or similarly sensitive and specific test.

12. The British Paediatric Surveillance Unit is soon to publish the findings of a nationwide survey of GBS neonatal disease. It is apparent that accurate UK data are required on the incidence of neonatal GBS infection.

13. The development of a vaccine against toxoplasmosis should be supported.

14. A placebo-controlled trial in pregnant women with primary CMV infection should determine if selected antivirals with safe preclinical profiles can decrease intrauterine transmission.

15. A CMV vaccine should be developed and used for universal vaccination.

16. Research is needed on the long-term follow-up of infants who have developed fetal varicella syndrome.

17. Further research is required on fetal effects when parvovirus B19 infection occurs after 20 weeks, whether monitoring is necessary beyond 30 weeks, and whether cardiac sampling with or without transfusion is practical at less than 17 weeks of gestation.

18. Further information is required as to whether transmission of hepatitis C from mother to infant may be reduced by elective caesarean section.

19. The timing of administration of antibiotic prophylaxis needs further investigation, particularly in relation to cord clamping with respect to the patterns of neonatal sepsis and antibiotic resistance.

20. Alternative approaches to preventing post caesarean section infection need urgent evaluation, particularly surgical technique, use of antiseptic agents for vaginal examinations in labour and general infection control measures.

21. Antibiotic regimens currently used for treating endometritis in the UK should be compared with the current best regimen in future randomised controlled trials.

Recommendations for education and health policy

General

1. Mechanisms must continue to allow monitoring of the prevalence of clinically important infections among the pregnant population.

2. Quality assurance for current screening programmes is required.

3. Current routine screening programmes in the UK include testing for rubella, syphilis, hepatitis B and human immunodeficiency viruses. Any alterations or additions to these programmes must be based on sound scientific evidence, and reviewed by the National Screening Committee.

4. Doctors and midwives should be aware of the diverse technologies that are available in the modern laboratory for the diagnosis of infections in the pregnant women and the fetus.

5. Good communication between laboratory staff and doctors/midwives is essential to provide comprehensive care to the infected pregnant woman.

6. Consideration must be given to keeping appropriate samples of placenta and membrane for research into congenital and neonatal infection.

7. Consideration is needed of the role of screening for blood-borne viruses (HIV, hepatitis B virus, hepatitis C virus) prior to prenatal invasive diagnostic procedures. Any existing positive results should be noted and discussed with the woman because of the potential risk of fetal infection.

8. Puerperal sepsis is not a disease of the past and general practitioners and midwives must be aware of the signs and be prepared to institute immediate treatment and referral of any recently delivered woman with a fever and/or offensive vaginal discharge.

9. Clinicians must remain vigilant for early signs of invasive streptococcal disease. The signs of necrotising fasciitis are high fever plus swelling and marked tenderness localised to a muscle mass. Early treatment with antibiotics still seems to be the best way to prevent death.

10. Over 150000 women die each year from puerperal sepsis. Medical treatment is often straightforward and inexpensive. Urgent action is needed by governments to make treatment available and accessible.

11. Worldwide about 100000 women die each year from sepsis following abortion. Provision for safe abortion should be available to all women.

Specific to particular organisms

12. GBS disease is the most frequent cause of infection in the neonate. Assessment of the risks of GBS disease for an individual mother and baby should be made by obstetricians and midwives, and timely and appropriate antibiotic prophylaxis considered where necessary. Guidelines should be in place and regularly audited.

13. There is insufficient evidence at present to recommend universal antenatal screening for GBS in the UK.

14. Any antibiotic administration to the mother in labour for GBS disease may have significant implications for the neonate and their subsequent management. Antibiotic choice and dose and timing should be considered carefully and the rationale and details communicated to the paediatricians caring for the neonate.

15. Clinicians must keep alert to the possibility of tuberculosis, particularly because of the difficulties in diagnosis, the high infectivity and the poor outcome if tuberculosis during pregnancy is not treated.

16. World Health Organization recommendations are that pregnant women (particularly those in their first and second pregnancies) living in malaria-endemic areas should receive antimalarial chemoprophylaxis or intermittent treatment with an effective antimalarial.

17. In observational studies, bacterial vaginosis is associated with second-trimester loss and preterm birth. Bacterial vaginosis can be diagnosed by composite (Amsel) criteria or Gram stain (Nugent score).

18. Appropriate health information about toxoplasmosis should be given to all pregnant women.

19. Reconsideration should be given to using hepatitis B immunoglobulin if the mother is of low infectivity, i.e. hepatitis Be antibody-positive.

20. Hepatitis E should be considered if a pregnant woman develops acute hepatitis after recently returning from an endemic area.

21. Pregnant women who develop a rash or have known exposure to parvovirus B19 should be seen promptly to assess serological status.

22. When fetal hydrops is found, the possibility of parvovirus B19 as a treatable cause must be considered.

Index